Clinical Applications of Pathophysiology

Assessment, Diagnostic Reasoning, and Management

Clinical Applications of Pathophysiology
Assessment, Diagnostic Reasoning, and Management

Valentina L. Brashers, MD
Assistant Professor of Nursing;
Clinical Assistant Professor of Medicine
University of Virginia
Charlottesville, Virginia

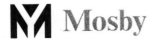

A Harcourt Health Sciences Company
St. Louis   London   Philadelphia   Sydney   Toronto

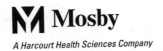

Mosby

A Harcourt Health Sciences Company

Publisher: Sally Schrefer
Developmental Editor: Michele D. Hayden
Project Manager: Gayle May Morris
Cover Design: David Zielinski
Design and Layout: Sue Anne Meeks
Manufacturing Manager: Linda Ierardi

A NOTE TO THE READER:
The author and publisher have made every attempt to check dosages and nursing content for accuracy. Because the science of pharmacology is continually advancing, knowledge base continues to expand. Therefore we recommend that the reader alway check product information for changes in dosage or administration before administeri any medication. This is particularly important with new or rarely used drugs.

Printed in the United States of America

Mosby, Inc
11830 Westline Industrial Drive
St. Louis, Missouri 63146

ISBN 0-323-00149-1

00 01 02 / 9 8 7 6 5 4 3 2

Contributors

Kathryn Ballenger, RN, MSN, CCRN, FNP
Instructor of Nursing
University of Virginia School of Nursing
Charlottesville, Virginia

Leslie Buchanan, RN, MSN, ENP
Clinician 4, Emergency Nurse Practitioner
Department of Emergency Medicine
University of Virginia Health System
Charlottesville, Virginia

Suzanne M. Burns, RN, MSN, RRT, ACNP-CS, CCRN
Clinician 5;
Associate Professor of Nursing
University of Virginia Health Sciences Center
Charlottesville, Virginia

Lucy R. Deivert, RN, BA, BSN
Registered Nurse
Pediatric Intensive Care Unit
The Children's Mercy Hospital
Kansas City, Missouri

Mikel Gray, PhD, CUNP, CCCN, FAAN
Associate Professor of Nursing
University of Virginia School of Nursing;
Nurse Practitioner
Department of Urology
University of Virginia
Charlottesville, Virginia

Kathleen R. Haden, RN, CS, MSN, ANP, OCN
Adult Nurse Practitioner
University of Virginia Cancer Center;
Clinical Instructor
University of Virginia School of Nursing
Charlottesville, Virginia

Gail L. Kongable-Beckman, RN, MSN
Assistant Professor, Research;
Clinical Scientist
Virginia Neurologic Institute
University of Virginia
Charlottesville, Virginia

Patrice Y. Neese, RN, MSN, CS, ANP
Nurse Practitioner
Breast & Melanoma Teams
Department of Surgery/Oncology
University of Virginia
Charlottesville, Virginia

Juanita Reigle, RN, MSN, ACNP-CS, CCRN
Clinician 5, Practitioner-Teacher
Heart Center
University of Virginia Health System
Charlottesville, Virginia

Reviewers

Charlé C.F. Avery, RN, CS, MSN, ANP
Advanced Practice Nurse
Baylor Senior Health Center - Hillside
Dallas, Texas

Janie B. Butts, RN, DSN
Instructor
University of Southern Mississippi
College of Nursing
Hattiesburg, Mississippi

Sue E. Huether, RN, PhD
Associate Professor
University of Utah College of Nursing
Salt Lake City, Utah

Kathryn L. McCance, RN, PhD
Professor
University of Utah College of Nursing
Salt Lake City, Utah

Kristynia M. Robinson, RN, PhD, FNPc
Associate Professor
Department of Nursing
Idaho State University
Pocatello, Idaho

Lorraine M. Wilson, RN, PhD
Professor of Nursing
Pathophysiology Instructor;
Director, MSN Program - Adult Health
Eastern Michigan University
Ypsilanti, Michigan

Preface

The purpose of this book is to provide a summary of the pathophysiology of selected common diseases, and apply that information to clinical assessment, diagnosis and management. Case studies are provided to reinforce the skills learned in each chapter, and an extensive up-to-date bibliography is included.

This text is designed to be used by the health care clinician, student, and educator. By understanding the underlying pathophysiologic processes, the reader can better predict clinical manifestations, choose evaluative studies, initiate appropriate therapies, and anticipate potential complications. In addition, insights into the underlying disease processes can prepare the practitioner for the use of new and innovative interventions and drugs.

This book is organized by body system, and 25 selected diagnoses have been included that are not only common to clinical practice, but represent concepts of pathophysiology, evaluation, and management that can be applied to many other illnesses. Each chapter has two distinct sections.

Section I contains a concise summary of the disease, including Definition, Epidemiology, Pathophysiology, Patient Presentation, Differential Diagnosis, Keys to Evaluation and Keys to Management. Algorithms and tables illustrate important points. This information is followed by a unique "Pathophysiology → Clinical Link" diagram that emphasizes how an understanding of the pathophysiologic principles can guide patient care. A bibliography of selected recent articles is included for each chapter.

Section II of each chapter contains a representative case study in a "fill-in-the-blank" format that can be used by clinicians and students to practice their skills and by educators to evaluate their students. Suggested solutions and rationales for the case study questions can be found in the back of the book.

Acknowledgments

This book would not exist without the generous and kind support of Dr. Kathy McCance and Dr. Sue Huether at the University of Utah. Having used their nationally-renowned Pathophysiology textbook in my classes for years, I was amazed when they welcomed me into their world, allowing me to see how they have achieved their well-deserved reputations as the finest of professional nurses, scholars and writers. They went out on a limb and gave me the chance to contribute to their outstanding texts, to participate in national conferences, and to essentially move into their homes during the development of this book. They continue to be the very best of mentors, role models, and friends.

They also introduced me to Sally Schrefer, Publisher of Academic Nursing at Mosby, who has been incredibly supportive and encouraging throughout this project. Developmental Editors Gail Brower and Shelly Hayden have gotten me through all the rough spots with endless patience and with a reassuring commitment to turning out the very best and most accurate book possible. Sue Meeks put in endless hours finalizing the chapters while overcoming the most amazing of computer-generated problems.

I am endlessly grateful to the expert clinical nurses who contributed many of the case studies for this book. Their expertise has guided my teaching, my writing, and my practice for many years. I would also like to thank my students for their enthusiasm for pathophysiology; they are my inspiration and my reason for coming to work each day. I would like to especially thank Lucy Deivert for her hard work and scholarly contribution to two chapters. I am convinced that her name will appear on many important publications in the future.

My colleagues at the University of Virginia School of Nursing have been supportive in both word and deed of my unique role in the School. It is my privilege to work with so knowledgeable, dedicated, and caring a group of professionals. I would like to especially thank Dr. Sharon Utz, who is my mentor, my boss, and my constant support in helping me grow professionally and personally as a part of nursing education. I would also like to thank my Dean, Dr. Jeanette Lancaster, who has always given me the opportunity to express my energies and ideas in creative ways.

Finally, I would like to thank my family and friends, especially Patty, for putting up with my long hours and distracted ways for so long.

Contents

CHAPTER 1

HYPERTENSION

DEFINITION

- Hypertension (HTN) is defined as sustained abnormal elevation of the arterial blood pressure.
- The Sixth Report of the Joint National Committee on Detection, Evaluation, and Treatment of High Blood Pressure (JNC VI) defines high blood pressure in adults as follows:

Category	Systolic, mmHg	Diastolic, mmHg
Optimal	<120	<80
Normal	<130	<85
High normal	130-139	85-89
Hypertension		
Stage 1 (mild)	140-159	90-99
Stage 2 (moderate)	160-179	100-109
Stage 3 (severe)	$\geq$180	$\geq$110

- The new category "Optimal" indicates the group at lowest cardiovascular risk.
- The category "High normal" indicates the group at risk for developing HTN for which there is an opportunity to prevent progression with lifestyle modification.
- 95% is essential HTN; 5% is secondary HTN.
- There are many contributing processes to essential HTN (see below).
- Secondary HTN can be caused by renal parenchymal disease, renal vascular disease, adrenocortical disease (Cushings or hyperaldosteronism), pheochromocytoma, hyperthyroidism, hyperparathyroidism, and some drugs.

EPIDEMIOLOGY

- Overall, 29% whites, 38% African Americans, and 60% of people over 65 have HTN.
- HTN is a risk factor for atherosclerotic coronary disease, congestive heart failure, stroke, and renal failure.
- African Americans tend to develop more severe HTN at an earlier age and have nearly twice the risk of stroke and myocardial infarction (MI) as whites.

1

- Children who have HTN are more likely to have secondary HTN if the blood pressure (BP) is greater than the 99th percentile for age.

- The elderly population tends to have more isolated systolic HTN, which has been clearly associated with an increased risk for MI and stroke.

- Risk factors in all populations include age, obesity, sedentary lifestyle, family history, smoking, alcohol, high sodium intake (especially in African Americans, the elderly, and diabetics), and low potassium or magnesium intake (especially in African Americans).

PATHOPHYSIOLOGY

- Extremely complicated interaction of genetics and the environment mediated by a host of neurohormonal mediators.

- Generally caused by increased peripheral resistance and/or increased blood volume.

- Current theories include:

  - Increased activity of the sympathetic nervous system (SNS).

  - Increased activity of the renin/angiotensin/aldosterone (RAA) system.

  - Altered activity of atrial natriuretic peptide (ANF), adrenomedullin, urodilatin, and endothelin.

  - Decreased synthesis or increased breakdown of nitric oxide.

- Each of these theories would explain an increase in peripheral resistance due to an increase in vasoconstrictors (SNS, RAA) or a decrease in vasodilators (ANF, adrenomedullin, urodilatin, nitric oxide) and are believed to mediate changes in what is called the "pressure-natriuresis relationship," which states that hypertensive individuals tend to have less renal sodium excretion for a given increase in blood pressure (Figure 1-1).

Figure 1-1.
Pressure-Natriuresis Relationship

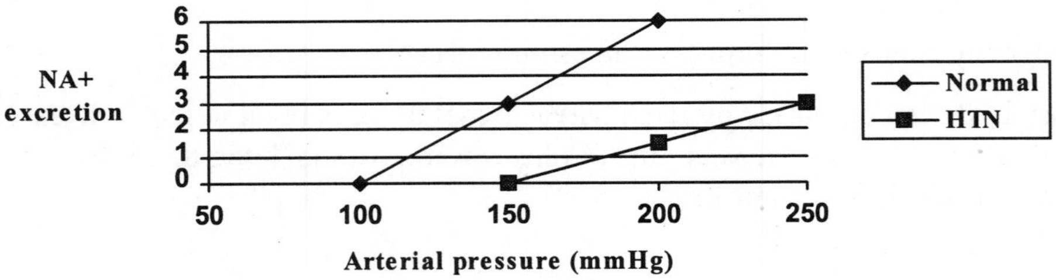

From Crowley, A. W., & Roman, R. J. (1996). The role of the kidney in hypertension. *Journal of the American Medical Association, 275,* 1581.

- Other theories include intracellular hypomagnesemia, decreased potassium or calcium intake, insulin resistance that interferes with insulin-mediated nitric oxide production, and an unclear genetic/environmental link between HTN and hyperinsulinemia, glucose intolerance, obesity, and hyperlipidemia.

- An understanding of this pathophysiology supports the current interventions employed in the management of HTN such as salt restriction, weight loss and diabetic control, SNS blockers, RAA blockers, nonspecific vasodilators, diuretics, and new experimental drugs that modulate ANF and endothelin.

PATIENT PRESENTATION

- History:

  Family history; childhood history of increased BP; other cardiac risk factors such as diabetes or dyslipidemia; history of stroke; smoking; alcohol abuse; high salt intake; recent changes in weight or obesity; medications, herbal remedies, or illicit drugs.

- Symptoms:

  Usually asymptomatic in early stages; if BP rises acutely, patient may develop epistaxis, headache, blurred vision, tinnitus, dizziness, transient neurologic deficits, or angina; if more slowly progressive, the patient may present with symptoms related to end-organ damage such as congestive heart failure, stroke, renal failure, or retinopathy.

- Examination:

  Systolic or diastolic HTN; skin for striae; retinopathy with vasoconstriction, arterial nicking, hemorrhages or exudates; focal neurologic deficits; cardiomegaly (displaced point of maximal impulse [PMI]), heave, gallops (S_3 or S_4); decreased peripheral pulses or bruits; abdominal bruits or masses; peripheral or pulmonary edema; if severe or sudden HTN, look for encephalopathic changes with cerebral edema and papilledema.

DIFFERENTIAL DIAGNOSIS

- First differentiate isolated increase in blood pressure from true HTN (see Keys to Assessment below).
- Then rule out secondary HTN:

  - Renal parenchymal disease

  - Renal vascular disease

  - Cushing disease or primary hyperaldosteronism

  - Pheochromocytoma

  - Hyperthyroidism

  - Hyperparathyroidism

KEYS TO ASSESSMENT

- Goals of evaluation are to establish the true diagnosis of HTN, rule out secondary HTN, assess for end-organ damage, and evaluate for overall cardiovascular and neurovascular risk profile.

- Diagnosis requires the measurement of blood pressure on at least three separate occasions averaging two readings at least 2 minutes apart, with the patient seated, the arm supported at heart level, after 5 minutes rest, with no smoking or caffeine intake in the past 30 minutes.

- 24-hour ambulatory blood pressure monitoring has a better correlation with end-organ damage, helps to screen out "white coat HTN" (occurs only in the clinic), and aids in the selection of antihypertensive therapy; it is recommended for patients with drug resistance, hypotensive symptoms with medications, episodic HTN, and autonomic dysfunction.

- Examine for abdominal masses, bruits, manifestations of Cushings (truncal obesity, striae), manifestations of pheochromocytoma (tachycardia, sweating, tremor).

- Funduscopic, vascular, cardiac, pulmonary, extremity and neurologic exam.

- Laboratory: urinalysis, chemistries including sodium, potassium, fasting glucose, blood urea nitrogen (BUN) and creatinine (Cr), serum calcium and magnesium, lipid profile, 12-lead electrocardiogram (ECG).

- Consider more specific tests such as renin, cortisol, urine catecholamines, renal ultrasound, echocardiogram, and vascular studies if history, physical, and severity of HTN indicate possible secondary cause or significant end-organ involvement.

KEYS TO MANAGEMENT

- Prevention—target persons with high-normal blood pressure, a family history of HTN, and one or more lifestyle contributors to age related increases in BP such as obesity, high sodium intake, physical inactivity, and excessive alcohol intake.

- Decisions on therapy for hypertensive patients are based on the following (Table 1-1):

  - The degree of blood pressure elevation

  - The presence of target organ damage

  - The presence of clinical cardiovascular disease or other risk factors

- Lifestyle modification:

  - Weight reduction (individualized and monitored program)

  - Exercise (regular aerobic exercise to achieve moderate physical fitness)

  - Low-salt diet (goal of <6 gm sodium chloride per day)

  - Low-fat, low-cholesterol diet

  - Decrease alcohol intake (no more than 2 beers, 10 oz of wine, or 2 oz of whiskey per day for men; half that amount for women)

  - Cessation of smoking

  - Increase potassium, calcium, and magnesium intake

- Pharmacologic (Figure 1-2).

  - Pharmacologic therapy is indicated for patients who have failed lifestyle modification alone, have blood pressure stage 2 or 3, have target organ damage, or have other significant cardiovascular risk factors.

  - JNC VI continues to recommend diuretics or β-blockers as first line agents for uncomplicated HTN.

  - Other conditions are associated with compelling indications for certain antihypertensive choices.

- A general principle is to fit the choice of antihypertensive to the individual patient.

- There is a new class of drugs known as angiotensin II receptor blockers—these agents have fewer side effects than the classic angiotensin converting enzyme (ACE) inhibitors and are effective in controlling blood pressure in many patients, but their long-term protection against target organ damage is unknown.

- Fixed-dose combinations of 2 agents from different classes often contain very low doses of each agent thus minimizing adverse effects while providing good antihypertensive efficacy (e.g., low dose diuretic + ACE inhibitor).

- After 1 year of successful blood pressure control, especially if there has been significant lifestyle modification, patients with uncomplicated HTN can be considered for step-down therapy including the following.

  - Medication reductions should be made slowly with close follow-up.

  - Patient should continue to be checked regularly as HTN can return even months or years after discontinuance.

Table 1-1. Risk Stratification and Treatment*

Blood Pressure Stages (mmHG)	Risk Group A (no risk factors; no TOD/CDD)[1]	Risk Group B (at least 1 risk factor not including diabetes; no TOD/CDD)	Risk Group C (TOD/CDD and/or diabetes with or without other risk factors)
High normal (130-139/85-89)	Lifestyle modification	Lifestyle modification	Drug therapy[2]
Stage 1 (140-159/90-99)	Lifestyle modification[3] (up to 12 months)	Lifestyle modification (up to 6 months)	Drug therapy
Stages 2 and 3 ($\geq$160/$\geq$110)	Drug therapy	Drug therapy	Drug therapy

* Lifestyle modification should be adjunctive therapy for all patients recommended for pharmacologic therapy.

[1] TOD/CCD indicates target-organ disease/clinical cardiovascular disease.
[2] For those with heart failure, renal insufficiency, or diabetes.
[3] For multiple risk factors, clinicians should consider drugs as initial therapy plus lifestyle modifications.

From: The Sixth Report of the Joint National Committee on Prevention, Detection, Evaluation, and Treatment of High Blood Pressure. (1997). *Archives of Internal Medicine 157*, 2420.

Figure 1-2.

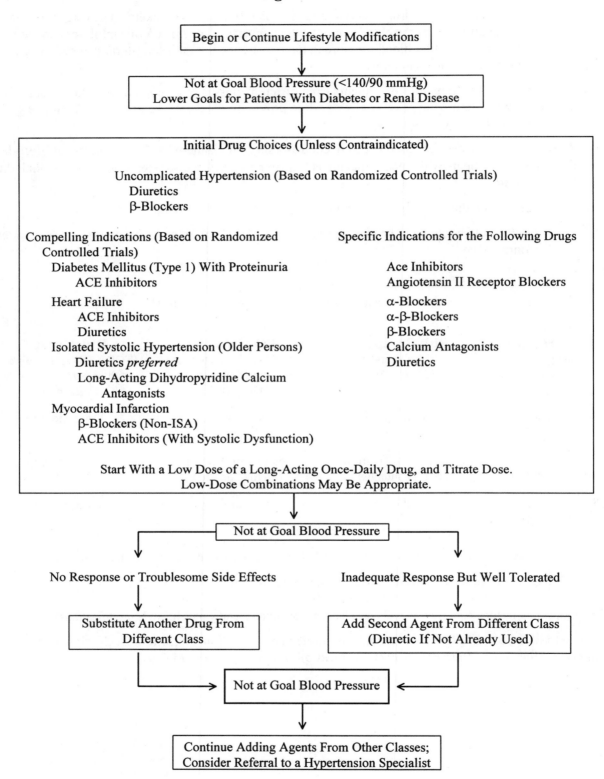

Begin or Continue Lifestyle Modifications

Not at Goal Blood Pressure (<140/90 mmHg)
Lower Goals for Patients With Diabetes or Renal Disease

Initial Drug Choices (Unless Contraindicated)

Uncomplicated Hypertension (Based on Randomized Controlled Trials)
  Diuretics
  β-Blockers

Compelling Indications (Based on Randomized Controlled Trials)
  Diabetes Mellitus (Type 1) With Proteinuria
    ACE Inhibitors
  Heart Failure
    ACE Inhibitors
    Diuretics
  Isolated Systolic Hypertension (Older Persons)
    Diuretics *preferred*
    Long-Acting Dihydropyridine Calcium
      Antagonists
  Myocardial Infarction
    β-Blockers (Non-ISA)
    ACE Inhibitors (With Systolic Dysfunction)

Specific Indications for the Following Drugs
    Ace Inhibitors
    Angiotensin II Receptor Blockers
    α-Blockers
    α-β-Blockers
    β-Blockers
    Calcium Antagonists
    Diuretics

Start With a Low Dose of a Long-Acting Once-Daily Drug, and Titrate Dose.
Low-Dose Combinations May Be Appropriate.

Not at Goal Blood Pressure

No Response or Troublesome Side Effects

Inadequate Response But Well Tolerated

Substitute Another Drug From Different Class

Add Second Agent From Different Class (Diuretic If Not Already Used)

Not at Goal Blood Pressure

Continue Adding Agents From Other Classes;
Consider Referral to a Hypertension Specialist

From: The Sixth Report of the Joint National Committee on Prevention, Detection, Evaluation, and Treatment of High Blood Pressure. (1997). *Archives of Internal Medicine, 157,* 2430.

Pathophysiology → ## Clinical Link

What is going on in the disease process that influences how the patient presents and how he or she should be managed?

What should you do now that you understand the underlying pathophysiology?

Patients whose blood pressures fall between 130 to 139 mmHG systolic and 85 to 89 mmHg diastolic are at increased risk for developing HTN.	It is critical to identify at-risk patients (family history, race, older age, smoker, high-salt diet, diabetes, dyslipidemia) and intervene with lifestyle modification.
The pathophysiology of the hemodynamic manifestations of HTN includes increased peripheral resistance and increased circulating volume.	HTN results in increased work for the heart, making cardiac complications (such as hypertrophy and ischemia) likely; the blood pressure will usually respond to vasodilators and diuresis.
Renal parenchyma disease, renal artery stenosis, and adrenal diseases result in hormonally-induced increases in peripheral resistance and circulating volume and therefore HTN.	The initial assessment of a patient with HTN should include evaluation for possible secondary causes, including a careful physical exam (rule out abdominal bruits or masses, striae) and selected laboratory tests (chemistries, urinalysis, BUN, and Cr).
One of the most important putative mediators of essential HTN is the over activity of the RAA system; angiotensin II has been implicated in the pathogenesis of other HTN-related diseases such as congestive heart failure, MI, and diabetic renal disease.	Angiotensin-converting enzyme inhibitors (and possibly the new angiotensin II receptor blockers) are effective in many patients with HTN and are specifically indicated in patients with congestive heart failure, MI with systolic dysfunction, and diabetes.
Another proposed mechanism of essential HTN is an abnormal pressure/natriuresis relationship.	Recent studies have reconfirmed the importance of salt restriction for most patients (especially African Americans, older people, and diabetics) and support the use of diuretics as first-line agents in uncomplicated HTN.
HTN is usually asymptomatic and target organ damage develops slowly.	Patient education about the seriousness of HTN and its potential complications improves adherence to therapy.

BIBLIOGRAPHY

Adcock, B. B., & Ireland, R. B. J. (1997). Secondary hypertension: A practical diagnostic approach [review, 23 refs]. *American Family Physician, 55*(4), 1263-1270.

Aitken, L., & Addison, C. (1996). The cost-effectiveness of ambulatory blood pressure monitoring. *Professional Nurse, 12*(3), 198-202.

Alderman, M. H., Madhavan, S., & Cohen, H. (1996). Antihypertensive drug therapy. The effect of JNC criteria on prescribing patterns and patient status through the first year [published erratum appears in *American Journal of Hypertension, 1996, 9*(8), 840]. *American Journal of Hypertension, 9*[5], 413-418.

Alderman, M. H., Ooi, W. L., Cohen, H., Madhavan, S., Sealey, J. E., & Laragh, J. H. (1997). Plasma renin activity: A risk factor for myocardial infarction in hypertensive patients. *American Journal of Hypertension, 10*(1), 1-8.

Anonymous. (1996). Update on the 1987 Task Force Report on High Blood Pressure in Children and Adolescents: A working group report from the National High Blood Pressure Education Program. National High Blood Pressure Education Program Working Group on hypertension control in children and adolescents [see comments]. *Pediatrics, 98*(4 Pt 1), 649-658.

Anonymous. (1997). Effects of weight loss and sodium reduction intervention on blood pressure and hypertension incidence in overweight people with high-normal blood pressure. The Trials of Hypertension Prevention, phase II. The trials of Hypertension Prevention Collaborative Research Group [see comments]. *Archives of Internal Medicine, 157*(6), 657-667.

Anonymous. (1997). Five-year findings of the hypertension detection and follow-up program. I. Reduction in mortality of persons with high blood pressure, including mild hypertension. Hypertension Detection and Follow-up Program Cooperative Group. 1979 [classical article, see comments]. *Journal of the American Medical Association, 277*(2), 157-166.

Anonymous. (1997) The Sixth Report of the Joint National Committee on Prevention, Detection, Evaluation, and Treatment of High Blood Pressure. *Archives of Internal Medicine 157*, 2413-2446.

Aono, T., Kuwajima, I., Suzuki, Y., & Ozawa, T. (1997). Relation between left ventricular remodeling and nocturnal blood pressure in the elderly with systemic hypertension. *American Journal of Cardiology, 80*(1), 81-84.

Appel, L. J., Moore, T. J., Obarzanek, E., Vollmer, W. M., Svetkey, L. P., Sacks, F. M., Bray, G. A., Vogt, T. M., Cutler, J. A., Windhauser, M. M., Lin, P. H., & Karanja, N. (1997). A clinical trial of the effects of dietary patterns on blood pressure. DASH Collaborative Research Group. *New England Journal of Medicine, 336*(16), 1117-1124.

Arauz-Pacheco, C., Lender, D., Snell, P. G., Huet, B., Ramirez, L. C., Breen, L., Mora, P., & Raskin, P. (1996). Relationship between insulin sensitivity, hyperinsulinemia, and insulin-mediated sympathetic activation in normotensive and hypertensive subjects. *American Journal of Hypertension, 9*(12 Pt 1), 1172-1178.

Bloem, L. J., Foroud, T. M., Ambrosius, W. T., Hanna, M. P., Tewksbury, D. A., & Pratt, J. H. (1997). Association of the angiotensinogen gene to serum angiotensinogen in blacks and whites. *Hypertension, 29*(5), 1078-1082.

Cengiz, E., Unalan, H., Tugrul, A., & Ekerbicer, H. (1997). Biofeedback assisted relaxation in essential hypertension: Short-term follow-up of contributing effects of pharmacotherapy on blood pressure and heart rate [Brief communication]. *Yonsei Medical Journal, 38*(2), 86-90.

Chalmers, J. (1996). Treatment guidelines in hypertension: Current limitations and future solutions [review, 38 refs]. *Journal of Hypertension, 14*(Suppl 4), S3-8.

Chobanian, A. V., & Alexander, R. W. (1996). Exacerbation of atherosclerosis by hypertension. Potential mechanisms and clinical implications [see comments] [review, 54 refs]. *Archives of Internal Medicine, 156*(17), 1952-1956.

Cowan, T. (1997). Ambulatory blood pressure monitors [review, 13 refs]. *Professional Nurse, 12*(5), 373-376.

Cowley, A. W. J. (1997). Genetic and nongenetic determinants of salt sensitivity and blood pressure [review, 50 refs]. *American Journal of Clinical Nutrition, 65*(2 Suppl), 587S-593S.

Curb, J. D., Pressel, S. L., Cutler, J. A., Savage, P. J., Applegate, W. B., Black, H., Camel, G., Davis, B. R., Frost, P. H., Gonzalez, N., Guthrie, G., Oberman, A., Rutan, G. H., & Stamler, J. (1996). Effect of diuretic-based antihypertensive treatment on cardiovascular disease risk in older diabetic patients with isolated systolic hypertension. Systolic Hypertension in the Elderly Program Cooperative Research Group [published erratum appears in *Journal of the American Medical Association, 1997, 277*[17], 1356] [see comments]. *Journal of the American Medical Association, 276*(23), 1886-1892.

Curzen, N., & Purcell, H. (1997). Matching the treatment to the patient in hypertension. *Practitioner, 241*(1572), 152-156.

Cutler, J. A. (1996). High blood pressure and end-organ damage [review, 24 refs]. *Journal of Hypertension (Supplement), 14*(6), S3-6.

Eaton, L., Buck, E. A., & Catanzaro, J. E. (1996). The nurse's role in facilitating compliance in clients with hypertension [review, 19 refs]. *MEDSURG Nursing, 5*(5), 339-345.

Elliott, H. L. (1996). Benefits of twenty-four-hour blood pressure control [review, 8 refs]. *Journal of Hypertension (Supplement), 14*(4), S15-9.

Ellis, M. L., & Patterson, J. H. (1996). A new class of antihypertensive therapy: Angiotensin II receptor antagonists [review, 55 refs]. *Pharmacotherapy, 16*(5), 849-860.

Epstein, M., & Bakris, G. (1996). Newer approaches to antihypertensive therapy. Use of fixed-dose combination therapy [see comments] [review, 88 refs]. *Archives of Internal Medicine, 156*(17), 1969-1978.

Ferro, C. J., & Webb, D. J. (1997). Endothelial dysfunction and hypertension [review, 102 refs]. *Drugs, 53*(Suppl 1), 30-41.

Fish, A. F., Smith, B. A., Frid, D. J., Christman, S. K., Post, D., & Montalto, N. J. (1997). Step treadmill exercise training and blood pressure reduction in women with mild hypertension. *Progress in Cardiovascular Nursing, 12*(1), 4-12.

Fogo, A., & Kon, V. (1996). Treatment of hypertension [review, 114 refs]. *Seminars in Nephrology, 16*(6), 555-566.

Frishman, W. H., & Michaelson, M. D. (1997). Use of calcium antagonists in patients with ischemic heart disease and systemic hypertension [review, 36 refs]. *American Journal of Cardiology, 79*(10A), 33-38, discussion 47-48.

Gifford, R. W. J. (1997). What's new in the treatment of hypertension [review, 41 refs]. *Cleveland Clinic Journal of Medicine, 64*(3), 143-150.

Glen, S. K., Elliott, H. L., Curzio, J. L., Lees, K. R., & Reid, J. L. (1996). White-coat hypertension as a cause of cardiovascular dysfunction [see comments]. *Lancet, 348*(9028), 654-657.

Goa, K. L., & Wagstaff, A. J. (1996). Losartan potassium: A review of its pharmacology, clinical efficacy and tolerability in the management of hypertension [review, 138 refs]. *Drugs, 51*(5), 820-845.

Gordon, N. F., Scott, C. B., & Levine, B. D. (1997). Comparison of single versus multiple lifestyle interventions: Are the antihypertensive effects of exercise training and diet-induced weight loss additive? *American Journal of Cardiology, 79*(6), 763-767.

Grimm, R. H. J., Grandits, G. A., Cutler, J. A., Stewart, A. L., McDonald, R. H., Svendsen, K., Prineas, R. J., & Liebson, P. R. (1997). Relationships of quality-of-life measures to long-term lifestyle and drug treatment in the Treatment of Mild Hypertension Study. *Archives of Internal Medicine, 157*(6), 638-648.

Gueyffier, F., Boutitie, F., Boissel, J. P., Pocock, S., Coope, J., Cutler, J., Ekbom, T., Fagard, R., Friedman, L., Perry, M., Prineas, R., & Schron, E. (1997). Effect of antihypertensive drug treatment on cardiovascular outcomes in women and men. A meta-analysis of individual patient data from randomized, controlled trials. The INDANA Investigators. *Annals of Internal Medicine, 126*(10), 761-767.

Haffner, S. M. (1997). Epidemiology of hypertension and insulin resistance syndrome [review, 88 refs]. *Journal of Hypertension (Supplement), 15*(1), S25-S30.

Hall, J. E. (1997). Mechanisms of abnormal renal sodium handling in obesity hypertension [review, 48 refs]. *American Journal of Hypertension, 10*(5 Pt 2), 49S-55S.

Hansson, L. (1996). Hypertension in the elderly [review, 31 refs]. *Journal of Hypertension (Supplement), 14*(3), S17-S21.

Hansson, L. (1996). The optimal blood pressure reduction [review, 22 refs]. *Journal of Hypertension (Supplement), 14*(2), S55-S58, discussion S58-S59.

Hansson, L. (1997). Issues in the treatment of hypertension: Current and future perspectives [review, 45 refs]. *Cardiology, 88*(Suppl 1), 47-53, discussion 54-55.

Harrap, S. B. (1996). An appraisal of the genetic approaches to high blood pressure [review, 20 refs]. *Journal of Hypertension (Supplement), 14*(5), S111-S115.

Higashi, Y., Oshima, T., Sasaki, N., Ishioka, N., Nakano, Y., Ozono, R., Yoshimura, M., Ishibashi, K., Matsuura, H., & Kajiyama, G. (1997). Relationship between insulin resistance and endothelium-dependent vascular relaxation in patients with essential hypertension. *Hypertension, 29*(1 Pt 2), 280-285.

Hunyor, S. N., Henderson, R. J., Lal, S. K., Carter, N. L., Kobler, H., Jones, M., Bartrop, R. W., Craig, A., & Mihailidou, A. S. (1997). Placebo-controlled biofeedback blood pressure effect in hypertensive humans. *Hypertension, 29*(6), 1225-1231.

Johnston, C. I. (1996). Future management of high blood pressure [review, 29 refs]. *Journal of Cardiovascular Pharmacology, 27*(Suppl 3), S55-S60.

Jones, D. W. (1996). Body weight and blood pressure. Effects of weight reduction on hypertension. *American Journal of Hypertension, 9*(8), 50s-54s.

Julius, S. (1996). The Hypertension Optimal Treatment (HOT) Study in the United States [review, 2 refs]. *American Journal of Hypertension, 9*(8), 41S-44S.

Julius, S., & Nesbitt, S. (1996). Sympathetic overactivity in hypertension. A moving target [review, 64 refs]. *American Journal of Hypertension, 9*(11), 113S-120S.

Kamide, K., Nagano, M., Nakano, N., Yo, Y., Kobayashi, R., Rakugi, H., Higaki, J., & Ogihara, T. (1996). Insulin resistance and cardiovascular complications in patients with essential hypertension. *American Journal of Hypertension, 9*(12 Pt 1), 1165-1171.

Kohno, M., Yokokawa, K., Yasunari, K., Kano, H., Minami, M., Hanehira, T., & Yoshikawa, J. (1997). Changes in plasma cardiac natriuretic peptides concentrations during 1 year treatment with angiotensin-converting enzyme inhibitor in elderly hypertensive patients with left ventricular hypertrophy. *International Journal of Clinical Pharmacology & Therapeutics, 35*(1), 38-42.

Kostis, J. B., Davis, B. R., Cutler, J., Grimm, R. H. J., Berge, K. G., Cohen, J. D., Lacy, C. R., Perry, H. M. J., Blaufox, M. D., Wassertheil-Smoller, S., Black, H. R., Schron, E., Berkson, D. M., Curb, J. D., Smith, W. M., McDonald, R., & Applegate, W. B. (1997). Prevention of heart failure by antihypertensive drug treatment in older persons with isolated systolic hypertension. SHEP Cooperative Research Group. *Journal of the American Medical Association, 278*(3), 212-216.

Kotchen, T. A., & Kotchen, J. M. (1997). Dietary sodium and blood pressure:Interactions with other nutrients [review, 61 refs]. *American Journal of Clinical Nutrition, 65*(2 Suppl), 708S-711S.

Mark, A. L. (1996). The sympathetic nervous system in hypertension: A potential long-term regulator of arterial pressure [review, 37 refs]. *Journal of Hypertension (Supplement), 14*(5), S159-65.

McCarron, D. A. (1997). Role of adequate dietary calcium intake in the prevention and management of salt-sensitive hypertension [review, 24 refs]. *American Journal of Clinical Nutrition, 65*(2 Suppl), 712S-716S.

Midgley, J. P., Matthew, A. G., Greenwood, C. M., & Logan, A. G. (1996). Effect of reduced dietary sodium on blood pressure: A meta-analysis of randomized controlled trials [see comments]. *Journal of the American Medical Association, 275*(20), 1590-1597.

Moore, C. R., Krakoff, L. R., & Phillips, R. A. (1997). Confirmation or exclusion of stage I hypertension by ambulatory blood pressure monitoring. *Hypertension, 29*(5), 1109-1113.

Mountokalakis, T. D. (1997). The renal consequences of arterial hypertension [review, 109 refs]. *Kidney International, 51*(5), 1639-1653.

Mulvany, M. J. (1996). Effects of angiotensin converting enzyme inhibition on vascular remodelling of resistance vessels in hypertensive patients [review, 38 refs]. *Journal of Hypertension (Supplement), 14*(6), S21-4.

Myers, M. G. (1996). Twenty-four-hour blood pressure control: A brief review of aspects of target-organ protection [review, 17 refs]. *Journal of Hypertension (Supplement), 14*(6), S7-S10.

Neutel, J., Abernethy, D. R., Moser, M., Gifford, R. W. J., & Frishman, W. H. (1997). Discussion: Recent data on the safety and efficacy of newer therapies in the management of hypertension. *American Journal of Hypertension, 10*(3), 24S-26S.

Nowson, C. A., McMurchie, E. J., Burnard, S. L., Head, R. J., Boehm, J., Hoang, H. N., Hopper, J. L., & Wark, J. D. (1997). Genetic factors associated with altered sodium transport in human hypertension: A twin study. *Clinical and Experimental Pharmacology & Physiology, 24*(6), 424-426.

Oalmann, M. C., Strong, J. P., Tracy, R. E., & Malcom, G. T. (1997). Atherosclerosis in youth: Are hypertension and other coronary heart disease risk factors already at work? [Review, 84 refs]. *Pediatric Nephrology, 11*(1), 99-107.

Opie, L. H. (1997). Calcium channel blockers for hypertension: Dissecting the evidence for adverse effects [review, 84 refs]. *American Journal of Hypertension, 10*(5 Pt 1), 565-577.

Osborne, C. G., McTyre, R. B., Dudek, J., Roche, K. E., Scheuplein, R., Silverstein, B., Weinberg, M. S., & Salkeld, A. A. (1996). Evidence for the relationship of calcium to blood pressure [review, 169 refs]. *Nutrition Reviews, 54*(12), 365-381.

Palombo, V., Scurti, R., Muscari, A., Puddu, G. M., Di, I. A., Zito, M., & Abate, G. (1997). Blood pressure and intellectual function in elderly subjects. *Age & Aging, 26*(2), 91-98.

Paolisso, G., & Barbagallo, M. (1997). Hypertension, diabetes mellitus, and insulin resistance: The role of intracellular magnesium [see comments] [review, 74 refs]. *American Journal of Hypertension, 10*(3), 346-355.

Paran, E., Anson, O., & Neumann, L. (1996). The effects of replacing beta-blockers with an angiotensin converting enzyme inhibitor on the quality of life of hypertensive patients. *American Journal of Hypertension, 9*(12 Pt 1), 1206-1213.

Parrinello, G., Scaglione, R., Pinto, A., Corrao, S., Cecala, M., Di, S. G., Amato, P., Licata, A., & Licata, G. (1996). Central obesity and hypertension: The role of plasma endothelin. *American Journal of Hypertension, 9*(12 Pt 1), 1186-1191.

Rahman, M., Douglas, J. G., & Wright, J. T. J. (1997). Pathophysiology and treatment implications of hypertension in the African-American population [Review, 177 refs]. *Endocrinology and Metabolism Clinics of North America, 26*(1), 125-144.

Resnick, L. M. (1997). Magnesium in the pathophysiology and treatment of hypertension and diabetes mellitus: Where are we in 1997? [editorial; comment]. *American Journal of Hypertension, 10*(3), 368-370.

Robertson, J. I. (1997). Risk factors and drugs in the treatment of hypertension [review, 38 refs]. *Journal of Hypertension (Supplement), 15*(1), S43-S46.

Schmieder, R. E., Martus, P., & Klingbeil, A. (1996). Reversal of left ventricular hypertrophy in essential hypertension. A meta-analysis of randomized double-blind studies [see comments]. *Journal of the American Medical Association, 275*(19), 1507-1513.

Schmieder, R. E., Rockstroh, J. K., Gatzka, C. D., Ruddel, H., & Schachinger, H. (1997). Discontinuation of antihypertensive therapy: Prevalence of relapses and predictors of successful withdrawal in a hypertensive community. *Cardiology, 88*(3), 277-284.

Schmieder, R. E., Rockstroh, J. K., Luchters, G., Hammerstein, U., & Messerli, F. H. (1997). Comparison of early target organ damage between blacks and whites with mild systemic arterial hypertension. *American Journal of Cardiology, 79*(12), 1695-1698.

Seals, D. R., Silverman, H. G., Reiling, M. J., & Davy, K. P. (1997). Effect of regular aerobic exercise on elevated blood pressure in postmenopausal women. *American Journal of Cardiology, 80*(1), 49-55.

Sleight, P. (1996). Primary prevention of coronary heart disease in hypertension [review, 29 refs]. *Journal of Hypertension (Supplement), 14*(2), S35-S38, discussion S38-S39.

Smulyan, H., & Safar, M. E. (1997). Systolic blood pressure revisited [review, 57 refs]. *Journal of the American College of Cardiology, 29*(7), 1407-1413.

Strandgaard, S. (1996). Hypertension and stroke [review, 40 refs]. *Journal of Hypertension (Supplement), 14*(3), S23-S27.

Strickland, C. (1997). Safety and efficacy of first-line antihypertensives. *Journal of Family Practice, 44*(6), 530-531.

Tonkin, A., & Wing, L. (1996). Management of isolated systolic hypertension [review, 47 refs]. *Drugs, 51*(5), 738-749.

Valvo, E., D'Angelo, A., & Maschio, G. (1997). Diuretics in hypertension [review, 26 refs]. *Kidney International (Supplement), 59*, S36-8.

van, P. P., de, Z. D., Navis, G., & de, J. P. E. (1996). Does the renin-angiotensin system determine the renal and systemic hemodynamic response to sodium in patients with essential hypertension? [see comments]. *Hypertension, 27*(2), 202-208.

Vanhoutte, P. M. (1996). Endothelial dysfunction in hypertension [review, 136 refs]. *Journal of Hypertension - Supplement, 14*(5), S83-93.

Wang, W. Y., Zee, R. Y., & Morris, B. J. (1997). Association of angiotensin II type 1 receptor gene polymorphism with essential hypertension. *Clinical Genetics, 51*(1), 31-34.

Whelton, P. K., Kumanyika, S. K., Cook, N. R., Cutler, J. A., Borhani, N. O., Hennekens, C. H., Kuller, L. H., Langford, H., Jones, D. W., Satterfield, S., Lasser, N. L., & Cohen, J. D. (1997). Efficacy of nonpharmacologic interventions in adults with high-normal blood pressure: Results from phase 1 of the Trials of Hypertension Prevention. Trials of Hypertension Prevention Collaborative Research Group. *American Journal of Clinical Nutrition, 65*(2 Suppl), 652S-660S.

Zanchetti, A. (1997). Antihypertensive therapy: How to evaluate the benefits [review, 26 refs]. *American Journal of Cardiology, 79*(10A), 3-8, discussion 47-8.

CASE STUDY

HYPERTENSION

INITIAL HISTORY:
- Age 47, male, African American
- Coming in for physical exam after having his blood pressure checked at a health fair and being told it was high
- Works as an executive for an insurance firm
- No specific complaints

Question 1.
What questions would you like to ask this patient?

ADDITIONAL HISTORY:
- No other health problems, on no medications
- Father and older brother both have hypertension
- History of MI and stroke at young ages in paternal grandparents
- Denies cardiac or neurologic symptoms

Question 2.
Are there other questions you would like to ask this patient?

MORE HISTORY:
- Eats significant amounts of prepackaged foods and snack foods
- Nonsmoker, drinks an average of 3 to 4 beers most evenings
- Has gained 12 pounds over the past year due to physical inactivity
- Last cholesterol checked 3 years ago; can only remember that his total cholesterol was 252 mg/dl; has "tried" to watch his diet

Question 3.
What are his risk factors for HTN?

PHYSICAL EXAMINATION:
- Mildly obese male in no distress
- T=37 orally; P = 95 and regular; RR = 14; BP = 156/98 in both arms, sitting

HEENT, Neck
- PERRLA, fundi with vasoconstriction but with no nicking, hemorrhages, or exudates
- Pharynx clear
- Neck supple without bruits or thyromegaly

Lungs
- Good lung expansion bilaterally
- Percussion without dullness throughout
- Breath sounds clear

Cardiac
- RRR, PMI 5th ICS at midclavicular line
- No murmurs
- Soft S$_4$ gallop heard at apex

Abdomen
- Mildly obese
- No abdominal bruits heard
- Soft without tenderness or organomegaly, liver 8 cm at midclavicular line
- No masses felt

Extremities
- No edema; no clubbing; no bruits
- Pulses full in all extremities

Neurological
- Alert and oriented
- Strength 5/5 throughout
- DTR 2+ and symmetrical
- Sensory intact to pin prick and light touch throughout
- Proprioception normal
- Gait steady

Question 4.
What are the pertinent positives and negatives on the physical exam and what might they mean?

Question 5.
What should be done now?

Question 6.
How should he prepare for his next visit, and how should his blood pressure be measured when he returns?

PATIENT'S RETURN VISIT:
- Patient continues to feel well, no complaints
- BP 160/100 both arms, sitting with arm elevated to heart level
- Rest of exam unchanged

Question 7.
What now?

PATIENT RETURNS FOR HIS THIRD VISIT:
- Still no complaints
- BP = 158/102
- Rest of exam unchanged

Question 8.
What now? Would you order laboratory tests? If so, what?

LABORATORY:
- All blood chemistries, including sodium, potassium, BUN, Cr, and calcium are normal.
- Complete blood count normal.
- Urinalysis negative for protein or glucose, microscopy without cells or cellular casts.
- Total cholesterol and LDL elevated; HDL slightly low.
- ECG shows increased QRS voltage in the chest leads.

Question 9.

What do the lab results mean?

Question 10.

How should this patient be managed?

CHAPTER 2

DYSLIPIDEMIA AND ATHEROSCLEROSIS

DEFINITION

- Dyslipidemia includes those changes in the lipid profile that are associated with an increased risk for atherosclerosis.

	Desirable	Borderline Risk	High Risk
Total Cholesterol, (mg/dl)	<200	200 to 239	≥240
LDL Cholesterol, (mg/dl)	<130	130 to 159	≥160
HDL Cholesterol (mg/dl)	≥50	35 to 49	<35
LDL/HDL ratio			>3.1
Triglycerides (TG, mg/dl)	>250 (fasting) considered probable risk		

- Atherosclerosis is a chronic disease characterized by thickening and hardening of the arterial wall. Lesions contain lipid deposits and become calcified, leading to vessel obstruction, platelet aggregation, and abnormal vasoconstriction.

EPIDEMIOLOGY

- Hyperlipidemia:
  - Estimates of the overall incidence of dyslipidemia in the United States range from 38% to 50%.
  - Relative dyslipidemia with changes in the vascular wall are common in children in the United States.
  - 1/500 persons has an identifiable heterozygous or homozygous familial hypercholesterolemia.
  - There is a high incidence of dyslipidemia in persons with diabetes, hypertension, and in African Americans.
  - The causes of dyslipidemia include the following: (1) common (polygenic) hypercholesterolemia; (2) familial hypercholesterolemias; (3) a diet high in saturated fats and/or cholesterol; diabetes; renal failure; (6) drugs (thiazides, steroids); smoking; and hypothyroidism.

- Atherosclerosis:
  - Atherosclerotic coronary disease is the leading cause of death in the United States.
  - Atherosclerotic cerebrovascular disease is the leading cause of stroke in the United States.

- Peripheral vascular disease is an important cause of disability.

- The risk factors include the following:
    1) Hyperlipidemia—increased total cholesterol or LDL cholesterol (especially small dense LDL), decreased HDL, increased triglycerides; increased lipoprotein(a) [Lp(a)]
        - Every 1% increase in cholesterol increases the risk of coronary disease by 3%
    2) Smoking
    3) Hypertension
    4) The male sex or the female after menopause
    5) Age >50
    6) Diabetes (insulin resistance)
    7) Increased serum fibrinogen
    8) Increased serum homocysteine (recently identified as being a very important independent indicator of coronary risk)
    9) High-fat diet, obesity, sedentary lifestyle
    10) Family history

PATHOPHYSIOLOGY

- Dyslipidemia, hypertension, smoking, autoimmune processes, diabetes, hyperhomocystinemia, and possibly, infections (such as chlamydia) cause arterial endothelial injury.

- The injured endothelial cells become more permeable, have increased levels of oxygen radicals, and become inflamed with recruitment of leukocytes and macrophages that adhere to the area of injury and produce more oxygen radicals (Figure 2-1).

- These leukocytes and macrophages release a host of inflammatory cytokines and mitogens that stimulate smooth muscle proliferation and inhibit the endothelial cells from excreting endogenous vasodilators such as nitric oxide.

- LDL is oxidized by the oxygen radicals, is phagocytosed by the macrophages, and then is carried into the vessel wall.

- Macrophages that are filled with oxidized LDL are called foam cells. Accumulations of these cells form a pathologic lesion called a fatty streak that induces further immunologic and inflammatory changes that result in progressive vessel damage.

- Fibrous tissue and damaged smooth muscle cells migrate into the area overlying the foam cells, forming a cap called a fibrous plaque.

- Further endothelial dysfunction and necrosis of tissue results in calcification of the lesion and protrusion into the vessel lumen; as the plaque progresses, it can ulcerate or rupture due to mechanical shear forces and continued necrosis of the vessel wall.

- Platelets aggregate and adhere to the surface of the ruptured plaque, the coagulation cascade is initiated, and a thrombus forms over the lesion that may completely obstruct the lumen of the vessel.

- The overall result is an artery that is narrowed and vulnerable to abnormal vasoconstriction and thrombosis.

- Lifestyle and pharmacologic interventions are possible at every step in this cascade of events that may prevent or reverse the process (see "Pathophysiology → Clinical Link").

Figure 2-1.

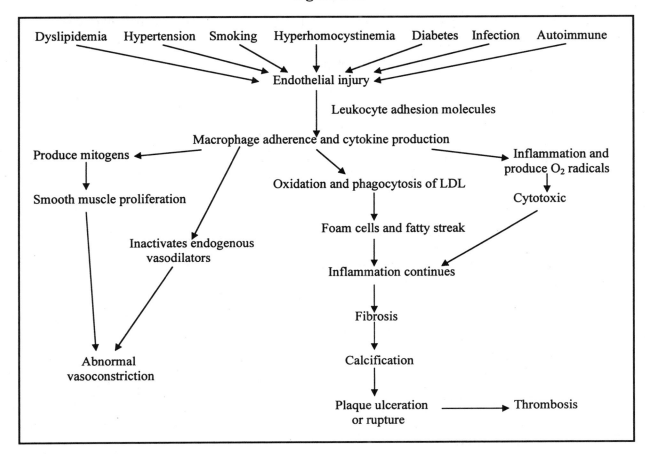

PATIENT PRESENTATION

- Dyslipidemia and atherosclerosis are often asymptomatic, and the decision to assess a patient is based on a history of risk factors.

- If the patient does present with symptoms, the symptoms are most often the result of atherosclerotic obstruction of major vessels with ischemia of target organs such as the heart, the kidneys, the brain, or the extremities.

- History

  High-fat diet; weight gain; sedentary lifestyle; age; gender; race; postmenopausal; smoking; diabetes; hypertension; family history; past medical history of high blood pressure or cardiac, cerebrovascular, or peripheral vascular disease.

- Symptoms

  Chest pain; shortness of breath; transient or permanent neurologic deficits; intermittent claudication (pain in leg with walking, relieved with rest); hair loss and skin ulcers on extremities; worsening headaches, dizziness, or epistaxis

- Examination

  Corneal arcus; xanthomas; increased blood pressure; abdominal bruits; bruits and decreased pulses in extremity arteries; obesity; evidence of congestive heart failure; focal neurologic deficits

DIFFERENTIAL DIAGNOSIS

- Familial dyslipidemia vs common polygenic dyslipidemia vs secondary dyslipidemia (renal failure, diabetes, drug-induced, hypothyroidism)
- Hypertension (primary as a risk factor, secondary due to renal vascular disease as a target organ effect)
- Ischemic heart disease
- Cerebrovascular disease
- Peripheral vascular disease

KEYS TO ASSESSMENT

- The goals are to identify modifiable risk factors and to assess for target organ effects.
- Remember, if one arterial system is diseased, it is likely that others are too.
- Lipid profile:
    - Current recommendations include a screening of total cholesterol in all adults over 20 years old every 5 years; the initial measurement should include an HDL.
    - The patient should be seated for 30 minutes, after fasting for 12 hours, and have had no recent major changes in weight, exercise, smoking, or blood pressure.
    - If the total cholesterol is <200, the patient should return for a repeat screening in 5 years.
    - If the total cholesterol is >200, a repeat measurement should be obtained and the results should be averaged to guide subsequent care decisions.
    - If the total cholesterol is 200 to 239 (borderline) and the patient has no coronary risk factors, he or she should be given diet guidelines and should return in 1 year.
    - If the total cholesterol is 200 to 239 and the patient has definite coronary artery disease or coronary risk factors, or if the total cholesterol is ≥240, he or she should receive a complete lipoprotein analysis and consideration for pharmacologic therapy.
        1) Lp(a) is a genetically determined risk factor especially in women and diabetics; a test should be ordered if there is advanced atherosclerosis without the conventional risk factors.
        2) Fasting blood glucose or glycosylated hemoglobin
        3) Serum electrolytes and blood urea nitrogen (BUN) and creatinine (Cr)
        4) Thyroid stimulating hormone (TSH)
        5) Liver function tests (aspartate aminotransferase [AST], alanine aminotransferase [ALT], alkaline phosphatase, lactate dehydrogenase [LDH])
        6) Serum homocysteine—not yet recommended for routine screening
        7) Electrocardiogram (ECG)
        8) Doppler ultrasound evaluation of selected arterial systems (popliteal, femoral, carotid) is done if the physical exam and history suggest involvement.
        9) Evaluation for evidence of coronary artery disease (see Chapter 3) or cerebrovascular disease (see Chapter 19).

KEYS TO MANAGEMENT

- Prevention

  - There is increasing evidence that atherosclerosis begins in childhood. Good diet habits and exercise with weight control should begin early in life and continue throughout the aging process.

  - Smoking cessation and exercise are associated with increased HDL.

  - Aggressive recognition and management of risk factors such as familial dyslipidemia, obesity, hypertension and diabetes.

  - Increase folate intake that lowers homocysteine levels, and increased antioxidant intake (especially vitamin E). Both have been associated with decreased risk of atherosclerosis and heart disease.

  - Consider hormone replacement therapy in postmenopausal women (it has been shown to decrease incidence of ischemic heart disease by as much as 50%).

- Diet therapy

  - A stepwise approach as recommended by National Cholesterol Education Program.

Nutrient	Step I	Step II
Total fat	≤30% of total calories	
Saturated fat	8% to 10%, of total calories	≤7% or total calories
Polyunsaturated fat	≤10% of total calories	
Monounsaturated fat	≤15% of total calories	
Carbohydrates	≥ 55% of total calories	
Protein	~15% of total calories	
Cholesterol	<300 mg/dl	<200 mg/dl
Total calories	Sufficient to achieve and maintain desirable weight	

  - Recent evidence suggests that a modest increase in the percentage of monounsaturated and ω-3 and ω-6 polyunsaturated fats is as important as reducing total saturated fats.

- Pharmacologic intervention

  - **Lipid lowering**:
    1) HMG-CoA reductase inhibitors (pravastatin, lovastatin) lower serum total cholesterol and LDL quickly and raise HDL with few side effects. Their long-term safety, efficacy, and ability to cause regression of atherosclerotic lesions are well-established, and most experts consider them firstline drug therapy.
       - Gastrointestinal distress occurs in about 5% of patients, and a reversible elevation in liver transaminase levels occurs in less than 2%. There is a rare incidence of myositis, primarily in patients who are also taking gemfibrozil.
    2) Fibric acid derivatives (gemfibrozil) decrease cholesterol slowly but are more effective than HMG-CoA reductase inhibitors in decreasing triglycerides.
       - There is a higher incidence of gastrointestinal distress, but fabric acid derivatives are safe, long-term, and effective in reducing coronary risk.

3) <u>Nicotinic acid</u> reduces total cholesterol, triglycerides and LDL, and raises HDL.
-   It causes flushing, gastrointestinal upset, and can impair glucose tolerance in prediabetic patients, but it has been shown to be effective in reducing coronary risk.

4) <u>Bile acid sequestrants</u> (cholestyramine and colestipol) decrease LDL slowly.
-   They increase triglycerides and have significant gastrointestinal side effects. They have been shown to reduce the incidence of coronary disease in hypercholesterolemia, but they should be avoided in patients with increased triglycerides.

- **Anticoagulation**—may be indicated to prevent thrombus formation on established plaques; aspirin, dipyridamole, clopidrogel, ticlopidine, anti-platelet GPIIb/IIIa receptor antibodies (integrelin, abciximab), warfarin and heparin are options.

- **Others**
1) Probucol and other antioxidants such as vitamin E have been shown to alter lipids and reduce atherosclerosis.
2) Estrogens have been shown to have a beneficial effect on lipid profiles and reduce coronary disease by up to 50% in postmenopausal women.
3) Soy protein, oat fiber, fish oils, and garlic have all been found to reduce cholesterol in some studies.
4) Angiotensin converting enzyme (ACE) inhibitors increase endogenous vasodilators, reduce smooth muscle hypertrophy, and decrease fibrosis in arterial walls and reduce the risk of coronary events in hypertension.
5) Antiinflammatories—aspirin's effect in reducing coronary events is now believed to be in part due to its antiinflammatory effects as well as its antithrombotic effects.

•   <u>Specific interventions for vascular systems</u>

- Once vessel obstruction becomes significant (by plaque rupture or superimposed thrombus formation), there may not be time to wait for diet and drugs to cause atherosclerotic regression.

- Alternatives for reestablishing vessel patency include percutaneous transluminal angioplasty, atherectomy, laser, or bypass grafting.

- In the event of acute thrombus formation, thrombolysis may be indicated.

Pathophysiology →

What is going on in the disease process that influences how the patient presents and how he or she should be managed?

Clinical Link

What should you do now that you understand the underlying pathophysiology?

There is a high incidence of dyslipidemia in the United States population, including children.	Patient screening should begin early in life with measurement of total cholesterol HDL initially, with further evaluation if indicated by a total cholesterol >200.
Serum plasma lipoprotein levels are determined by many factors including genetics, diet, drugs, gender, age, and other diseases such as diabetes.	A careful history with attention to modifiable risk factors can improve the lipoprotein profile, and patients should be evaluated for diet therapy, exercise, estrogen replacement, and lipid-lowering drugs when appropriate.
Endothelial injury begins the whole process of atherosclerosis.	Risk factor modification can prevent the initiation of atherosclerosis.
Macrophages and leukocytes are involved in inflammatory and immune processes that promote the atherosclerotic lesion, especially via the production of toxic oxygen radicals.	Antiinflammatories, immune modulators, and antioxidants are all current or future therapies for the prevention and treatment of atherosclerosis.
Abnormal smooth muscle hypertrophy and inactivation of endogenous vasodilators result in vasoconstriction which is an important contributor to arterial ischemic syndromes.	Modulation of the role that macrophages and leukocytes play in atherogenesis not only reduce plaque formation but also prevent additional vessel obstruction due to vasoconstriction.
Oxidation of LDL is a vital step in atherogenesis and results in the formation of the fatty streak as well as promotes further inflammation and plaque generation.	Reduction in LDL and antioxidant therapy markedly reduce atherogenesis and can result in regression of established lesions.

Pathophysiology → Clinical Link

Pathophysiology	Clinical Link
Once fibrosis begins in the fatty streak, the atherosclerotic process becomes less reversible and more likely to result in plaque ulceration and rupture.	Antiinflammatories may also help prevent maturation of the plaque, making the lesion more responsible to lipid-lowering and other risk factor reductions, as well as reduce the risk of sudden vessel occlusion.
Endothelial dysfunction due to plaques result in superimposed thrombosis which is the major cause of complete vessel obstruction and infarction of distal tissues.	Antiplatelet drugs help prevent the adhesion of platelets to the injured endothelium, thus preventing thrombus formation and reducing the risk of infarction.

BIBLIOGRAPHY

Anonymous. (1996). A randomised, blinded, trial of clopidogrel versus aspirin in patients at risk of ischaemic events (CAPRIE). CAPRIE Steering Committee. *Lancet, 348*(9038), 1329-1339.

Barter, P. J., & Rye, K. A. (1996). High density lipoproteins and coronary heart disease [review, 96 refs]. *Atherosclerosis, 121*(1), 1-12.

Basha, B. J., & Sowers, J. R. (1996). Atherosclerosis: An update [review, 107 refs]. *American Heart Journal, 131*(6), 1192-1202.

Bjelajac, A., Goo, A. K., & Weart, C. W. (1996). Prevention and regression of atherosclerosis: Effects of HMG-CoA reductase inhibitors [review, 53 refs]. *Annals of Pharmacotherapy, 30*(11), 1304-1315.

Blasi, F., Denti, F., Erba, M., Cosentini, R., Raccanelli, R., Rinaldi, A., Fagetti, L., Esposito, G., Ruberti, U., & Allegra, L. (1996). Detection of Chlamydia pneumoniae but not *Helicobacter pylori* in atherosclerotic plaques of aortic aneurysms. *Journal of Clinical Microbiology, 34*(11), 2766-2769.

Blum, A., & Miller, H. I. (1996). The role of inflammation in atherosclerosis [review, 79 refs]. *Israel Journal of Medical Sciences, 32*(11), 1059-1065.

Bult, H. (1996). Nitric oxide and atherosclerosis: Possible implications for therapy [review, 47 refs]. *Molecular Medicine Today, 2*(12), 510-518.

Busse, R., & Fleming, I. (1996). Endothelial dysfunction in atherosclerosis [review, 185 refs]. *Journal of Vascular Research, 33*(3), 181-194.

Chobanian, A. V., & Alexander, R. W. (1996). Exacerbation of atherosclerosis by hypertension. Potential mechanisms and clinical implications [see comments] [review, 54 refs]. *Archives of Internal Medicine, 156*(17), 1952-1956.

Cook, P. J., & Lip, G. Y. (1996). Infectious agents and atherosclerotic vascular disease [review, 127 refs]. *QJM, 89*(10), 727-735.

Cox, D. A., & Cohen, M. L. (1996). Effects of oxidized low-density lipoprotein on vascular contraction and relaxation: Clinical and pharmacological implications in atherosclerosis [review, 182 refs]. *Pharmacological Reviews, 48*(1), 3-19.

De, Meyer, G. R., & Herman, A. G. (1997). Vascular endothelial dysfunction [review, 187 refs]. *Progress in Cardiovascular Diseases, 39*(4), 325-342.

Devaraj, S., & Jialal, I. (1996). Oxidized low-density lipoprotein and atherosclerosis [review, 86 refs]. *International Journal of Clinical and Laboratory Research, 26*(3), 178-184.

Durand, P., Fortin, L. J., Lussier-Cacan, S., Davignon, J., & Blache, D. (1996). Hyperhomocysteinemia induced by folic acid deficiency and methionine load—Applications of a modified HPLC method. *Clinica Chimica Acta, 252*(1), 83-93.

Dusting, G. J. (1996). Nitric oxide in coronary artery disease: Roles in atherosclerosis, myocardial reperfusion and heart failure [review, 108 refs]. *EXS, 76*, 33-55.

Everson, S. A., Lynch, J. W., Chesney, M. A., Kaplan, G. A., Goldberg, D. E., Shade, S. B., Cohen, R. D., Salonen, R., & Salonen, J. T. (1997). Interaction of workplace demands and cardiovascular reactivity in progression of carotid atherosclerosis: Population based study. *British Medical Journal, 314*(7080), 553-558.

Fallest-Strobl, P. C., Koch, D. D., Stein, J. H., & McBride, P. E. (1997). Homocysteine: A new risk factor for atherosclerosis [see comments] [review, 21 refs]. *American Family Physician, 56*(6), 1607-1612.

Ferrari, R., Ceconi, C., Curello, S., Pepi, P., Mazzoletti, A., & Visioli, O. (1996). Cardioprotective effect of angiotensin-converting enzyme inhibitors in patients with coronary artery disease [review, 132 refs]. *Cardiovascular Drugs and Therapy, 10*(Suppl 2), 639-647.

Fitzpatrick, L. A. (1996). Gender-related differences in the development of atherosclerosis: Studies at the cellular level. *Clinical and Experimental Pharmacology and Physiology, 23*(3), 267-269.

Galton, D. J. (1997). Genetic determinants of atherosclerosis-related dyslipidemias and their clinical implications. *Clinica Chimica Acta, 257*(2), 181-197.

Ganz, P., Creager, M. A., Fang, J. C., McConnell, M. V., Lee, R. T., Libby, P., & Selwyn, A. P. (1996). Pathogenic mechanisms of atherosclerosis: Effect of lipid lowering on the biology of atherosclerosis [review, 87 refs]. *American Journal of Medicine, 101*(4A), 4A10S-16S.

Glasser, S. P., Selwyn, A. P., & Ganz, P. (1996). Atherosclerosis: Risk factors and the vascular endothelium [review, 56 refs]. *American Heart Journal, 131*(2), 379-384.

Graier, W. F., & Kostner, G. M. (1997). Glycated low-density lipoprotein and atherogenesis: The missing link between diabetes mellitus and hypercholesterolaemia? [editorial] [review, 32 refs]. *European Journal of Clinical Investigation, 27*(6), 457-459.

Gupta, S., & Leatham, E. W. (1997). The relation between Chlamydia pneumoniae and atherosclerosis [editorial]. *Heart, 77*(1), 7-8.

Hamilton, C. A. (1997). Low-density lipoprotein and oxidised low-density lipoprotein: Their role in the development of atherosclerosis [review, 152 refs]. *Pharmacology and Therapeutics, 74*(1), 55-72.

Hardman, A. E. (1996). Exercise in the prevention of atherosclerotic, metabolic and hypertensive diseases: A review [review, 145 refs]. *Journal of Sports Sciences, 14*(3), 201-218.

Hassig, A., Wen-Xi, L., & Stampfli, K. (1996). The pathogenesis and prevention of atherosclerosis [review, 24 refs]. *Medical Hypotheses, 47*(5), 409-412.

Hebert, P. R., Gaziano, J. M., Chan, K. S., & Hennekens, C. H. (1997). Cholesterol lowering with statin drugs, risk of stroke, and total mortality. An overview of randomized trials [review, 53 refs]. *Journal of the American Medical Association, 278*(4), 313-321.

Heitzer, T., Yla-Herttuala, S., Luoma, J., Kurz, S., Munzel, T., Just, H., Olschewski, M., & Drexler, H. (1996). Cigarette smoking potentiates endothelial dysfunction of forearm resistance vessels in patients with hypercholesterolemia. Role of oxidized LDL. *Circulation, 93*(7), 1346-1353.

Hoeg, J. M. (1996). Can genes prevent atherosclerosis? *Journal of the American Medical Association, 276*(12), 989-992.

Iribarren, C., Belcher, J. D., Jacobs, D. R. J., Gross, M. D., Schreiner, P. J., & Sidney, S. (1996). Relationship of lipoproteins, apolipoproteins, triglycerides and lipid ratios to plasma total cholesterol in young adults: The CARDIA Study. Coronary Artery Risk Development in Young Adults. *Journal of Cardiovascular Risk, 3*(4), 391-396.

Jensen-Urstad, K. J., Reichard, P. G., Rosfors, J. S., Lindblad, L. E., & Jensen-Urstad, M. T. (1996). Early atherosclerosis is retarded by improved long-term blood glucose control in patients with IDDM. *Diabetes, 45*(9), 1253-1258.

Kowala, M. C. (1997). The role of endothelin in the pathogenesis of atherosclerosis [review, 159 refs]. *Advances in Pharmacology, 37*, 299-318.

Kronenberg, F., Steinmetz, A., Kostner, G. M., & Dieplinger, H. (1996). Lipoprotein(a) in health and disease [review, 238 refs]. *Critical Reviews in Clinical Laboratory Sciences, 33*(6), 495-543.

Kwiterovich, P. O. J. (1997). The effect of dietary fat, antioxidants, and pro-oxidants on blood lipids, lipoproteins, and atherosclerosis [review, 75 refs]. *Journal of the American Dietetic Association, 97*(7 Suppl), S31-S41.

Lassila, H. C., Tyrrell, K. S., Matthews, K. A., Wolfson, S. K., & Kuller, L. H. (1997). Prevalence and determinants of carotid atherosclerosis in healthy postmenopausal women. *Stroke, 28*(3), 513-517.

Lee, R. T., & Libby, P. (1997). The unstable atheroma [review, 75 refs]. *Arteriosclerosis, Thrombosis and Vascular Biology, 17*(10), 1859-1867.

Liao, W. (1996). Endotoxin: Possible roles in initiation and development of atherosclerosis [review, 101 refs]. *Journal of Laboratory and Clinical Medicine, 128*(5), 452-460.

Luscher, T. F., Tanner, F. C., & Noll, G. (1996). Lipids and endothelial function: Effects of lipid-lowering and other therapeutic interventions [review, 67 refs]. *Current Opinion Lipidology, 7*(4), 234-240.

Mancini, G. B. (1996). Emerging concepts: Angiotensin-converting enzyme inhibition in coronary artery disease [review, 22 refs]. *Cardiovascular Drugs and Therapy, 10*(Suppl 2), 609-612.

Mantov, S., & Raev, D. (1996). Additive effect of diabetes and systemic hypertension on the immune mechanisms of atherosclerosis. *International Journal of Cardiology, 56*(2), 145-148.

Martin, A. J., Ryan, L. K., Gotlieb, A. I., Henkelman, R. M., & Foster, F. S. (1997). Arterial imaging: Comparison of high-resolution US and MR imaging with histologic correlation. *Radiographics, 17*(1), 189-202.

Massy, Z. A., & Keane, W. F. (1996). Pathogenesis of atherosclerosis [review, 65 refs]. *Seminars in Nephrology, 16*(1), 12-20.

McCully, K. S. (1996). Homocysteine and vascular disease [review, 20 refs]. *Nature Medicine, 2*(4), 386-389.

McGill, H. C. J., McMahan, C. A., Malcom, G. T., Oalmann, M. C., & Strong, J. P. (1997). Effects of serum lipoproteins and smoking on atherosclerosis in young men and women. The PDAY Research Group. Pathobiological Determinants of Atherosclerosis in Youth. *Arteriosclerosis, Thrombosis and Vascular Biology, 17*(1), 95-106.

Minchoff, L. E., & Grandin, J. A. (1996). Syndrome X. Recognition and management of this metabolic disorder in primary care [review, 30 refs]. *Nurse Practitioner, 21*(6), 74-75.

Mlot, C. (1996). Chlamydia linked to atherosclerosis [news]. *Science, 272*(5267), 1422

Nathan, L., & Chaudhuri, G. (1997). Estrogens and atherosclerosis [review, 279 refs]. *Annual Review of Pharmacology and Toxicology, 37*, 477-515.

Nielsen, L. B. (1996). Transfer of low density lipoprotein into the arterial wall and risk of atherosclerosis [review, 102 refs]. *Atherosclerosis, 123*(1-2), 1-15.

Nieto, F. J., Adam, E., Sorlie, P., Farzadegan, H., Melnick, J. L., Comstock, G. W., & Szklo, M. (1996). Cohort study of cytomegalovirus infection as a risk factor for carotid intimal-medial thickening, a measure of subclinical atherosclerosis [see comments]. *Circulation, 94*(5), 922-927.

Olsson, A. G., & Yuan, X. M. (1996). Antioxidants in the prevention of atherosclerosis [review, 45 refs]. *Current Opinion In Lipidology, 7*(6), 374-380.

Ong, G., Thomas, B. J., Mansfield, A. O., Davidson, B. R., & Taylor-Robinson, D. (1996). Detection and widespread distribution of Chlamydia pneumoniae in the vascular system and its possible implications. *Journal of Clinical Pathology, 49*(2), 102-106.

Peeling, R. W., & Brunham, R. C. (1996). Chlamydiae as pathogens: New species and new issues [review, 78 refs]. *Emerging Infectious Diseases, 2*(4), 307-319.

Pettersson, K. S., Ostlund-Lindqvist, A. M., & Westerlund, C. (1996). The potential of antioxidants to prevent atherosclerosis development and its clinical manifestations [review, 47 refs]. *EXS, 76*, 21-31.

Pitt, B. (1995). Potential role of angiotensin converting enzyme inhibitors in treatment of atherosclerosis [review, 37 refs]. *European Heart Journal, 16*(Suppl K), 49-54.

Raman, M., & Nesto, R. W. (1996). Heart disease in diabetes mellitus [review, 64 refs]. *Endocrinology & Metabolism Clinics of North America, 25*(2), 425-438.

Saikku, P. (1997). *Chlamydia pneumoniae* and atherosclerosis—An update [review, 41 refs]. *Scandinavian Journal of Infectious Diseases—Supplementum, 104,* 53-56.

Sander, D., & Klingelhofer, J. (1996). Diurnal systolic blood pressure variability is the strongest predictor of early carotid atherosclerosis. *Neurology, 47*(2), 500-507.

Sarrel, P. M. (1996). Cardiovascular disease in women: Implications of hormone replacement therapy [review, 20 refs]. *International Journal of Fertility & Menopausal Studies, 41*(2), 90-93.

Schell, W. D., & Myers, J. N. (1997). Regression of atherosclerosis: A review [review, 46 refs]. *Progress in Cardiovascular Diseases, 39*(5), 483-496.

Schroeder, A. P., & Falk, E. (1996). Pathophysiology and inflammatory aspects of plaque rupture [review, 94 refs]. *Cardiology Clinics, 14*(2), 211-220.

Selwyn, A. P., Kinlay, S., Creager, M., Libby, P., & Ganz, P. (1997). Cell dysfunction in atherosclerosis and the ischemic manifestations of coronary artery disease [review, 106 refs]. *American Journal of Cardiology, 79*(5A), 17-23.

Semenkovich, C. F., & Heinecke, J. W. (1997). The mystery of diabetes and atherosclerosis: Time for a new plot [review, 121 refs]. *Diabetes, 46*(3), 327-334.

Simon, A., Megnien, J. L., & Levenson, J. (1997). Detection of preclinical atherosclerosis may optimize the management of hypertension [review, 95 refs]. *American Journal of Hypertension, 10*(7 Pt 1), 813-824.

Sloop, G. D. (1996). A unifying theory of atherogenesis [review, 35 refs]. *Medical Hypotheses, 47*(4), 321-325.

Smith, E. B. (1996). Haemostatic factors and atherogenesis [review, 80 refs]. *Atherosclerosis, 124*(2), 137-143.

Sniderman, A. D., Pedersen, T., & Kjekshus, J. (1997). Putting low-density lipoproteins at center stage in atherogenesis. *American Journal of Cardiology, 79*(1), 64-67.

Steinberg, D. (1997). Lewis A. Conner Memorial Lecture. Oxidative modification of LDL and atherogenesis [review, 96 refs]. *Circulation, 95*(4), 1062-1071.

Susic, D. (1997). Hypertension, aging, and atherosclerosis. The endothelial interface [review, 55 refs]. *Medical Clinics of North America, 81*(5), 1231-1240.

Sutton-Tyrrell, K., Evans, R. W., Meilahn, E., & Alcorn, H. G. (1996). Lipoprotein(a) and peripheral atherosclerosis in older adults. *Atherosclerosis, 122*(1), 11-19.

Swain, R. A., & St. Clair, L. (1997). The role of folic acid in deficiency states and prevention of disease [review, 53 refs]. *Journal of Family Practice, 44*(2), 138-144.

Tawakol, A., Omland, T., Gerhard, M., Wu, J. T., & Creager, M. A. (1997). Hyperhomocyst(e)inemia is associated with impaired endothelium-dependent vasodilation in humans. *Circulation, 95*(5), 1119-1121.

Tenaglia, A. N., Buda, A. J., Wilkins, R. G., Barron, M. K., Jeffords, P. R., Vo, K., Jordan, M. O., Kusnick, B. A., & Lefer, D. J. (1997). Levels of expression of P-selectin, E-selectin, and intercellular adhesion molecule-1 in coronary atherectomy specimens from patients with stable and unstable angina pectoris. *American Journal of Cardiology, 79*(6), 742-747.

Vogel, R. A. (1997). Coronary risk factors, endothelial function, and atherosclerosis: A review [review, 79 refs]. *Clinical Cardiology, 20*(5), 426-432.

Watanabe, T., Haraoka, S., & Shimokama, T. (1996). Inflammatory and immunological nature of atherosclerosis [review, 55 refs]. *International Journal of Cardiology, 54*(Suppl), S51-S60.

Welch, G. N., Upchurch, G. J., & Loscalzo, J. (1997). Hyperhomocyst(e)inemia and atherothrombosis [review, 64 refs]. *Annals of the New York Academy of Sciences, 811,* 48-58, discussion 58-59.

Westhuyzen, J. (1997). The oxidation hypothesis of atherosclerosis: An update [review, 90 refs]. *Annals of Clinical & Laboratory Science, 27*(1), 1-10.

Zanchetti, A. (1996). Trials investigating the anti-atherosclerotic effects of antihypertensive drugs [review, 14 refs]. *Journal of Hypertension—Supplement, 14*(2), S77-S80, discussion S80-S81.

CASE STUDY[*]

DYSLIPIDEMIA AND ATHEROSCLEROSIS

INITIAL HISTORY:
- 69-year-old white male
- Complains of excruciating left leg pain
- Reports sudden onset 45 minutes ago while sitting on a bench at the shopping mall, unrelieved with massage/rest, pain is nonradiating
- Reports has previously had occasional left leg aching discomfort when walking long distances

Question 1.
  What other questions would you like to ask about his medical, family, and social history?

PREVIOUS MEDICAL HISTORY AND HOME MEDICATIONS:
- Denies any history of chest pain or focal neurological symptoms
- No significant previous medical history; does not think he has ever been told he has hypertension, diabetes or dyslipidemia
- 75 pack/year smoking history—continues to smoke
- Uses alcohol occasionally
- He is not on any medications and he has no allergies.

ADDITIONAL FAMILY AND SOCIAL HISTORY:
- Father died of myocardial infarction at age 78; mother is alive and suffers from hypertension and cerebrovascular disease; 1 brother, age 62, 1 sister, age 58—both alive and well
- Patient lives with wife of 45 years, is a retired civil engineer (retired 4 years ago), and enjoys gardening and travel.
- He feels healthy overall and does not seek regular medical care.

* Kathryn Ballenger, RN, MSN, CCRN, FNP, contributed this case study.

INITIAL PHYSICAL FINDINGS:
- Left leg is mottled and cyanotic, distal to the knee, cool to touch.
- Right leg is pink and warm.
- Doppler of the left dorsalis pedis (DP) and posterior tibialis (PT) pulses reveal decreased pulses with faint bruits heard.
- Right DP and PT pulses are palpable

Question 2.
What is your initial diagnosis?

Question 3.
What are the possible causes of this patient's problem?

Question 4.
What are the potential general sequelae if this problem is not resolved?

PHYSICAL EXAMINATION
- T = 36.9 PO; sitting BP = 160/90 mmHg left arm, 166/92 mmHg right arm; P = 96 beats/minute, regular rate; RR = 20 breaths/minute, unlabored
- Slightly obese man complaining of left lower leg and calf aching/throbbing pain, "8" on a scale of 1 to 10

HEENT, Neck, Lungs, Cardiac
- Unremarkable, fundi without lesions
- Supple, no adenopathy or thyromegaly, no bruits
- Bilateral and symmetrical chest expansion with clear breath sounds
- S_1 S_2 clear; no rub, gallop, or murmur; regular rate

Abdomen, Neurological
- Abdomen with +bowel sounds throughout, nontender, nondistended.
- Alert and oriented, appropriately anxious; cranial nerves X to XII intact; strength 5/5 throughout, DTRs 2+ and symmetrical, sensation intact

Skin, Extremities
- Skin intact, warm, pink except for left leg (cool and mottled distal to knee)
- Peripheral pulses all palpable except for left DP and PT
- Faint bruits by doppler
- No edema

Question 5.
What are the immediate therapeutic alternatives for restoring perfusion to this man's leg, and which do you feel would be most appropriate in this case?

Question 6.
What studies would you initiate at this time?

LABORATORY RESULTS:
- Glucose = 225; urine myoglobin = negative
- Triglycerides = 315; cholesterol = 353; HDL = 40; LDL = 165
- All other blood work within normal limits; 12-lead ECG is normal
- Rectal exam—guaiac negative

Question 7.
What risk factors for atherosclerotic peripheral vascular disease do you identify for this man?

PATIENT UPDATE:
- The patient is admitted to the hospital, is anticoagulated, and undergoes urokinase therapy. Resolution of his blood clot is noted on fluoroscopy, as well as improved distal pulses. Two hours later, however, his status changes as follows:
    - Left DP is absent by doppler; left PT is unchanged
    - Left leg is increasingly mottled
    - Left leg demonstrates increased calf size, edema, and tightness
    - Urine is positive for myoglobin
    - Patient reports numbness and tingling in his left leg and foot

Question 8.
Based on these new findings, what complications is this patient exhibiting and what precautions must be taken?

PATIENT UPDATE:
- A left calf fasciotomy is performed with the following results:
    - Left DP pulse improves to present pulsatile flow by doppler; left PT pulse also is present by doppler
    - Patient reports resolving numbness and tingling
    - Mottled appearance of the left leg begins to disappear

PATIENT COURSE:
- The patient's left femoral artery clot is successfully dissolved with urokinase therapy, and normal perfusion is restored to his left leg. The fasciotomy site is sutured and closed 2 days later.
- The angiographic findings of a severe distal femoral artery stenosis is successfully opened through percutaneous transluminal angioplasty. Angiography findings are consistent with peripheral atherosclerotic vascular disease.
- The patient's diastolic blood pressure remains 88 to 98 mmHg and his blood glucose levels remain 150 to 270 during his hospital course.

Question 9.
What are the priorities for medical aspects of care now that this patient's acute problem has been resolved?

Question 10.
What essential information and education do you need to provide this patient prior to discharge?

CHAPTER 3

ISCHEMIC HEART DISEASE

DEFINITION

- An imbalance between the demand for myocardial perfusion and the supply of oxygenated blood by the coronary arteries

- Results in either transient myocardial ischemia (angina) or prolonged ischemia resulting in permanent muscle damage (myocardial infarction [MI])

- Most commonly caused by obstruction of coronary flow by atherosclerotic disease of the coronary vessels, especially when accompanied by an increase in myocardial demand (e.g., exercise) and/or thrombus formation superimposed on a ruptured atherosclerotic plaque

EPIDEMIOLOGY

- Number 1 killer of adults in the United States (~700,000 deaths/year).

- Over 1 million MIs per year in the United States.

- Cardiovascular deaths have decreased 50% in the past 3 decades.

- It is estimated that over 2 million Americans have silent myocardial ischemia with an increased risk of MI and sudden death.

- Risk factors are the same as those for atherosclerosis:

    - The male gender or female after menopause

    - Smoking

    - Dyslipidemia

    - Hypertension

    - Diabetes

    - Family history of ischemic heart disease, especially before age 50

    - Hyperhomocystinemia

    - Obesity

    - Sedentary lifestyle

    - Stress

PATHOPHYSIOLOGY

- Atherosclerotic lesions form in coronary vessels (see Chapter 2).

- As the lesion begins to obstruct coronary flow, increases in myocardial demand for blood (exercise, stress, etc.) result in transient ischemia relieved with rest (stable angina).

- As the plaque becomes more complicated, small fissures in the surface of the lesion attract platelets and transient thrombotic occlusions of the coronary vessel can occur even at rest (unstable angina).

- If the plaque ruptures, exposure of more of the thrombogenic plaque material leads to rapid thrombus formation that occludes the vessel for a prolonged period resulting in infarction of the distal tissue (MI).

- Each of the stages of coronary artery disease also has components of abnormal vasoconstriction caused by endothelial dysfunction; in rare cases, coronary spasm is adequate to cause infarction in the absence of significant atherosclerotic lesions.

- Recent evidence suggests that the atherothrombotic events have an inflammatory component that contributes to platelet aggregation as evidenced by high levels of C-reactive protein in patients suffering from acute coronary ischemia.

- When infarction occurs, inflammatory cells infiltrate the necrotic tissue and eventually fibroblasts lay down scar tissue.

- Myocytes in the vicinity of the actual area of infarction may develop one of two other changes:

  - Myocardial "stunning" during which myocytes lose their normal conductive and contractile function for prolonged periods even after perfusion has been restored.

  - Myocardial "remodeling" is a process mediated in part by the renin/angiotensin/aldosterone (RAA) system that causes myocyte hypertrophy and abnormal contractile function in the areas surrounding the infarcted area; this process contributes to the development of chronic congestive heart failure (CHF) (see Chapter 4).

- Myocardial ischemia and the resultant anaerobic metabolism by the myocytes release lactic acid, which causes stimulation of sympathetic afferents giving the sensation of pain in the substernal area; cross stimulation of other sympathetic afferents results in the "radiation" of pain to the neck, jaw, left shoulder, or left arm. Elderly patients, patients with diabetes, postoperative patients, and a significant number of men aged 45 to 65 have "silent" ischemia or infarction due to autonomic dysfunction.

- During the ischemic episode, ventricular function is abnormal and ejection fraction falls with transient (angina) or permanent (infarction) increases in ventricular end-diastolic volume (VEDV). If the coronary obstruction involves the perfusion to the left ventricle then pulmonary venous congestion ensues; if the right ventricle is ischemic then increases in systemic venous pressures occur.

- Conduction disturbances with ischemia or infarction result in electrocardiogram (ECG) changes that are diagnostic in approximately 70% of patients; additional conductive abnormalities can result in bradycardia and heart block, tachyarrhythmias, ventricular fibrillation, or asystole.

- Angina.

  - Transient ischemia without infarction—angina can be stable (predictable pain with exercise relieved with rest), silent, or unstable (pain at increasing frequency, duration, or severity or occurring at rest).

- Slowly increasing atherosclerotic coronary obstructions allow for collateral perfusion such that there is little risk of infarction and overall prognosis is fairly good; however, risk of MI and death increases as the number of affected vessels and the severity of the obstructions increase with time.

- Silent ischemia is associated with an increased risk of MI and sudden death especially in postinfarction patients.

- Unstable angina is associated with a high risk of MI and death and must be recognized and treated promptly.

- There is increasing evidence that repeated episodes of transient ischemia result, even without infarction, in myocardial remodeling and an increased risk of heart failure.

- Myocardial infarction.

    - Prolonged ischemia with infarction is almost always due to thrombus formation over a fractured plaque; this has led to the use of thrombolytic therapy in MI.

    - Changes in the ventricular wall with necrosis and then fibrosis after infarction result in altered ventricular compliance, decreased contractility, and possible ventricular aneurysm formation.

    - Cardiogenic shock may occur if contractility is severely compromised, if there is rupture of the septal or ventricular wall, if there is infarction of the chordae tendinea with abrupt regurgitation of the mitral valve, or if there are arrhythmias that prevent adequate ventricular filling and ejection.

PATIENT PRESENTATION

- History:

    Previous coronary disease; family history of heart disease; hypertension; smoking; dyslipidemia; diabetes; recent stress; previous episodes of dyspnea on exertion or edema; light-headed or syncopal episodes.

- Symptoms:

    Substernal pressure/pain or chest tightness with or without radiation to the neck, jaw, left shoulder, or arm; dyspnea; nausea or vomiting; diaphoresis; light-headedness or loss of consciousness; onset of symptoms associated with exercise, cold exposure, or stress; pain relieved with rest versus prolonged and persistent.

- Examination:

    Between ischemic episodes, the exam may be normal or reveal evidence of underlying risk factors such as hypertension, manifestations of dyslipidemia such as xanthelasma, corneal arcus, or diabetic manifestations such as intertrigo or neuropathy. There may be signs of atherosclerotic disease in the other arteries as evidenced by bruits, decreased pulses, or neurologic findings. Some patients will exhibit the signs of CHF from previous ischemic events (see Chapter 4). During acute ischemic episodes, the patient is usually anxious, tachycardic, tachypneic, with possible pulmonary rales, S_3, S_4, or murmurs. If there is cardiogenic shock, then hypotension with poor tissue perfusion occurs. Finally, acute arrhythmias may manifest with ectopic beats or the absence of a detectable pulse, shock, and loss of consciousness.

DIFFERENTIAL DIAGNOSIS

- Peptic ulcer disease with or without perforation
- Gastroesophageal reflux
- Pericarditis
- Costochondritis
- Aortic dissection
- Mitral valve prolapse
- Pulmonary embolus
- Other pulmonary disease
- Panic attack

KEYS TO ASSESSMENT

- <u>Acute chest pain</u>

    - Remember that elderly patients and diabetics may not have any of the classic symptoms and present with a feeling of unease or dyspnea only.

    - Rapid assessment is important while initiating supportive care measures.

    - The first decision is whether the patient is experiencing cardiac or noncardiac symptomatology, then if there is transient angina or MI. Symptoms correlated with a high likelihood of MI include symptoms less than 48 hours but more than 1 hour and pain radiating to the neck or left arm; symptoms correlated with low risk for MI include radiation of the pain to the abdomen or back and stabbing pain (versus pressure or heaviness).

    - If this is noncardiac pain, the physical exam may show evidence of primary lung or gastrointestinal disease or there may be reproduction of the chest pain with palpation of the rib cage consistent with costochondritis.

    - Blood should be drawn immediately for complete blood count (CBC), coagulation parameters, electrolytes, creatinine phosphokinase MB (CPK-MB), and troponin I. (Troponin I is more specific than CPK-MB for myocardial damage. If it is positive, there is some myocardial ischemia and the prognosis is worse; if it is negative, one still cannot "rule out" MI. The CPK-MB must be repeated at 4, 8, and 12 hours to "rule out" MI.)

    - An ECG should be done immediately, and if possible, both with pain and after pain relief. ST segment elevation with T wave inversion is highly suggestive of MI. ST depression can be seen in transient ischemia, but remember that the ECG is neither sensitive (~30% will be nondiagnostic even with ischemia) nor specific. Bundle branch blocks make the interpretation of the ECG for ischemia more difficult and may themselves indicate myocardial damage. The presence of a new Q wave is diagnostic for MI; many will not develop a Q wave (non-Q wave MI), which indicates that not all of the myocardium in the distribution of that artery has been infarcted and that the patient is at high risk for recurrent infarction.

    - Patients referred to hospitals where specialized cardiology care is available may undergo immediate noninvasive testing such as echocardiography or technetium scanning. If a patient presents in shock he or she may undergo immediate coronary catheterization.

- Nonacute symptoms or MI "ruled out"
    - Evaluation focuses on risk factors and character of the pain to determine likelihood that a history of chest pain was cardiac in origin.
    - If the history is consistent with cardiac pain and the symptoms occurred at rest, were more severe than in the past, or are occurring more frequently, then the diagnosis of unstable angina must be considered and the patient should be referred for immediate hospitalization and evaluation with probable catheterization.
    - If the history is consistent with cardiac pain but it is predictable, relieved with rest, and of normal severity and duration compared to any previous episodes, this most likely represents stable angina and the patient should undergo one of many possible diagnostic studies to determine the extent of coronary disease and the possible need for invasive therapy. Each of the following tests has been found to be useful in the evaluation of patients for coronary disease; the choice rests on the local availability of the test:
        1) Stress ECG with thallium—increases sensitivity over stress ECG alone, is safe, and correlates with amount of myocardium at risk and prognosis.
        2) Single photon emission computed tomography (SPECT) done at rest or with exercise is highly sensitive for coronary disease and has been correlated with prognosis.
        3) Dipyridamole, dobutamine, or arbutamine echocardiography is highly sensitive and specific for the detection of coronary disease.
        4) Coronary angiography should be considered if the noninvasive testing suggests significant coronary obstruction or myocardium at risk for ischemia.
        5) Other tests include magnetic resonance imaging (MRI) and computed tomography (CT) scanning.

KEYS TO MANAGEMENT

- Prevention
    - Diet—decreasing dietary fat and cholesterol decreases cardiac risk (see Chapter 2). Intake of increased fiber, fish oils, and garlic have all been suggested. Increasing antioxidants is still controversial, some studies show as much as a 40% decrease in coronary risk with the intake of 200 to 800 IU of vitamin E daily; other studies show no clear risk reduction with vitamin E, beta-carotene, or vitamin C. More studies are needed. Increasing folate decreases serum homocysteine and significantly lowers coronary risk. Finally, moderate alcohol intake has been shown to reduce cardiac risk by as much as 40%.
    - Exercise decreases risk by as much as 45%, weight reduction decreases risk by as much as 55%.
    - Smoking cessation can decrease risk by 50% to 70% after 5 years.
    - Blood pressure control by lifestyle, diet, and medication can decrease risk by 20%.
    - Pharmacologic:
        1) Antiplatelet drugs such as aspirin (325 mg per day or every other day), ticlopidine, clopidrogel, integrelin, or abciximab (see Chapter 2) reduce risk by 30% to 50%.
        2) Cholesterol lowering drugs, especially the HMG-CoA reductase inhibitors, greatly reduce risk in patients with dyslipidemias and can cause regression of atherosclerotic lesions (see Chapter 2).

3) Secondary prevention after MI includes beta-blockers, aspirin and lipid lowering drugs; in patients with CHF following MI, the use of angiotensin converting enzyme (ACE) inhibitors, nitrates, and warfarin have been associated with decreased MI recurrence and mortality.

- Acute myocardial infarction

    - Admit to the hospital.

    - Oxygen, intravenous (IV) access, support ventilation and circulation if indicated (CPR).

    - Immediate administration of aspirin; ticlopidine if allergic to aspirin.

    - Morphine and nitrates.

    - If ECG is diagnostic for ischemia (>1 mm ST elevation in $\geq$ 2 leads or chest pain and ST depression in anterior precordial leads) and there are no contraindications, then administer intravenously (IV) thrombolytics plus heparin OR perform emergent catheterization with percutaneous transluminal coronary angioplasty (PTCA) with or without coronary artery stenting and heparin (as effective if not more so than thrombolytics but requires experienced staff and proper support facilities).

    - If contraindications to thrombolysis or nondiagnostic ECG, but MI ruled in by enzymes, use IV nitrates for refractory ischemia and pain only.

    - IV beta-blockers reduce mortality; they must be used cautiously to avoid CHF and bradycardia.

    - Trials are underway with low-molecular weight heparin for acute MI in patients who cannot receive thrombolytics; early results are encouraging.

    - ACE inhibitors begin at 6 to 8 hours in patients with an ejection fraction less than 40%; controversial whether to begin all patients at 3 to 10 days if stable—studies are ongoing.

    - Calcium channel blockers—only diltiazem in patients with normal left ventricle (LV) function and non-Q wave infarction has shown any benefit; however, a new third generation calcium channel blocker shows promise.

    - Antiarrhythmics are not indicated prophylactically at this time; studies with amiodarone look promising.

    - Magnesium is controversial, there is not enough evidence to support its use at this time.

    - New anticoagulant drugs such as hirulog and hirudin are being tested; preliminary results are mixed.

    - Prior to discharge, most patients should undergo noninvasive testing such as thallium or SPECT imaging to assess risk for recurrent ischemia and the need for angioplasty or coronary bypass grafting.

    - Patient teaching prior to discharge is vital to recovery and risk reduction.

    - After discharge, patients should be enrolled in a cardiac rehabilitation program.

- Unstable angina

    - Patients should be admitted to the hospital.

    - Aspirin is given immediately on admission.

- Acute management with IV heparin, thrombolytics, or emergent PTCA have been shown to reduce the risk of MI.

- When stable, the patient should undergo noninvasive testing or catheterization for definitive diagnosis and to aid in selecting surgical or medical therapy.

- Stable angina

  - Risk reduction and antiplatelet drugs are most important: treat hypertension, diabetes, and dyslipidemia; smoking cessation; and assess for contributing factors such as anemia or hyperthyroidism and treat appropriately.

  - If noninvasive testing reveals three vessel or left main coronary disease, then PTCA or coronary artery bypass grafting (CABG) is indicated.

  - If coronary disease is less severe, then medical therapy has a good prognosis (although at least one study shows that quality of life was improved after PTCA or CABG in patients with mild to moderate coronary obstruction).

  - Lifestyle changes: avoid excessive fatigue, modify early morning activities due to an increased risk of angina in the morning, eat several smaller meals, avoid anxiety-provoking situations, engage in stepped exercise program.

  - Aspirin 80 to 325 mg/day or every other day.

  - Sublingual nitrates or spray for episodes of pain or as prophylaxis against activities known to precipitate angina; topical or oral nitrates if angina occurs more than 3 to 4 times per week with nitrate-free intervals to avoid tolerance.

  - Beta-blocker for most patients especially if tachycardic or hypertensive; avoid in the elderly and patients with obstructive airways disease.

  - Calcium channel blocker for those with intolerance to beta blockers or add to beta blockers if pain persists.

  - If pain persists or worsens, then catheterization and possible PTCA or CABG is necessary.

Pathophysiology   →   ## Clinical Link

What is going on in the disease process that influences how the patient presents and how he or she should be managed?

What should you do now that you understand the underlying pathophysiology?

The spectrum of ischemic heart disease includes all of the stages in the pathogenesis of atherosclerosis and has the same risk factors, with superimposed threat of thrombosis.	Prevention of coronary artery disease rests on the reduction in risk factors for atherosclerosis plus antiplatelet drugs and/or anticoagulant drugs.
Ischemic myocardium produces lactic acid that stimulates the sympathetic nervous system.	Elderly patients and those with diabetes may not have pain with myocardial ischemia. The examiner must have a high index of suspicion in patients with risk factors.
Myocardial ischemia can be transient or prolonged with actual necrosis of heart muscle; myocyte death results in the release of the cardiac enzymes CPK-MB and troponin I.	Measurement of serum cardiac enzymes differentiates angina or noncardiac pain from true MI, but the serum levels of these markers may take hours to rise, thus delaying the definitive diagnosis.
Cardiac ischemia results in decreased LV contractility with increased LVEDV and pulmonary venous congestion.	Dyspnea and transient or persistent CHF and pulmonary edema are common features of MI and carry a negative impact on prognosis.
Transient ischemia with exercise or stress occurs when there is a fixed but partial coronary obstruction such that demand exceeds supply for coronary perfusion.	Stable angina has predictable precipitating factors and is relieved with rest; lifestyle modification can reduce anginal symptoms.
MI occurs when a coronary atherosclerotic plaque ruptures and thrombus forms.	In patients without contraindications, the rapid administration of antiplatelet or thrombolytic drugs can restore perfusion, limit infarct size, and reduce mortality.

Pathophysiology $\longrightarrow$ **Clinical Link**

Unstable angina occurs when a coronary atherosclerotic plaque is beginning to crack and platelets begin sticking to the lesion.	$\rightarrow$	Unstable angina is essentially one step from MI in its pathophysiology and must be treated aggressively to avoid MI.
Some of the effects of myocardial ischemia include remodeling and stunning; these have deleterious effects on LV function.	$\rightarrow$	Treatment of ischemic disease with ACE inhibitors and beta-blockers may prevent future CHF.

BIBLIOGRAPHY

Albarran, J. W., & Bridger, S. (1997). Problems with providing education on resuming sexual activity after myocardial infarction: Developing written information for patients [review, 42 refs]. *Intensive and Critical Care Nursing, 13*(1), 2-11.

Ambrosio, G., Betocchi, S., Pace, L., Losi, M. A., Perrone-Filardi, P., Soricelli, A., Piscione, F., Taube, J., Squame, F., Salvatore, M., Weiss, J. L., & Chiariello, M. (1996). Prolonged impairment of regional contractile function after resolution of exercise-induced angina. Evidence of myocardial stunning in patients with coronary artery disease. *Circulation, 94*(10), 2455-2464.

Amos, D. J., & White, H. D. (1997). Remodeling after myocardial infarction: An opportunity for early intervention [review, 10 refs]. *Basic Research in Cardiology, 92*(2), 69-71.

Amsterdam, E. A. (1996). Controlled trials comparing reteplase with alteplase and streptokinase in patients with acute myocardial infarction [review, 9 refs]. *Pharmacotherapy, 16*(5 Pt 2), 137S-140S.

Anderson, J. L. (1996). Post-myocardial infarction trials: Beta blockers, antiarrhythmics, thrombolytics [review, 35 refs]. *Controlled Clinical Trials, 17*(3 Suppl), 17S-27S.

Anonymous. (1996). Acute myocardial infarction: Pre-hospital and in-hospital management. The Task Force on the Management of Acute Myocardial Infarction of the European Society of Cardiology [review, 127 refs]. *European Heart Journal, 17*(1), 43-63.

Anonymous. (1996). Early and six-month outcome in patients with angina pectoris early after acute myocardial infarction (the GISSI-3 APPI [angina precoce post-infarto] study). The GISSI-3 APPI Study Group. *American Journal of Cardiology, 78*(11), 1191-1197.

Anonymous. (1997). Coronary angioplasty versus medical therapy for angina: The second Randomized Intervention Treatment of Angina (RITA-2) Trial. RITA-2 trial participants. *Lancet, 350*(9076), 461-468.

Antman, E. M. (1996). Magnesium in acute myocardial infarction: Overview of available evidence [review, 53 refs]. *American Heart Journal, 132*(2 Pt 2 Su), 487-495, discussion 496-502.

Arnstein, P. M., Buselli, E. F., & Rankin, S. H. (1996). Women and heart attacks: Prevention, diagnosis, and care [review, 67 refs]. *Nurse Practitioner, 21*(5), 57-58.

Bates, D. W., Miller, E., Bernstein, S. J., Hauptman, P. J., & Leape, L. L. (1997). Coronary angiography and angioplasty after acute myocardial infarction [review, 121 refs]. *Annals of Internal Medicine, 126*(7), 539-550.

Borghi, C., & Ambrosioni, E. (1996). Primary and secondary prevention of myocardial infarction [review, 22 refs]. *Clinical and Experimental Hypertension, 18*(3-4), 547-558.

Brand, F. N., Larson, M., Friedman, L. M., Kannel, W. B., & Castelli, W. P. (1996). Epidemiologic assessment of angina before and after myocardial infarction: The Framingham study. *American Heart Journal, 132*(1 Pt 1), 174-178.

Brann, W. M., & Tresch, D. D. (1997). Management of stable & unstable angina in elderly patients. *Comprehensive Therapy, 23*(1), 49-56.

Burger, A. J., Kamalesh, M., Kumar, S., & Nesto, R. (1996). Effect of beta adrenergic receptor blockade on cardiac autonomic tone in patients with chronic stable angina. *Pacing and Clinical Electrophysiology, 19*(4 Pt 1), 411-417.

Camargo, C. A. J., Stampfer, M. J., Glynn, R. J., Grodstein, F., Gaziano, J. M., Manson, J. E., Buring, J. E., & Hennekens, C. H. (1997). Moderate alcohol consumption and risk for angina pectoris or myocardial infarction in U.S. male physicians. *Annals of Internal Medicine, 126*(5), 372-375.

Cleland, J. G., Cowburn, P. J., & Morgan, K. (1996). Neuroendocrine activation after myocardial infarction: Causes and consequences [review, 68 refs]. *Heart, 76*(3 Suppl 3), 53-59.

Collins, R., Peto, R., Baigent, C., & Sleight, P. (1997). Aspirin, heparin, and fibrinolytic therapy in suspected acute myocardial infarction [review, 97 refs]. *New England Journal of Medicine, 336*(12), 847-860.

Cornock, M. A. (1996). Psychological approaches to cardiac pain [review, 18 refs]. *Nursing Standard, 11*(12), 34-38.

Dargie, H. J. (1996). Angina and left ventricular dysfunction [review, 25 refs]. *European Heart Journal, 17*(Suppl G), 2-7.

Davies, G. J., Kobrin, I., Caspi, A., Reisin, L. H., de, A. D. C., Armagnijan, D., Coelho, O. R., & Schneeweiss, A. (1997). Long-term antianginal and antiischemic effects of mibefradil, the novel T-type calcium channel blocker: A multicenter, double-blind, placebo-controlled, randomized comparison with sustained-release diltiazem. *American Heart Journal, 134*(2 Pt 1), 220-228.

Davies, G. J., Tzivoni, D., & Kobrin, I. (1997). Mibefradil in the treatment of chronic stable angina pectoris: Comparative studies with other calcium antagonists. *American Journal of Cardiology, 80*(4B), 34C-39C.

Doughty, R. N., & Sharpe, N. (1996). Optimal treatment of angina in older patients [review, 39 refs]. *Drugs and Aging, 8*(5), 349-357.

Eisenberg, M. J., & Topal, E. J. (1996). Prehospital administration of aspirin in patients with unstable angina and acute myocardial infarction [review, 34 refs]. *Archives of Internal Medicine, 156*(14), 1506-1510.

Fleischmann, K. E., Lee, T. H., Come, P. C., Goldman, L., Cook, E. F., Caguoia, E., Johnson, P. A., Albano, M. P., & Lee, R. T. (1997). Echocardiographic prediction of complications in patients with chest pain. *American Journal of Cardiology, 79*(3), 292-298.

Futterman, L. G., & Lemberg, L. (1997). SGOT, LDH, HBD, CPK, CK-MB, MB1MB2, cTnT, cTnC, cTnI [review, 6 refs]. *American Journal of Critical Care, 6*(4), 333-338.

Gambhir, D. S. (1996). Amiodarone in high-risk post-infarction patients, Lessons from EMIAT and CAMIAT. European Myocardial Infarct Amiodarone Trial and Canadian Amiodarone Myocardial Infarction Arrhythmia Trial [review, 14 refs]. *Indian Heart Journal, 48*(4), 339-341.

Goodkin, K., & Appels, A. (1997). Behavioral-neuroendocrine-immunologic interactions in myocardial infarction [review, 45 refs]. *Medical Hypotheses, 48*(3), 209-214.

Hedges, J. R., Gibler, W. B., Young, G. P., Hoekstra, J. W., Slovis, C., Aghababian, R., Smith, M., & Rubison, M. (1996). Multicenter study of creatine kinase-MB use: Effect on chest pain clinical decision making. *Academic Emergency Medicine, 3*(1), 7-15.

Howell, J. M. (1996). Acute myocardial infarction and congestive heart failure [review, 36 refs]. *Emergency Medicine Clinics of North America, 14*(1), 83-91.

Huber, K., Runge, M. S., Bode, C., & Gulba, D. (1996). Thrombolytic therapy in acute myocardial infarction—Update 1996 [review, 99 refs]. *Annals of Hematology, 73*(Suppl 1), S29-S38.

Jackson, G. (1996). Current approaches to stable angina. *Practitioner, 240*(1568), 642-644.

Jackson, G. (1997). Stable angina: Drugs, angioplasty or surgery? [review, 20 refs]. *European Heart Journal, 18*(Suppl B), B2-B10.

Jesse, R. L., & Kontos, M. C. (1997). Evaluation of chest pain in the emergency department [review, 289 refs]. *Current Problems in Cardiology, 22*(4), 149-236.

Juhan-Vague, I., Pyke, S. D., Alessi, M. C., Jespersen, J., Haverkate, F., & Thompson, S. G. (1996). Fibrinolytic factors and the risk of myocardial infarction or sudden death in patients with angina pectoris. ECAT Study Group. European Concerted Action on Thrombosis and Disabilities [see comments]. *Circulation, 94*(9), 2057-2063.

Just, H., Frey, M., & Zehender, M. (1996). Calcium antagonist drugs in hypertensive patients with angina pectoris [review, 27 refs]. *European Heart Journal, 17*(Suppl G), 20-24.

Kegel, L. M. (1996). Case management, critical pathways, and myocardial infarction [review, 46 refs]. *Critical Care Nurse, 16*(2), 97-104.

Klemsdal, T. O., & Gjesdal, K. (1996). Intermittent or continuous transdermal nitroglycerin: Still an issue, or is the case closed? [review, 61 refs]. *Cardiovascular Drugs and Therapy, 10*(1), 5-10.

Kubzansky, L. D., Kawachi, I., Spiro, A., Weiss, S. T., Vokonas, P. S., & Sparrow, D. (1997). Is worrying bad for your heart? A prospective study of worry and coronary heart disease in the Normative Aging Study. *Circulation, 95*(4), 818-824.

Kynman, G. (1997). Thrombolysis: The development of unit guidelines [review, 43 refs]. *Intensive & Critical Care Nursing, 13*(1), 30-41.

Lee, H. O. (1997). Typical and atypical clinical signs and symptoms of myocardial infarction and delayed seeking of professional care among blacks [review, 56 refs]. *American Journal of Critical Care, 6*(1), 7-13, quiz 14-15.

Maggioni, A. P., Sessa, F., Latini, R., & Tognoni, G. (1997). Treatment of acute myocardial infarction today [review, 29 refs]. *American Heart Journal, 134*(2 Pt 2), S9-S14.

Mittleman, M. A. (1996). Angina in patients with an active lifestyle [review, 33 refs]. *European Heart Journal, 17*(Suppl G), 30-35.

Miura, T., Miki, T., Tsuchihashi, K., & Iimura, O. (1996). Ischemic preconditioning against infarction: Its mechanism and clinical implications [review, 63 refs]. *EXS, 76*, 365-382.

Moliterno, D. J., & Topol, E. J. (1997). Conjunctive use of platelet glycoprotein IIb/IIIa antagonists and thrombolytic therapy for acute myocardial infarction [review, 41 refs]. *Thrombosis and Haemostasis, 78*(1), 214-219.

Noble, S., & McTavish, D. (1996). Reteplase. A review of its pharmacological properties and clinical efficacy in the management of acute myocardial infarction [review, 55 refs]. *Drugs, 52*(4), 589-605.

O'Rourke, R. A. (1996). Cost-effective management of chronic stable angina [review, 22 refs]. *Clinical Cardiology, 19*(6), 497-501.

Olson, H. G., & Aronow, W. S. (1996). Medical management of stable angina and unstable angina in the elderly with coronary artery disease [review, 72 refs]. *Clinics in Geriatric Medicine, 12*(1), 121-140.

Peterson, E. D., Shaw, L. J., & Califf, R. M. (1997). Risk stratification after myocardial infarction [review, 280 refs]. *Annals of Internal Medicine, 126*(7), 561-582.

Pinto, J. V. J., Ramani, K., Neelagaru, S., Kown, M., & Gheorghiade, M. (1997). Amiodarone therapy in chronic heart failure and myocardial infarction: A review of the mortality trials with special attention to STAT-CHF and the GESICA trials. Grupo de Estudio de la Sobrevida en la Insuficiencia Cardiaca en Argentina [review, 34 refs]. *Progress in Cardiovascular Diseases, 40*(1), 85-93.

Pocock, S. J., Henderson, R. A., Seed, P., Treasure, T., & Hampton, J. R. (1996). Quality of life, employment status, and anginal symptoms after coronary angioplasty or bypass surgery. 3-year follow-up in the Randomized Intervention Treatment of Angina (RITA) Trial. *Circulation, 94*(2), 135-142.

Popovic, A. D., & Thomas, J. D. (1997). Detecting and preventing ventricular remodeling after MI [review, 26 refs]. *Cleveland Clinic Journal of Medicine, 64*(6), 319-325.

Rakugi, H., Yu, H., Kamitani, A., Nakamura, Y., Ohishi, M., Kamide, K., Nakata, Y., Takami, S., Higaki, J., & Ogihara, T. (1996). Links between hypertension and myocardial infarction [review, 67 refs]. *American Heart Journal, 132*(1 Pt 2 Su), 213-221.

Rapaport, E., & Gheorghiade, M. (1996). Pharmacologic therapies after myocardial infarction [review, 61 refs]. *American Journal of Medicine, 101*(4A), 4A61S-69S, discussion 4A69S.

Rapola, J. M., Virtamo, J., Haukka, J. K., Heinonen, O. P., Albanes, D., Taylor, P. R., & Huttunen, J. K. (1996). Effect of vitamin E and beta carotene on the incidence of angina pectoris. A randomized, double-blind, controlled trial. *Journal of the American Medical Association, 275*(9), 693-698.

Reeder, G. S., & Gersh, B. J. (1996). Modern management of acute myocardial infarction [review, 136 refs]. *Current Problems in Cardiology, 21*(9), 585-667.

Renkin, J. (1996). Clinical benefit of angiotensin converting enzyme inhibition after acute myocardial infarction: Myocardial reperfusion revisited [review, 40 refs]. *Journal of Hypertension (Supplement), 14*(6), S15-S19.

Rich, M. W. (1996). Therapy for acute myocardial infarction [review, 148 refs]. *Clinics in Geriatric Medicine, 12*(1), 141-168.

Rosado, A., & Lamas, G. A. (1997). Left ventricular remodeling: Clinical significance and therapy [review, 18 refs]. *Basic Research in Cardiology, 92*(2), 66-68.

San, R. J. A., Vilacosta, I., Castillo, J. A., Rollan, M. J., Peral, V., Sanchez-Harguindey, L., & Fernandez-Aviles, F. (1996). Dipyridamole and dobutamine-atropine stress echocardiography in the diagnosis of coronary artery disease. Comparison with exercise stress test, analysis of agreement, and impact of antianginal treatment. *Chest, 110*(5), 1248-1254.

Schlaifer, J. D., & Kerensky, R. A. (1997). Ischemic preconditioning: Clinical relevance and investigative studies [review, 24 refs]. *Clinical Cardiology, 20*(7), 602-606.

Shechter, M., Hod, H., Kaplinsky, E., & Rabinowitz, B. (1996). The rationale of magnesium as alternative therapy for patients with acute myocardial infarction without thrombolytic therapy [review, 39 refs]. *American Heart Journal, 132*(2 Pt 2 Su), 483-486, discussion 496-502.

Silvestry, F. E., & Kimmel, S. E. (1996). Calcium-channel blockers in ischemic heart disease [review, 45 refs]. *Current Opinion in Cardiology, 11*(4), 434-439.

Swedberg, K., & Sharpe, N. (1996). The value of angiotensin converting enzyme inhibitors for the treatment of patients with left ventricular dysfunction, heart failure or after acute myocardial infarction [review, 31 refs]. *European Heart Journal, 17*(9), 1306-1311.

Talbert, R. L. (1996). Strategies in the management of acute myocardial infarction [review, 52 refs]. *Pharmacotherapy, 16*(5 Pt 2), 127S-136S.

Torp-Pedersen, C., Kober, L., & Burchardt, H. (1997). The place of angiotensin-converting enzyme inhibition after acute myocardial infarction [review, 24 refs]. *American Heart Journal, 134*(2 Pt 2), S25-S30.

van, B. A. J., Jukema, J. W., Zwinderman, A. H., Crijns, H. J., Lie, K. I., & Bruschke, A. V. (1996). Reduction of transient myocardial ischemia with pravastatin in addition to the conventional treatment in patients with angina pectoris. REGRESS Study Group. *Circulation, 94*(7), 1503-1505.

Verthein, U., & Kohler, T. (1997). The correlation between everyday stress and angina pectoris: A longitudinal study. *Journal of Psychosomatic Research, 43*(3), 241-245.

Wallentin, L. (1996). Low molecular weight heparins: A valuable tool in the treatment of acute coronary syndromes [review, 90 refs]. *European Heart Journal, 17*(10), 1470-1476.

Weaver, W. D. (1996). The role of thrombolytic drugs in the management of myocardial infarction. Comparative clinical trials [review, 36 refs]. *European Heart Journal, 17*(Suppl F), 9-15.

Whisenant, B. K., & Wolfe, C. L. (1997). Acute myocardial infarction. Recommendations for medical management and primary angioplasty [review, 29 refs]. *Postgraduate Medicine, 102*(3), 159-160.

Wilcox, T. (1997). Angina: Improving the outcome. *RN, 60*(7), 34-39, quiz 40.

Yusuf, S., Anand, S., Avezum, A. J., Flather, M., & Coutinho, M. (1996). Treatment for acute myocardial infarction. Overview of randomized clinical trials [review, 77 refs]. *European Heart Journal, 17*(Suppl F), 16-29.

CASE STUDY

ISCHEMIC HEART DISEASE

INITIAL HISTORY:
- 40-year-old male complaining of substernal chest pain that began approximately 90 minutes before he came to the emergency room.
- The pain has eased slightly but is still present; was 8/10 in severity, now 5/10.

Question 1.
   Based on this history alone, what is your differential diagnosis?

Question 2.
   What other symptoms would you like to ask him about?

ADDITIONAL HISTORY:
- He can also feel the pain in his left shoulder.
- He also feels short of breath and somewhat sick to his stomach, but he has not vomited.
- He denies coughing, fever, or change in the nature of the pain with deep breathing.

Question 3.
   What risk factors would you like to ask him about?

ADDITIONAL HISTORY:

- 40 pack/year history of smoking.
- His blood pressure has been a little elevated on his last 2 visits to his nurse practitioner at 148/92.
- He eats a lot of fatty foods but says his cholesterol doesn't change no matter what he eats; it was 242 last month.
- His father has angina that began at age 53.
- He denies diabetes.
- He exercises regularly and has not gained weight.

Question 4.

What else would you like to know about his past medical history?

PAST MEDICAL HISTORY:

- He says he has had a couple of episodes of shortness of breath while jogging but attributed it to "growing old."
- He has never been hospitalized except for one case of influenza complicated by pneumonia 3 years ago.
- He perceives himself as very healthy, is on no medications, and has no known allergies.

Question 5.

Based on the history, now what is your differential diagnosis?

PHYSICAL EXAMINATION:

- Alert, moderately anxious man in mild distress
- T = 37 orally; P = 100 with occasional premature beat; RR = 24; BP = 160/98 in both arms sitting

HEENT, Skin, Neck

- Skin warm and diaphoretic without cyanosis
- PERRLA, fundi benign, pharynx clear
- Neck supple without thyromegaly, adenopathy, or bruits
- <2 cm jugular venous distension

Lungs
- Tachypneic, mild use of accessory muscles of respiration
- No tenderness upon palpation of the chest wall
- No dullness to percussion
- Slight inspiratory crackles (rales) heard at both bases without egophony
- No rubs

Cardiac
- Tachycardia with occasional premature beat
- Apical pulse at 5th intercostal space just lateral to the midclavicular line
- Soft S_3, no S_4, no murmurs
- No rubs

Abdomen, Extremities, Neurological
- Abdomen with bowel sounds heard throughout; no organomegaly or tenderness; no bruits; rectal guaiac negative
- Extremities with full and symmetrical pulses; slight bruit over left femoral artery; no pedal edema
- Alert and oriented; neurologic exam in tact to cognition, strength, sensation, gait, and deep tendon reflexes

Question 6.
What are the pertinent positives and negatives on the exam and what might they mean?

Question 7.
What diagnostics would you like to obtain now?

INITIAL DIAGNOSTICS:
- ECG shows 4 mm ST elevation with T-wave inversion in the anterior precordial leads with occasional premature ventricular contraction
- Arterial blood gases on room air: pH = 7.46, $PaCO_2$ = 32, PaO_2 = 90
- Chest x-ray with borderline cardiomegaly and mild pulmonary congestion without acute infiltrates or pleural disease and no widening of the mediastinum

Question 8.
What do these initial diagnostic results indicate?

Question 9.
What therapeutic interventions would you like to initiate while obtaining additional the diagnostic data?

INITIAL MANAGEMENT:
- Patient is placed on nasal cannulae and an IV D_5W at KVO is started.
- He is given aspirin, 325 mg/PO.
- He receives 2 mg/IV morphine, 40 mg/IV furosemide, and topical nitrates.
- He is reassured and kept up-to-date with his diagnosis and care.

MORE DIAGNOSTICS:
- Electrolytes and CBC normal
- PT and PTT normal
- CPK-MB normal
- Troponin I normal

Question 10.
What now?

RE-EVALUATION OF THE PATIENT:
- Pain is now 2/10 in severity, dyspnea is better.
- P = 98; RR = 20; BP = 148/92
- Lungs are now clear.
- Cardiac with continued occasional PCV, S_3 is gone, no new murmurs.
- Repeat ECG with ST elevation now down to 2 mm and new Q-waves in anterior leads.

Question 11.
What interventions should be considered now?

FURTHER MANAGEMENT:
- Patient is given 2 mg morphine and the amount of topical nitrate is increased.
- ECG reveals wall motion abnormality of the anterior left ventricle; ejection fraction is now 55%.
- History reveals no contraindications to thrombolysis.

Question 12.
What medications should be given now?

ADDITIONAL MANAGEMENT:
- Patient receives accelerated tPA followed by heparin.
- He receives IV beta-blockers.
- His blood pressure normalizes and he has no more pain so no IV nitrates are given.
- His ECG normalized over time except for small Q-waves anteriorly.
- He is admitted to the CCU.

HOSPITAL COURSE:
- Patient continues to do well without recurrence of chest pain or dyspnea.
- Telemetry reveals no more ectopy.
- Patient is started on an ACE inhibitor on day 3 post-MI.
- He undergoes SPECT evaluation and is found to have no additional myocardium at risk consistent with single-vessel disease and completed infarction.
- He is gradually ambulated and is ready for discharge by day 6.

Question 13.

What should this patient be told and what medications should he be given before he is discharged?

CHAPTER 4

CONGESTIVE HEART FAILURE

DEFINITION

- Congestive heart failure (CHF) is a pathophysiologic condition in which the heart is unable to generate an adequate cardiac output such that there is inadequate perfusion of tissues, and/or increased diastolic filling pressure of the left ventricle, such that pulmonary capillary pressures are increased.

- CHF refers to primary dysfiunction of the left ventricle (LV).

- CHF may be systolic, diastolic, or both.

- Primary dysfunction of the right ventricle is associated most commonly with pulmonary disease (see Chapter 6) and is not considered congestive heart failure.

EPIDEMIOLOGY

- 1.5% to 2% of all adults in the United States are affected; 700,000 hospitalizations occur per year.

- The most common risk factor for the development of heart failure is age.

- CHF is the most common reason for the elderly to be admitted to the hospital (75% of patients admitted with CHF are between 65 and 75 years old).

- 44% of Medicare patients that are hospitalized for CHF will be readmitted within 6 months.

- There are 2 million outpatient visits per year for CHF; the costs are estimated at $10 billion annually.

- 80% 6-year mortality in men; 65% 6-year mortality in women

- Risk factors other than age include ischemic heart disease, hypertension, cardiomyopathy, renal failure, diabetes, and valvular heart disease.

PATHOPHYSIOLOGY

- CHF results from a complex interaction between factors that affect the contractility, afterload, preload, or lusitropic function of the heart, and the subsequent neurohumoral and hemodynamic responses that seek to create circulatory compensation.

- Although the hemodynamic consequences of heart failure respond to standard pharmacologic interventions, there are critical neurohumoral interactions whose combined effect is to exacerbate and perpetuate the syndrome.

- **Renin/angiotensin/aldosterone (RAA) system**—Angiotensin and aldosterone have been implicated in structural changes in the myocardium that are seen with ischemic injury and hypertensive hypertrophic cardiomyopathy. These changes include myocardial remodeling and sarcomere death, loss of the normal collagen matrix, and interstitial fibrosis. The resulting myocyte and sarcomere slippage, heart dilation, and scar formation with loss of normal myocardial compliance contribute to the hemodynamic and symptomatic features of CHF.

- **Sympathetic nervous system (SNS)**—Epinephrine and norepinephrine cause increased peripheral resistance with increased work for the heart, tachycardia, and increased oxygen consumption by the myocardium. They also appear to contribute to ventricular remodeling.

- **Endogenous vasodilators, such as endothelin and nitric oxide, cardiac peptides, and natriuretic peptides**—The roles in CHF are being defined and the interventions are being tested.

- The initial etiologic event influences the early responses of the myocardium, but as the syndrome progresses, common mechanisms emerge such that patients with advanced CHF share similar symptomatic presentations and respond to similar pharmacologic interventions irrespective of the initial cause of their CHF.

- Although many patients have both systolic and diastolic left ventricular dysfunction, these categories are best considered separately in order to understand their effects on circulatory homeostasis and their responses to various interventions.

  - Systolic left ventricular dysfunction.
    1) **Diminished cardiac output** due to decreased contractility, increased afterload, or increased preload results in a decreased ejection fraction and an increased left ventricular end diastolic volume (LVEDV). This increases the end diastolic pressures in the left ventricle (LVEDP) and causes pulmonary venous congestion and pulmonary edema.
    2) **Decreased contractility (ionotropy)** results from inadequate or uncoordinated myocardial function such that the LV cannot eject more than 60% of its end-diastolic volume (LVEDV). This causes a gradual increase in LVEDV (also called preload) resulting in an increase in LVEDP and pulmonary venous congestion. The most common cause of decreased contractility is ischemic heart disease, which not only results in actual necrosis of myocardial tissue, but also causes ventricular "remodeling." Remodeling is a process mediated in part by angiotensin II (ANG II) that causes scarring and sarcomere dysfunction in the heart surrounding the area of ischemic injury. Cardiac arrhythmias and primary cardiomyopathies such as those caused by alcohol and amyloidosis also cause decreased contractility. Decreased cardiac output leads to underperfusion of the systemic circulation and activation of the sympathetic nervous system and the RAA system, causing increased peripheral resistance and increased afterload.
    3) **Increased afterload** means there is increased resistance to LV ejection. This is usually due to the increased peripheral vascular resistance commonly seen in hypertension. It may also be due to aortic valvular stenosis. The LV responds to this increased work with myocardial hypertrophy, a response that increases LV muscle mass but at the same time increases LV demand for coronary perfusion. An energy-starved state is created that, in concert with ANG II and other neuroendocrine responses, causes deleterious changes in the myocytes such as fewer mitochondria for energy production, altered gene expression with production of abnormal contractile proteins (actin, myosin, and tropomyosin), interstitial fibrosis, and decreased myocyte survival. Over time, contractility begins to decline with decreased cardiac output and ejection fraction, increased LVEDV, and pulmonary congestion.

4) **Increased preload** means increased LVEDV, which can be increased directly by excess intravascular volume similar to that seen with an infusion of intravenous fluids or with renal failure. As LVEDV increases, it stretches the heart, putting the sarcomeres at a mechanical disadvantage and thus decreasing contractility. This decreased contractility, resulting in a decreased ejection fraction, contributes further to the increased LVEDV, thus creating a viscous cycle of worsening heart failure.

5) Thus a patient can enter this cycle of decreased contractility, increased afterload, and increased preload for a number of reasons (e.g., myocardial infarction [MI], hypertension, fluid overload) and will eventually develop all of the hemodynamic and neurohumoral features of CHF as one mechanism leads to the other (Figure 4-1).

Figure 4-1.

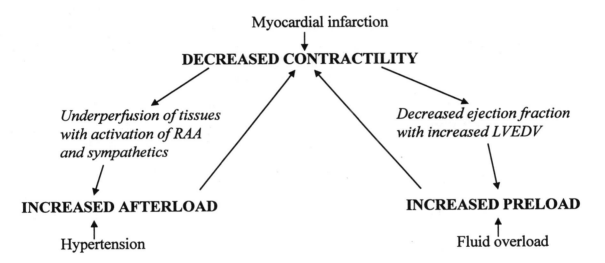

- Diastolic left ventricular dysfunction
    1) It causes up to 40% of all cases of CHF.
    2) It is defined as a condition with classic findings of congestive failure with abnormal diastolic but normal systolic function; pure diastolic dysfunction would be characterized by resistance to ventricular filling with an increase in LVEDP without an increase in LVEDV or a decrease in cardiac output.
    3) The resistance to left ventricular filling results from abnormal relaxation (lusitropy) of the LV and can be caused by any condition that stiffens the ventricular myocardium such as ischemic heart disease resulting in scarring, hypertension resulting in hypertrophic cardiomyopathy, restrictive cardiomyopathy, or pericardial disease.
    4) Increases in heart rate allow less time for diastolic filling and exacerbate the symptoms of diastolic dysfunction. Therefore exercise intolerance is common.
    5) Because treatment would require actually changing myocardial compliance, the effectiveness of currently available drugs is limited.

PATIENT PRESENTATION

- History:

  Previous myocardial infarction; risk factors for ischemic heart disease (smoking, hyperlipidemia, diabetes); hypertension; valvular disease; cardiomyopathy; pericardial disease; renal failure; excessive intravenous; recent high intake of salt (may increase symptoms in a patient with underlying LV dysfunction).

- Symptoms:

  Dyspnea especially on exertion; orthopnea; paroxysmal nocturnal dyspnea; cough; pedal edema; decreased urine output; fatigue; weight gain; chest pain.

- Examination:

  Weight gain; tachypnea; tachycardia; murmurs; cyanosis; inspiratory crackles (rales); frothy sputum production; edema; cold, clammy skin; weak peripheral pulses; jugular venous distension; hepatojugular reflux; **systolic dysfunction**: S_3, shift of apical pulse, hypotension during episodes of pulmonary edema; **diastolic dysfunction**: S_4, strong but nondisplaced apical pulse, hypertension during episodes of pulmonary edema; hepatosplenomegaly.

DIFFERENTIAL DIAGNOSIS

- CHF must be differentiated from the following:

  - Noncardiogenic pulmonary edema (acute respiratory distress syndrome [ARDS])

  - Chronic obstructive pulmonary disease (COPD)

  - Pneumonia

  - Asthma

  - Interstitial pulmonary fibrosis

  - Other primary lung diseases

- The underlying cause of the CHF must be established from the following:

  - Myocardial ischemia/infarction

  - Hypertensive hypertrophic cardiomyopathy

  - Valvular heart disease

  - Primary cardiomyopathy (idiopathic, alcohol, post infectious, amyloidosis, restrictive)

  - Pericardial disease

  - Fluid overload (iatrogenic versus renal failure)

KEYS TO ASSESSMENT

- CHF is a manifestation of an underlying cardiac insult; begin immediately to assess for the cause of LV dysfunction.

- A quick physical exam can often establish the diagnosis of CHF; therapeutic intervention can begin even as assessment progresses.

- Early electrocardiographic monitoring for ischemia or arrhythmias is vital.

- Obtain arterial blood gases immediately, then begin oxygen.

- Obtain serum electrolytes, blood urea nitrogen (BUN) and creatinine (Cr); complete blood count (CBC); and thyroid studies if age over 65 or atrial fibrillation.

- A chest x-ray may show cardiomegaly, pulmonary edema, and pleural effusions; the diagnosis of pericardial or valvular disease can often be made on the chest x-ray.

- Echocardiography (ECG) can estimate ejection fraction and cardiac output, demonstrate LV wall motion abnormalities consistent with ischemia, show hypertrophic cardiomyopathy, or diagnose valvular and pericardial disease.

- Emergent cardiac catheterization may be indicated in patients suspected of acute coronary artery disease and thrombosis.

- Hemodynamic monitoring (central venous catheter) remains controversial; current indications include the following:

    - Uncertainty about diagnosis

    - Deteriorating course

    - Lack of expected response to interventions

    - High dose intravenous nitrates or inotropics indicated

KEYS TO MANAGEMENT

- Acute CHF:

    - Let the patient sit up if not hypotensive.

    - Oxygen—get arterial blood gas on room air quickly, then put on a mask at 60%; intubate if there is ventilatory failure or if the patient is progressively cyanotic and has decreasing mental status.

    - Treat myocardial ischemia if indicated (see Chapter 3).

    - Adminsiter morphine, nitroglycerin, and IV diuretic (furosemide) if no significant hypotension.

    - Consider intravenous (IV) inotropics (dobutamine, dopamine)—use them early if hypotensive.

    - If necessary, switch to IV nitrates if there is a high peripheral vascular resistance (hypertensive). Nitroglycerin is safer than nitroprusside.

    - An intraaortic balloon pump is indicated if there is refractory hypotension (cardiogenic shock), refractory ischemia in preparation for emergency coronary bypass grafting (CABG), or acute mitral regurgitation in preparation for operative valvular repair or replacement.

    - Emergent coronary catheterization and balloon angioplasty or CABG is used in selected patients with ischemia.

- Chronic CHF:

    - Definitive management of underlying cause is optimal.

    - Lifestyle modification with salt restriction, exercise, and education about monitoring symptoms (daily weights, dyspnea, edema, chest pain) is recommended.

- A nurse-mediated home-based management system has been shown to improve outcomes and decrease hospitalizations.

- Diuretics, inotropics, and vasodilators remain the mainstay of therapy for CHF.
  1) **Diuretics:** furosemide remains the most commonly used diuretic along with bumetanide or torasemide. Diuretics clearly improve exercise intolerance and edema, but electrolyte imbalance and adverse effects on serum lipids and glucose must be watched.
  2) **Inotropics:**
     - Digoxin clearly improves exercise tolerance, increases cardiac output, slows the progression of CHF, downregulates sympathetic tone, and improves quality of life. It may decrease mortality when used with angiotensin converting enzyme (ACE) inhibitors. It is important to follow blood levels and avoid hypokalemia, which may lead to arrhythmias.
     - Phosphodiesterase inhibitors (milrinone, amrinone, enoximone, prioximone) have short-term benefits to cardiac output and exercise tolerance, but their long-term safety is unclear including increases in mortality, significant hypotension, syncope, and allergy.
     - Adrenergic agonists, such as intermittent IV dobutamine and xamoterol, have short-term benefits, but both can cause increased mortality.
     - New inotropics, such as vesnarinone, flosequinan, and pimobencan, have shown promise, but long-term safety has not yet been established.
  3) **Vasodilators:**
     - ACE inhibitors and angiotensin II receptor blockers improve hemodynamic and neurohumoral manifestations of CHF with improvements in symptoms and dramatic improvements in survival. Most are well tolerated except for first-dose hypotension, cough (especially with captopril) and risk of renal dysfunction in some patients. They are useful in both systolic and diastolic dysfunction.
     - Nitrates also improve hemodynamic and neurohumoral manifestations of CHF. They are associated with significant headache, and tolerance requires intermittent dosing.
  4) **Second and third generation calcium channel blockers** (amlodipine, felodipine) may be useful in diastolic dysfunction and late-stage systolic dysfunction. First generation calcium blockers increase sympathetic activity and do not reduce mortality in CHF.
  5) **Third generation beta-blockers** (carvedilol, bucindolol, labetalol) increase ejection fraction, decrease sympathetic tone with vasodilation and decreased myocardial oxygen consumption, and decrease ventricular remodeling. There is increasing evidence for decreased mortality and improved symptoms. A high dose results in pulmonary edema; a low dose causes clinical worsening for the first 4 to 10 weeks with improvement at about 10 to 12 weeks. Start with very low doses and increase slowly.
  6) **Antiarrhythmics** are generally not indicated, despite the high incidence of sudden death in CHF; both beta-blockers and ACE inhibitors decrease ventricular ectopy. Amiodarone is the only antiarrhythmic that has been associated with decreased mortality.
  7) **Anticoagulants** are indicated if there is atrial fibrillation, valvular disease, or a known intraventricular thrombus.
  8) **Surgery** for CHF includes heart transplant and cardiomyoplasty (transplanting latissimus dorsi muscle into the heart wall), as indicated for selected patients.

Pathophysiology

What is going on in the disease process that influences how the patient presents and how he or she should be managed?

Clinical Link

What should you do now that you understand the underlying pathophysiology?

→

CHF is a very common syndrome with age as the greatest risk factor along with underlying coronary or hypertensive heart disease.	A careful history and physical are important when evaluating elderly patients and those at risk for heart disease.
Acute congestive failure is a common complication of acute myocardial infarction, severe valvular disease, underlying fluid overload, and hypertensive crisis.	The management of acute CHF must include evaluation and therapy for the initiating process, not just for CHF.
Neurohumoral mechanisms contribute to the pathophysiology, especially RAA system and SNS.	Management should include ACE inhibitors and possibly beta-blockers.
Systolic LV dysfunction results in a vicious cycle of decreased contractility, increased afterload, and increased preload.	Once the full picture of CHF is established, most patients with systolic dysfunction will require inotropics, diuretics and vasodilators.
Diastolic LV dysfunction common and results from decreased LV compliance and abnormal lusitropy, most commonly from the effects of hypertension and the RAA system.	Diastolic function should be suspected in symptomatic patients with normal ejection fraction; current treatment and prevention includes ACE inhibitors. New calcium channel blockers are also being tried.

BIBLIOGRAPHY

Anonymous. (1997). ASHP therapeutic guidelines on angiotensin-converting-enzyme inhibitors in patients with left ventricular dysfunction. This official ASHP practice standard was developed through the ASHP Commission on Therapeutics and approved by the ASHP Board of Directors on November 16, 1996 [see comments] [review, 109 refs]. *American Journal of Health-System Pharmacy, 54*(3), 299-313.

Aronow, W. S. (1997). Treatment of congestive heart failure in older persons [review, 43 refs]. *Journal of the American Geriatrics Society, 45*(10), 1252-1257.

Bales, A. C., & Sorrentino, M. J. (1997). Causes of congestive heart failure. Prompt diagnosis may affect prognosis [review, 19 refs]. *Postgraduate Medicine, 101*(1), 44-49.

Bolotin, G., Van der Veen, F. H., Schreuder, J., Lorusso, R., Ben, D. J., & Uretzky, G. (1996). Cardiomyoplasty—The beginning of a new era [review, 40 refs]. *Israel Journal of Medical Sciences, 32*(5), 321-326.

Bonarjee, V. V., & Dickstein, K. (1996). Novel drugs and current therapeutic approaches in the treatment of heart failure [review, 122 refs]. *Drugs, 51*(3), 347-358.

Bulpitt, C. J. (1996). Quality of life with ACE inhibitors in chronic heart failure [review, 35 refs]. *Journal of Cardiovascular Pharmacology, 27*(Suppl 2), S31-S35.

Cash, L. A. (1996). Heart failure from diastolic dysfunction [review, 24 refs]. *Dimensions of Critical Care Nursing, 15*(4), 170-177, quiz 178-80.

Cleland, J. G. (1996). From left ventricular dysfunction to heart failure [review, 20 refs]. *Archives des Maladies du Coeur et des Vaisseaux, 89*(11), 1397-1402.

Cleland, J. G., & Habib, F. (1996). Assessment and diagnosis of heart failure [review, 20 refs]. *Journal of Internal Medicine, 239*(4), 317-325.

Cohn, J. N. (1996). The management of chronic heart failure [see comments] [review, 89 refs]. *New England Journal of Medicine, 335*(7), 490-498.

Cowie, M. R., Mosterd, A., Wood, D. A., Deckers, J. W., Poole-Wilson, P. A., Sutton, G. C., & Grobbee, D. E. (1997). The epidemiology of heart failure [review, 160 refs]. *European Heart Journal, 18*(2), 208-225.

Dahlen, R., & Roberts, S. L. (1996). Acute congestive heart failure: Preventing complications [review, 46 refs]. *Dimensions of Critical Care Nursing, 15*(5), 226-241, quiz 242-244.

Dargie, H. J., McMurray, J. J., & McDonagh, T. A. (1996). Heart failure—Implications of the true size of the problem [review, 30 refs]. *Journal of Internal Medicine, 239*(4), 309-315.

Dhalla, N. S., Kaura, D., Liu, X., & Beamish, R. E. (1996). Mechanisms of subcellular remodeling in post-infarct heart failure [review, 75 refs]. *EXS, 76,* 463-477.

Douban, S., Brodsky, M. A., Whang, D. D., & Whang, R. (1996). Significance of magnesium in congestive heart failure [review, 103 refs]. *American Heart Journal, 132*(3), 664-671.

Doughty, R. N., & Sharpe, N. (1997). Beta-adrenergic blocking agents in the treatment of congestive heart failure: Mechanisms and clinical results [review, 70 refs]. *Annual Review of Medicine, 48,* 103-114.

Dracup, K. (1996). Heart failure secondary to left ventricular systolic dysfunction. Therapeutic advances and treatment recommendations [review, 30 refs]. *Nurse Practitioner, 21*(9), 56-58.

Drexler, H. (1996). Endothelial function in heart failure: Some unsolved issues [editorial; comment] [review, 25 refs]. *European Heart Journal, 17*(12), 1775-1777.

Drexler, H., & Coats, A. J. (1996). Explaining fatigue in congestive heart failure [review, 83 refs]. *Annual Review of Medicine, 47,* 241-256.

Dusting, G. J. (1996). Nitric oxide in coronary artery disease: Roles in atherosclerosis, myocardial reperfusion and heart failure [review, 108 refs]. *EXS, 76,* 33-55.

Eichhorn, E. J., & Bristow, M. R. (1996). Medical therapy can improve the biological properties of the chronically failing heart. A new era in the treatment of heart failure [review, 156 refs]. *Circulation, 94*(9), 2285-2296.

Eichhorn, E. J., & Bristow, M. R. (1997). Practical guidelines for initiation of beta-adrenergic blockade in patients with chronic heart failure [editorial] [review, 55 refs]. *American Journal of Cardiology, 79*(6), 794-798.

Elkayam, U. (1996). Nitrates in the treatment of congestive heart failure [review, 56 refs]. *American Journal of Cardiology, 77*(13), 41C-51C.

Erhardt, L. (1996). ACE inhibitors before or after heart failure? [review, 73 refs]. *European Journal of Clinical Pharmacology, 49*(Suppl 1), S19-S28.

Forker, A. D. (1996). A cardiologist's perspective on evolving concepts in the management of congestive heart failure [review, 65 refs]. *Journal of Clinical Pharmacology, 36*(11), 973-984.

Funk, M., & Krumholz, H. M. (1996). Epidemiologic and economic impact of advanced heart failure [review, 33 refs]. *Journal of Cardiovascular Nursing, 10*(2), 1-10.

Gheorghiade, M., & Pitt, B. (1997). Digitalis Investigation Group (DIG) trial: A stimulus for further research [review, 136 refs]. *American Heart Journal, 134*(1), 3-12.

Guerra-Garcia, H., Taffet, G., & Protas, E. J. (1997). Considerations related to disability and exercise in elderly women with congestive heart failure [review, 86 refs]. *Journal of Cardiovascular Nursing, 11*(4), 60-74.

Howell, J. M. (1996). Acute myocardial infarction and congestive heart failure [review, 36 refs]. *Emergency Medicine Clinics of North America, 14*(1), 83-91.

Jaarsma, T., Abu-Saad, H. H., Halfens, R., & Dracup, K. (1997). 'Maintaining the balance'—Nursing care of patients with chronic heart failure [review, 32 refs]. *International Journal of Nursing Studies, 34*(3), 213-221.

Jaffe, R., Flugelman, M. Y., Halon, D. A., & Lewis, B. S. (1997). Ventricular remodeling: From bedside to molecule [review, 60 refs]. *Advances in Experimental Medicine and Biology, 430,* 257

Kjekshus, J., & Swedberg, K. (1996). Treatment of heart failure [review, 53 refs]. *Journal of Internal Medicine, 239*(4), 335-343.

Kleber, F. X., & Wensel, R. (1996). Current guidelines for the treatment of congestive heart failure [review, 70 refs]. *Drugs, 51*(1), 89-98.

Krum, H. (1997). Beta-adrenoceptor blockers in chronic heart failure—A review [review, 57 refs]. *British Journal of Clinical Pharmacology, 44*(2), 111-118.

Levin, T. N. (1997). Acute congestive heart failure. The need for aggressive therapy [review, 16 refs]. *Postgraduate Medicine, 101*(1), 97-100.

Love, M. P., & McMurray, J. J. (1996). Endothelin in congestive heart failure [review, 86 refs]. *Basic Research in Cardiology, 91*(Suppl 1), 21-29.

Massie, B. M., & Shah, N. B. (1997). Evolving trends in the epidemiologic factors of heart failure: Rationale for preventive strategies and comprehensive disease management [review, 52 refs]. *American Heart Journal, 133*(6), 703-712.

Mehra, M. R., Cassidy, C. A., deGruiter, H. G., & Ventura, H. O. (1997). The unique management of refractory advanced systolic heart failure [review, 30 refs]. *Heart and Lung, 26*(4), 280-288.

Mitamura, H. (1996). Ventricular arrhythmias in heart failure [review, 71 refs]. *Keio Journal of Medicine, 45*(1), 1-8.

Moser, D. K. (1996). Maximizing therapy in the advanced heart failure patient [review, 62 refs]. *Journal of Cardiovascular Nursing, 10*(2), 29-46.

Munger, M. A., & Furniss, S. M. (1996). Angiotensin II receptor blockers: Novel therapy for heart failure? [review, 86 refs]. *Pharmacotherapy, 16*(2 Pt 2), 59S-68S.

Nelson, K. M., & Yeager, B. F. (1996). What is the role of angiotensin-converting enzyme inhibitors in congestive heart failure and after myocardial infarction? [review, 44 refs]. *Annals of Pharmacotherapy, 30*(9), 986-993.

Nicholls, D. P., Onuoha, G. N., McDowell, G., Elborn, J. S., Riley, M. S., Nugent, A. M., Steele, I. C., Shaw, C., & Buchanan, K. D. (1996). Neuroendocrine changes in chronic cardiac failure [review, 140 refs]. *Basic Research in Cardiology, 91*(Suppl 1), 13-20.

Oka, R. K. (1996). Physiologic changes in heart failure—"What's new" [review, 93 refs]. *Journal of Cardiovascular Nursing, 10*(2), 11-28.

Packer, M. (1996). New concepts in the pathophysiology of heart failure: Beneficial and deleterious interaction of endogenous haemodynamic and neurohormonal mechanisms [review, 28 refs]. *Journal of Internal Medicine, 239*(4), 327-333.

Patterson, J. H., & Adams, K. F. J. (1996). Pathophysiology of heart failure: Changing perceptions [review, 26 refs]. *Pharmacotherapy, 16*(2 Pt 2), 27S-36S.

Pieper, J. A. (1996). Evolving role of calcium channel blockers in heart failure [review, 26 refs]. *Pharmacotherapy, 16*(2 Pt 2), 43S-49S.

Pinto, J. V. J., Ramani, K., Neelagaru, S., Kown, M., & Gheorghiade, M. (1997). Amiodarone therapy in chronic heart failure and myocardial infarction: A review of the mortality trials with special attention to STAT-CHF and the GESICA trials. Grupo de Estudio de la Sobrevida en la Insuficiencia Cardiaca en Argentina [review, 34 refs]. *Progress in Cardiovascular Diseases, 40*(1), 85-93.

Pinto, Y. M., Buikema, H., van Gilst, W. H., & Lie, K. I. (1996). Activated tissue renin-angiotensin systems add to the progression of heart failure [review, 25 refs]. *Basic Research in Cardiology, 91*(Suppl 2), 85-90.

Rahimtoola, S. H., & Tak, T. (1996). The use of digitalis in heart failure [review, 146 refs]. *Current Problems in Cardiology, 21*(12), 781-853.

Rich, M. W. (1997). Epidemiology, pathophysiology, and etiology of congestive heart failure in older adults [review, 48 refs]. *Journal of the American Geriatrics Society, 45*(8), 968-974.

Schwabauer, N. J. (1996). Retarding progression of heart failure: Nursing actions [review, 38 refs]. *Dimensions of Critical Care Nursing, 15*(6), 307-317.

Semeraro, C., Marchini, F., Ferlenga, P., Masotto, C., Morazzoni, G., Pradella, L., & Pocchiari, F. (1997). The role of dopaminergic agonists in congestive heart failure [review, 37 refs]. *Clinical and Experimental Hypertension, 19*(1-2), 201-215.

Sigurdsson, A., & Swedberg, K. (1996). The role of neurohormonal activation in chronic heart failure and postmyocardial infarction [review, 50 refs]. *American Heart Journal, 132*(1 Pt 2 Su), 229-234.

Sullivan, M. J., & Hawthorne, M. H. (1996). Nonpharmacologic interventions in the treatment of heart failure [review, 44 refs]. *Journal of Cardiovascular Nursing, 10*(2), 47-57.

Swedberg, K., & Sharpe, N. (1996). The value of angiotensin converting enzyme inhibitors for the treatment of patients with left ventricular dysfunction, heart failure or after acute myocardial infarction [review, 31 refs]. *European Heart Journal, 17*(9), 1306-1311.

Teerlink, J. R. (1996). Neurohumoral mechanisms in heart failure: A central role for the renin-angiotensin system [review, 70 refs]. *Journal of Cardiovascular Pharmacology, 27*(Suppl 2), S1-S8.

Tresch, D. D. (1997). The clinical diagnosis of heart failure in older patients [review, 38 refs]. *Journal of the American Geriatrics Society, 45*(9), 1128-1133.

van Veldhuisen, D. J., de Graeff, P. A., Remme, W. J., & Lie, K. I. (1996). Value of digoxin in heart failure and sinus rhythm: New features of an old drug? [review, 99 refs]. *Journal of the American College of Cardiology, 28*(4), 813-819.

Vanhoutte, P. M. (1996). Endothelium-dependent responses in congestive heart failure [review, 61 refs]. *Journal of Molecular & Cellular Cardiology, 28*(11), 2233-2240.

Vasan, R. S., & Levy, D. (1996). The role of hypertension in the pathogenesis of heart failure. A clinical mechanistic overview [review, 159 refs]. *Archives of Internal Medicine, 156*(16), 1789-1796.

Young, J. B. (1997). Carvedilol for heart failure: Renewed interest in beta blockers [review, 30 refs]. *Cleveland Clinic Journal of Medicine, 64*(8), 415-422.

CASE STUDY*

CONGESTIVE HEART FAILURE

INITIAL HISTORY:
- 66-year-old white male
- Increasing shortness of breath over last month
- Noticed feet and ankles swelling by end of the day
- Has occasional episodes of chest tightness
- Has been waking up in the middle of the night with acute shortness of breath
- Feels tired most of the time

Question 1.
What is your differential diagnosis based on the information you have now?

Question 2.
What other questions would you like to ask now?

ADDITIONAL HISTORY:
- History of transmural anterior wall; MI 7 years ago
- 3-vessel coronary artery bypass graft surgery 7 years ago
- 2 pack/day smoker for 40 years; quit after bypass surgery
- Positive family history of heart disease
- 15-year history of hypertension
- No history of a cough
- No palpitations
- Current medications: SL NTG 1/150 PRN; selective beta-adrenergic blocker once daily; and ASA 2 daily

* Juanita Reigle, RN, MSN, ACNP-CS, CCRN, contributed this case study.

Question 3.

Now what do you think about his history?

PHYSICAL EXAMINATION:
- BP = 110/60 (sitting); AP 118 and regular; RR = 24 (increases with minimal activity, such as walking to exam room); T = 37.2 orally; WT = 82 kg

HEENT, Skin, Neck
- Fundoscopic exam normal
- Skin is pale; cool extremities
- Neck supple, no bruits over carotid arteries
- No thyromegaly, no adenopathy
- + jugular venous distension (JVD)—increased 6 cm above sternal angle at 45°
- + hepato-jugular reflex (HJR)

Lungs
- Bibasilar crackles that do not clear with cough
- Right base dull to percussion

Cardiac
- Point of maximal impulse (PMI) sustained and displaced laterally
- Normal S_1 S_2; +S_3 at apex
- II/VI blowing holosystolic murmur at apex, radiating to axilla

Abdomen, Extremities, Neurological
- Liver percusses to 12 cm in midclavicular line; no bruits
- 2+ pitting edema in feet and ankles extending to midcalf bilaterally
- 2+ radial pulses, 1+ dorsalis pedis, and 1+ posterior tibial pulses bilaterally; cool skin
- Alert and oriented
- Cranial nerves intact, sensory intact
- Deep tendon reflexes (DTR) 2+ and symmetrical; strength 4/5 throughout

Question 4.

What abnormal physical findings support the diagnosis of heart failure?

Question 5.
What studies would you initiate while preparing your interventions?

Question 6.
What therapies would you initiate immediately while awaiting results of the laboratory studies?

LABORATORY RESULTS:
- NA = 134   WBC = 7.8
- K = 3.6   HCT = 40
- BUN = 48   HGB = 13.2
- Cr = 1.9   PLT = 219
- GLU = 97
- CA = 8.6   ALB = 3.2
- MG = 2.2   TSH = 0.64
- ALK PHOS = 60   T4 = 1.4
- AST = 15
- pH = 7.34; $PaCO_2$ = 48; PaO_2 = 90 (room air)

CHEST X-RAY AND READING:

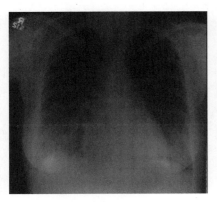
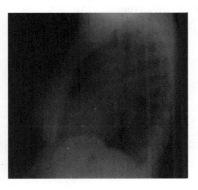

- Cardiomegaly
- Bilateral small pleural effusions (right > left)
- Perihilar infiltrates
- +Kerley B lines

Question 7.
What is this patient's estimated creatinine clearance?

ELECTROCARDIOGRAM:
- Sinus tachycardia
- Possible left atrial enlargement
- Poor R wave progression V1-V3
- No evidence of acute ischemia
- Left ventricular hypertrophy (LVH) with strain

Question 8.
What additional therapies would you initiate based on the laboratory values?

EMERGENCY ROOM COURSE:
- Pt diuresis 2500 cc clear yellow urine after administration of a loop diuretic
- Bibasilar crackles diminish
- Weight now 81.5 kg
- BP = 100/68; HR = 96

Question 9.
What discharge medications should be prescribed?

Question 10.
What referrals should be made for further follow-up?

Question 11.
What patient teaching should occur before discharge?

CHAPTER 5

ASTHMA

DEFINITION

- "A <u>chronic inflammatory disorder</u> of the airways in which many cells and cellular elements play a role, in particular, mast cells, eosinophils, T lymphocytes, macrophages, neutrophils, and epithelial cells. In susceptible individuals, this inflammation causes <u>recurrent episodes</u> of wheezing, breathlessness, chest tightness, and coughing, particularly at night or in the early morning. These episodes are usually associated with widespread but variable <u>airflow obstruction that is often reversible</u> either spontaneously or with treatment. The inflammation also causes an associated increase in the existing <u>bronchial hyperresponsiveness to a variety of stimuli</u>. Subbasement membrane <u>fibrosis</u> may occur in some patients with asthma and these changes contribute to persistent abnormalities in lung function."

- The scheme for asthma classification has been revised in the United States from one based on etiology and pathophysiology (allergic [extrinsic], idiopathic [intrinsic], exercise induced, occupational, and nocturnal) to one based on clinical severity (mild intermittent, mild persistent, moderate persistent, and severe persistent) (Table 5-1)

EPIDEMIOLOGY

- 5% of adults in the United States; 8% of children in the United States. It is estimated that 15 million people in the United States have asthma.

- The incidence has increased 60% during the past decade.

- There was a 6.2% annual increase in asthma mortality during the 1980s; there are approximately 5000 deaths annually in the United States.

- Childhood exposure to damp housing, cigarette smoke, and high levels of allergens has been associated with an increased risk for asthma.

- There is a familial association for asthma.

PATHOPHYSIOLOGY

- Genetics—abnormality in IL-4 gene leading to increased IgE synthesis; genetic tendency for airway obstruction in response to stimuli with increased immunologic and neurogenic stimulation.

- Bronchial hyperresponsiveness.

- Mast cell degranulation releases vasoactive, bronchospastic, and inflammatory mediators including histamine, prostaglandins, and leukotrienes (Figure 5-1).

- Bronchoconstriction and mucosal edema results in airway narrowing that is worse during expiration.

Table 5-1.
Asthma Classification

DISEASE CATEGORY	SYMPTOMS	NOCTURNAL SYMPTOMS	DAILY MEDICAL FOR LONG-TERM CONTROL	MEDICAL FOR QUICK RELIEF
STEP 4 Severe persistent	Continual symptoms Limited physical activity Frequent exacerbations	Frequent	**Two daily medications** Antiinflammatory agent (high-dose inhaled glucocorticoid) **and** Long-acting bronchodilator (inhaled or oral β_2-agonist or theophylline) **and** Oral glucocorticoid	Short-acting inhaled β_2-agonist Daily use or increasing use indicates need for additional long-term therapy
STEP 3 Moderate persistent	Daily symptoms Daily use of inhaled short-acting β_2-agonist Exacerbations affect activity Exacerbations at least twice weekly and may last for days	More frequent than once weekly	**One or two daily medications** Antiinflammatory agent (medium-dose inhaled glucocorticoid) **and/or** Medium-dose inhaled glucocorticoid plus long-acting bronchodilator	Short-acting inhaled β_2-agonist Daily use or increasing use indicates need for additional long-term therapy
STEP 2 Mild persistent	Symptoms more frequent than twice weekly but less than once a day Exacerbations may affect activity	More frequent than once weekly	**One daily medication** Antiinflammatory agent (low-dose inhaled glucocorticoid, cromolyn, or nedocromil) **or** Sustained-release theophylline *Note:* Leukotriene modifiers may be considered for patients at least 12 years old.	Short-acting inhaled β_2-agonist Daily use or increasing use indicates need for additional long-term therapy
STEP 1 Mild intermittent	Symptoms no more frequent than twice weekly Asymptomatic and with normal PEFR between exacerbations Exacerbations brief (hours to days) Intensity of exacerbations varies	No more frequent than twice monthly	No daily medication	Short-acting inhaled β_2-agonist Use more than twice weekly may indicate need to initiate long-term therapy

- Airway inflammation results in both acute mucosal edema and mucus production as well as persistent epithelial desquamation and the potential for long-term tissue damage (see Figure 5-1).

- Late asthmatic response—neuropeptides and lymphocytes combine to produce a recurrence of bronchoconstriction at 4 to 8 hours after the initial attack.

- Increased expiratory airway resistance leads to hyperinflation and ventilation/perfusion mismatching with resultant hypoxemia (Figure 5-2).

- During severe attacks, increased work of breathing and hypoventilation can lead to hypercapnia.

PATIENT PRESENTATION

- <u>History</u>:

    Asthma in past or history of frequent "colds" with wheezing (often seasonal); nighttime cough; history of allergies; intolerance to exercise, cold, drugs, smoke; dyspnea at work; family history of asthma.

- <u>Symptoms</u>:

    Intermittent dry cough, wheezing, chest tightness, dyspnea—often after a predictable stimulus (allergen, cold exposure, smoke, etc.); may be associated with rhinitis, postnasal drainage, pharyngitis, sputum production, or viral prodromal symptoms.

- <u>Examination</u>:

    Anxiety, cyanosis, tachypnea, tachycardia, accessory muscle use, chest hyperexpansion; expiratory wheezing with prolonged expiratory phase of breathing; impending respiratory failure.

DIFFERENTIAL DIAGNOSIS

- Bronchitis

- Exacerbation of chronic obstructive pulmonary disease (COPD)

- Pneumonia

- Pneumonitis

- Anaphylaxis

- Foreign body

- Upper airway obstruction

- Congestive heart failure

- Pulmonary embolus

- Bronchogenic carcinoma

- Bronchopulmonary aspergillosis

Figure 5-1.

Inflammatory Mechanisms in Asthma

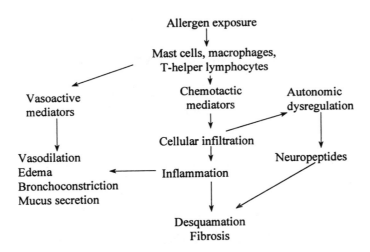

Figure 5-2.

Pathophysiology of Asthma Attack

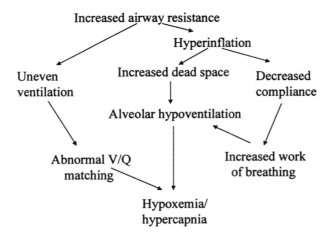

KEYS TO ASSESSMENT

- Level of consciousness, cyanosis

- Respiratory rate, heart rate, blood pressure

- Accessory muscles, lung expansion, expiratory phase, wheezing

- Peak flow—monitoring the severity of airflow obstruction contributes to management decisions; often a peak flow of <50% of predicted indicates the need for hospital admission

- Pulsus paradoxus

    - Drop in systolic blood pressure with inspiration of greater than 10 mmHg

- Oximetry—useful in mild to moderate attacks

- Arterial blood gases: indicated in severe attacks and when oxygen saturation falls to <91%

    - Calculate the A-a gradient

    - Expect respiratory alkalosis and mild hypoxemia

    - Normalization of arterial pH and carbon dioxide ($PaCO_2$) may indicate impending respiratory failure

- Chest x-ray

    - Only indicated if pneumothorax, pneumonia, or other complications are suspected

    - May appear completely normal except for hyperexpansion

    - Mucus plugging or infiltrates may be visible

- Sputum

    - Eosinophilia, infection, mucus, and mucoid casts

- Spirometry

    - Reduction in forced expiratory volume in 1 second (FEV_1) greater than 20% with acute attack or with methacholine challenge

KEYS TO MANAGEMENT

- **Prevention and nonpharmacologic management**

    - Rule out chronic sinusitis or gastroesophageal reflux disease

    - Limit allergen or irritant exposure

    - Home peak flow monitoring

    - Consider immunotherapy in the atopic patient

    - Treat infections early

    - Annual influenza vaccine

    - Patient education

- **Acute:** β-agonists remain the mainstay of therapy; steroids are crucial for treating the inflammatory process.
  - Must initiate management promptly without delaying for diagnostic tests.
  - Start oxygen; consider intubation at the first sign of hypercapnia.
  - Inhaled short-acting β-agonists: continuous nebulized vs q 20 min X 1 hour, then hourly.
  - Prednisone 60 to 80 mg orally.
  - Consider ipratropium MDI or nebulized as adjunctive therapy.
  - Aminophylline can be considered if FEV_1 <1 L/sec or if on chronic therapy and blood levels are subtherapeutic.
  - Monitor need for admission and for late asthmatic response (4 to 8 hrs).
- **Chronic:** Management is based on clinical severity (see Table 5-1).
  - In all patients, except those with mild intermittent symptoms (require use of a β-agonist inhaler less than twice per week), antiinflammatories are crucial for preventing long-term airway damage.
  - New recommendations include starting antiinflammatory therapy early, even in young children.
  - Inhaled steroids are safe and effective as first line antiinflammatory agents.
  - Cromolyn sodium and the new leukotriene receptor antagonists may be used as first line drugs for mild to moderate persistent asthma but their efficacy is not as clearly proven as with inhaled steroids.
  - β-agonists have been found to be safe and effective when used properly; new long-acting drugs (salmeterol) provide consistent control of symptoms.
  - Ipratropium may be additive but controversial in the United States.
  - "Quick relief" drugs are used in addition to the antiinflammatory and long-acting $beta_2$-agonists, and for acute exacerbations.
  - Consider theophylline if symptoms persist or the patient has nighttime attacks.
  - Use oral steroids as a last resort; leukotriene receptor antagonists may allow for decreased oral steroid dependence..
  - Peak flows tend to be lowest at 0400. For nocturnal symptoms, consider medication dosing in the evening (1600 to 1800).
  - Refer to asthma specialist for moderate to severe asthma.

Pathophysiology →

What is going on in the disease process that influences how the patient presents and how he or she should be managed?

Clinical Link

What should you do now that you understand the underlying pathophysiology?

Pathophysiology	Clinical Link
Genetic causes.	Family history, allergic history.
Allergen or irritating stimuli initiates attack.	History of exposure.
Mast cells release inflammatory mediators that cause bronchoconstriction, edema, and sputum production.	Management must include antiinflammatories as well as bronchodilators.
Eosinophils and neuropeptides cause late asthmatic response.	Recurrent symptoms after 4 to 8 hours; patient must be monitored.
A combination of inflammatory mediators, neuropeptides, and immune responses lead to epithelial desquamation and chronic inflammation.	Antiinflammatories MUST be used accurately and chronically to treat attack and to prevent long-term airway hyperresponsiveness and scarring.
V/Q mismatch and hypoxemia with hypocapnia early but increased work of breathing may lead to hypercapnia and sudden respiratory failure.	Arterial blood gases should be monitored carefully—oximetry is NOT adequate alone.

BIBLIOGRAPHY

Barnes, N. (1997). Leukotriene receptor antagonists: Clinical effects [review, 63 refs]. *Journal of the Royal Society of Medicine, 90*(4), 200-204

Barnes, P. J. (1997). Current therapies for asthma. Promise and limitations [Review, 95 refs]. *Chest, 111*(2 Suppl), 17S-26S.

Black, P. N., & Sharpe, S. (1997). Dietary fat and asthma: Is there a connection? [review, 72 refs]. *European Respiratory Journal, 10*(1), 6-12.

Bleecker, E. (1998). Inhaled corticosteroids: Current products and their role in patient care [review, 8 refs[, *Journal of Allergy and Clinical Immunology, 101*(2 Pt 2), S400-S4002.

Bloemen, P. G., Henricks, P. A., & Nijkamp, F. P. (1997). Cell adhesion molecules and asthma [review, 164 refs]. *Clinical and Experimental Allergy, 27*(2), 128-141.

Brenner, B., & Kohn, M. S. (1998). The acute asthmatic patient in the ED: To admit or discharge [review, 45 refs]. *American Journal of Emergency Medicine, 16*(1), 69-75.

British Asthma Guidelines Coordinating Committee. (1997) British guidelines on asthma management: 1995 review and position statement. *Thorax, 52*, S1-S24.

Burge, P. S. (1997). The relationship between peak expiratory flow and respiratory symptoms. *European Respiratory Journal,* (Suppl 24), 76S-68S.

Clark, D. R., & Lahren, K. M. (1997). Noninvasive positive pressure ventilation. *Southern Medical Journal, 90*(1), 72-74.

Corren, J. (1997). Allergic rhinitis and asthma: How important is the link? [review, 55 refs]. *Journal of Allergy and Clinical Immunology, 9*(2), S781-S786.

Cote, J., Cartier, A., Robichaud, P., Boutin, H., Malo, J. L., Rouleau, M., Fillion, A., Lavallee, M., Krusky, M., & Boulet, L. P. (1997). Influence on asthma morbidity of asthma education programs based on self-management plans following treatment optimization. *American Journal of Respiratory and Critical Care Medicine, 155*(5), 1509-1514.

Cross, S. (1997). Revised guidelines on asthma management [review] *Professional Nurse, 12*(6), 408-410.

Cross, S. (1997). Self-management of asthma [review, 10 refs]. *Professional Nurse, 12*(8), 561-562.

Cross, S. (1997). The management of acute asthma [review, 11 refs]. *Professional Nurse, 12*(7), 495-497.

Davies, R. J., Wang, J., Abdelaziz, M. M., Calderon, M. A., Khair, O., Devalia, J. L., & Rusznak, C. (1997). New insights into the understanding of asthma [review, 41 refs]. *Chest, 111*(2 Suppl), S2-10S.

Di Stefano, A., Lusuardi, M., Braghiroli, A., & Donner, C. F. (1997). Nocturnal asthma: Mechanisms and therapy [review, 60 refs]. *Lung, 175*(1), 53-61.

Diaz, J. E., Dubin, R., Gaeta, T. J., Pelczar, P., & Bradley, K. (1997). Efficacy of atropine sulfate in combination with albuterol in the treatment for acute asthma. *Academic Emergency Medicine, 4*(2), 107-113.

Djukanovic, R., Homeyard, S., Gratziou, C., Madden, J., Walls, A., Montefort, S., Peroni, D., Polosa, R., Holgate, S., & Howarth, P. (1997). The effect of treatment with oral corticosteroids on asthma symptoms and airway inflammation. *American Journal of Respiratory and Critical Care Medicine, 155*(3), 826-832.

Donahue, J. G., Weiss, S. T., Livingston, J. M., Goetsch, M. A., Greineder, D. K., & Platt, R. (1997). Inhaled steroids and the risk of hospitalization for asthma. *Journal of the American Medical Association, 277*(11). 887-891.

Doull, I. J., & Holgate, S. T. (1997). Asthma: Early predisposing factors [review, 42 refs]. *British Medical Bulletin, 53*(1), 71-80.

Ebell, M. (1997). Predicting need for hospitalization in adults with asthma. *Journal of Family Practice, 44*(5), 440-441.

Farber, H. J., Wattigney, W., & Berenson, G. (1997). Trends in asthma prevalence: The Bogalusa Heart Study. *Annals of Allergy, Asthma, and Immunology, 78*(3), 265-269.

Ganassini, A., & Rossi, A. (1997). Short-term regular beta 2-adrenergic agonists treatment is safe in mild asthmatics taking low doses of inhaled steroids. *Journal of Asthma, 34*(1), 61-66.

Geppert, E. F., & Collazo, S. (1998). Establishing a partnership with the patient with asthma [review, 19 refs]. *Journal of Allergy and Clinical Immunology, 101*(2 Pt 2), S405-S408.

Giangrasso, T. (1997). Potential for tolerance, morbidity, and mortality resulting from regular use of beta 2-adrenergic agonists in asthma [review, 31 refs]. *Southern Medical Journal, 90*(2), 173-179.

Harding, S. M., & Richter, J. E. (1997). The role of gastroesophageal reflux in chronic cough and asthma [review, 85 refs]. *Chest, 111*(5), 1389-1402.

Huovinen, E., Kaprio, J., Vesterinen, E., & Koskenvuo, M. (1997). Mortality of adults with asthma: A prospective cohort study. *Thorax, 52*(1), 49-54.

Jackevicius, C., Joyce, D. P., Kesten, S., & Chapman, K. R. (1997). Prehospitalization inhaled corticosteroid use in patients with COPD or asthma. *Chest, 111*(2), 296-302.

Jagoda, A., Shepherd, S. M., Spevitz, A., & Joseph, M. M. (1997). Refractory asthma, Part 1: Epidemiology, pathophysiology, pharmacologic interventions [review, 159 refs]. *Annals of Emergency Medicine, 29*(2), 262-274.

Jagoda, A., Shepherd, S. M., Spevitz, A., & Joseph, M. M. (1997). Refractory asthma, Part 2: Airway interventions and management [review, 59 refs]. *Annals of Emergency Medicine, 29*(2), 275-281.

Jain, P., & Kavuru, M. S. (1997). A practical guide for peak expiratory flow monitoring in asthma patients [review, 42 refs]. *Cleveland Clinic Journal of Medicine, 64*(4), 195-202.

Kay, A. B., Barata, L., Meng, Q., Durham, S. R., & Ying, S. (1997). Eosinophils and eosinophil-associated cytokines in allergic inflammation [review, 26 refs]. *International Archives of Allergy and Immunology, 113*(1-3), 196-199.

Keatings, V. M., O'Connor, B. J., Wright, L. G., Huston, D. P., Corrigan, C. J., & Barnes, P. J. (1997). Late response to allergen is associated with increased concentrations of tumor necrosis factor-alpha and IL-5 in induced sputum. *Journal of Allergy and Clinical Immunology, 99*(5), 693-698.

Kelly, H. W. (1997). Asthma pharmacotherapy: Current practices and outlook [review, 35 refs]. *Pharmacotherapy, 17*(1 Pt 2), 13S-21S.

Kleerup, E. C. (1997). Bronchodilators: New drugs and controversies [review, 26 refs]. *Current Opinions in Pulmonary Medicine, 3*(1), 17-22.

Klinnert, M. D., McQuaid, E. L., & Gavin, L. A. (1997). Assessing the family asthma management system. *Journal of Asthma, 34*(1), 77-88.

Koren, H. S. (1997). Environmental risk factors in atopic asthma [review, 27 refs]. *International Archives of Allergy and Immunology, 113*(1-3), 65-68.

Kraft, M., Wenzel, S. E., Bettinger, C. M., & Martin, R. J. (1997). The effect of salmeterol on nocturnal symptoms, airway function, and inflammation in asthma. *Chest, 111*(5), 1249-1254.

Leff, A. R. (1997). Future directions in asthma therapy. Is a cure possible? [review, 18 refs]. *Chest, 111*(2 Suppl), 61S-68S.

Leff, A. R. (1998). Pharmacologic management of asthma [review, 19 refs]. *Journal of Allergy and Clinical Immunology, 101*(2 Pt 2), S397-S399.

Li, J. T. (1997). Mechanisms of asthma [review, 47 refs]. *Current Opinions in Pulmonary Medicine, 3*(1), 10-16.

MacDonald, P. (1997). Asthma in older people. *Nursing Times, 93*(19), 42-43.

Madge, P., McColl, J., & Paton, J. (1997). Impact of a nurse-led home management training programme in children admitted to hospital with acute asthma: A randomised controlled study [see comments]. *Thorax, 52*(3), 223-228.

Marinkovich, V. A. (1997). Immunotherapy for asthma [letter]. *New England Journal of Medicine, 336*(26), 1912-1913.

Middleton, A. D. (1997). Managing asthma: It takes teamwork. *American Journal of Nursing, 97*(1), 39-43.

Monteleone, C. A., & Sherman, A. R. (1997). Nutrition and asthma [review, 61 refs]. *Archives of Internal Medicine, 157*(1), 23-34.

Nicklas, R. A. (1997). National and international guidelines for the diagnosis and treatment of asthma [review, 28 refs]. *Current Opinions in Pulmonary Medicine, 3*(1), 51-55.

Ober, C. (1998). Do genetics play a role in the pathogenesis of asthma? [review, 27 refs]. *Journal of Allergy and Clinical Immunology, 101*(2 Pt 2), S417-S410.

O'Byrne, P. M. (1997). Leukotrienes in the pathogenesis of asthma [review, 94 refs]. *Chest, 111*(2 Suppl), 27S-34S.

O'Byrne, P. M. (1997). Treatment of mild asthma. *Lancet, 349*(9055), 818.

Pollard, S. J., Spector, S. L., Yancey, S. W., Cox, F. M., & Emmett, A. (1997). Salmeterol versus theophylline in the treatment of asthma. *Annals of Allergy, Asthma, and Immunology, 78*(5), 457-464.

Ruffilli, A., & Bonini, S. (1997). Susceptibility genes for allergy and asthma [review, 176 refs]. *Allergy, 52*(3), 256-273.

Sears, M. R. (1997). Use of peak expiratory flow meters in adults: Practical aspects. *European Respiratory Journal,* (Suppl 24), 72S-74S.

Second Expert Panel on the Management of Asthma, National Heart, Lung and Blood Institute. (1997) Highlights of the Expert Panel Report 2: Guidelines for the Diagnosis and Management of Asthma. Bethesda (MD): National Institutes of Health; May (Publication No. NIH97-4051A).

Shi, H., Qin, S., Huang, G., Chen, Y., Xiao, C., Xu, H., Liang, G., Xie, Z., Qin, X., Wu, J., Li, G., & Zhang, C. (1997). Infiltration of eosinophils into the asthmatic airways caused by interleukin 5. *American Journal of Respiratory Cell and Molecular Biology, 16*(3), 220-224.

Singh, A. D., & Sanderson, C. J. (1997). Anti-interleukin 5 strategies as a potential treatment for asthma. *Thorax, 52*(5), 483-485.

Sly, R. M., & O'Donnell, R. (1997). Stabilization of asthma mortality [see comments] [review, 66 refs]. *Annals of Allergy, Asthma, and Immunology, 78*(4), 347-354.

Sorkness, C. A. (1997). The use of 5-lipoxygenase inhibitors and leukotriene receptor antagonists in the treatment of chronic asthma [review, 14 refs]. *Pharmacotherapy, 17*(1 Pt 2), 50S-54S.

Soutar, A., Seaton, A., & Brown, K. (1997). Bronchial reactivity and dietary antioxidants. *Thorax, 52*(2), 166-170.

Spahn, J. D., Leung, D. Y., Szefler, S. J. (1997). New insights into the pathogenesis and management of steroid-resistant asthma [review, 150 refs]. *Journal of Asthma, 34*(3), 177-194.

Suissa, S., Dennis, R., Ernst, P., Sheehy, O., & Wood-Dauphinee, S. (1997). Effectiveness of the leukotriene receptor antagonist zafirlukast for mild-to-moderate asthma. A randomized, double-blind, placebo-controlled trial. *Annals of Internal Medicine, 126*(3), 177-183.

Tashkin, D. P. (1998). New devices for asthma [review, 25 refs]. *Journal of Allergy and Clinical Immunology, 101*(2 Pt 2), S409-S416.

van der Palen, J., Klein, J. J., & Rovers, M. M. (1997). Compliance with inhaled medication and self-treatment guidelines following a self-management programme in adult asthmatics. *European Respiratory Journal, 10*(3), 652-657.

Ziment, I. (1997). Alternative therapies for asthma [review, 93 refs]. *Current Opinion in Pulmonary Medicine, 3*(1), 61-71.

CASE STUDY

ASTHMA

INITIAL HISTORY:
- 15-year-old girl
- Mowing lawn when symptoms develop
- Prodrome of rhinorrhea and tearing
- Dyspnea and chest tightness
- No better after going inside
- Now 1 hour later

Question 1.
What is your differential diagnosis based on the information you have now?

Question 2.
What other questions would you like to ask now?

ADDITIONAL HISTORY:
- History of asthma since childhood; mother and brother have asthma
- Allergic to grass, ragweed, cats
- Cough productive of clear phlegm
- Uses "blue" inhaler when needed for the past 6 months as often as twice a day
- No other medical history

Question 3.
Now what do you think about her history?

PHYSICAL EXAMINATION:
- Alert but anxious teenager; in some respiratory distress; using accessory muscle of respiration
- T = 37 orally; P = 105 beats/min and regular; RR = 30 breaths/min and labored; BP = 115/68 mmHg sitting

HEENT, Skin, Neck
- Conjunctiva inflamed and edematous, tearing; fundi without lesions; nasal mucosa edematous, clear discharge; pharynx with clear postnasal drainage
- Skin flushed and pink; diaphoretic; supple
- No adenopathy; no thyromegaly, no bruits

Lungs
- Chest expansion somewhat limited; diaphragms percuss low in posterior chest with 2 cm movement; prolonged expiratory phase; expiratory wheezes, scattered coarse rhonchi, no rales, or egophony

Cardiac
- Heart sounds distant; tachycardia but regular; slight systolic ejection murmur (SEM) LLSB without radiation; no gallops or clicks

Abdomen, Extremities, Neurological
- Abdomen nondistended; bowel sounds present and not hyperactive; liver percusses 2 cm below RCM but overall size 8 cm; no tenderness or masses
- Extremities clammy but good capillary refill at 3 seconds; no edema; no clubbing
- Alert, oriented but anxious; cranial nerves intact; strength 5/5 throughout; DTR 2+ and symmetrical; sensory intact to touch

Question 4.
What studies would you initiate now while preparing your interventions?

Question 5.
What therapies would you initiate immediately while awaiting results of the lab studies?

LABORATORY RESULTS:
- pH = 7.55, PaO_2 = 65, $PaCO_2$ = 30 (RA); peak flow = 200 (<50% of predicted); electrolytes normal
- HCT = 37%, WBC = 5500, PLTS = 340,000
- ECG = sinus tachycardia

Question 6.
What is her A-a gradient?

EMERGENCY ROOM COURSE:
- Patient becomes increasingly dyspneic despite nebulizer and O_2.
- Becoming more anxious and confused.

PHYSICAL EXAM NOW:
- P = 110 and regular; RR = 40 and labored; BP = 130/90
- Lungs with inspiratory and expiratory wheezes; early cyanosis
- Extremities cold and clammy; no longer alert or oriented

REPEAT LAB STUDIES:
- pH = 7.35, PaO_2 = 45, $PaCO_2$ = 42 (40% mask); peak flow = cannot cooperate
- Heart monitor = sinus tachycardia

Question 7.
What do you think is happening? Why is she more dyspneic? What does her lung exam suggest? Why are her extremities cold? Why is her color pink? Why is she confused? What do her blood gases mean?

Question 8.
What interventions should be initiated now?

RESPONSE TO THERAPY:
- Gradual return of respiratory rate to 35, pulse to 100; color improves; more alert
- Lungs with expiratory wheezes only; peak flow = 180
- pH = 7.48, PaO_2 = 90, $PaCO_2$ = 32 (60% mask)

Question 9.
Now what should be done and what can the patient expect?

HOSPITAL COURSE:
- Patient does well with normalization of labs.
- Tired but breathing normally after 3 days; discharged on 4th day.

Question 10.
What instructions and medications should this patient go home with?

Question 11.
What steps can she take to prevent future attacks?

CHAPTER 6

CHRONIC OBSTRUCTIVE PULMONARY DISEASE

DEFINITION

- Chronic obstructive pulmonary disease (COPD) is a syndrome characterized by abnormal tests of expiratory airflow that do not change markedly over periods of several months of observation.

- Pathologic lung changes are consistent with emphysema or chronic bronchitis.

- Airflow limitation is worse during expiration and does not show major reversibility in response to pharmacological agents.

- Results from Inflammation and structural damage to alveoli and airways.

- COPD may also include chronic asthmatic bronchitis which has a reversible component to the airflow limitation but progresses and becomes less reversible.

EPIDEMIOLOGY

- Fourth leading cause of death in the United States

- 100,000 deaths in the United States in 1996

- Smoking accounts for >90% of the risk for COPD.

- Other known risk factors include passive smoking and occupational exposures.

- Other putative risk factors include socioeconomic status, airway hyperresponsiveness, family history, and past respiratory illness.

- Genetic enzyme deficiencies (alpha$_1$-antitrypsin, and chymotrypsin) account for only a very small percentage of cases.

PATHOPHYSIOLOGY

- Many patients with COPD have characteristics of both emphysema and chronic bronchitis, with one or the other pathophysiologic processes predominating.

- **Emphysema:** reduced elastic recoil resulting in expiratory airway collapse and hyperinflation; disintegration of alveolar walls and bulla formation.

- In the lung, there is a normal balance between enzymes that promote lung remodeling (elastases) and those that inhibit lung remodeling (antielastases such as alpha$_1$-antitrypsin). Smoking and other putative environmental factors inhibit the activity of the antielastases thus shifting the balance to elastic fiber damage with loss of normal airway elasticity and destruction of alveolar walls.

- Airway collapse during expiration with airtrapping leads to hyperexpansion of the lung and chest wall, putting the muscles of respiration at a mechanical disadvantage and increasing the work of breathing—decreased ventilation with hypercapnia.

- Loss of alveolar surface area and abnormalities of the alveolar capillary barrier leading to decreased gas exchange—hypoxemia.

- **Chronic bronchitis:** chronic cough productive of phlegm for at least 3 months per year for at least 2 consecutive years

  - Increase in goblet cells in the airway mucosa with hypertrophy and hyperplasia of submucosal glands and production of copious amounts of tenacious sputum—organisms can adhere and grow with persistent bacterial colonization of the airways and cause recurrent infectious exacerbations.

  - Associated epithelial inflammation and smooth muscle hypertrophy lead to scarring.

- **Both emphysema and chronic bronchitis:**

  - Chronic hypercapnia can lead to decreased sensitivity of the respiratory center to changes in PaCO$_2$, making the patient dependent on chemoreception of low PaO$_2$ as the main stimulus to breathing. Supplemental oxygen may eliminate this stimulus resulting in decreased ventilatory response and additional carbon dioxide retention.

  - Diffuse pulmonary hypoxemia and hypercapnia results in widespread pulmonary arteriolar vasoconstriction and increased pulmonary artery pressures. The right ventricle responds poorly to this increased workload and may dilate and fail with increased pressures being transmitted to the systemic venous circulation and resultant peripheral edema (*cor pulmonale*).

PATIENT PRESENTATION

- Although there may be considerable overlap in the clinical presentations of emphysema and chronic bronchitis, it is useful to categorize the clinical manifestations by predominant disease process.

- History:

  - **Emphysema:** active or passive smoking history; occupational history; history of episodes of cough and dyspnea; progressive exercise limitation; possible family history especially if in nonsmoker.

  - **Chronic bronchitis:** history of smoking, recurrent pulmonary infections with copious sputum production of most days for at least 3 months per year for at least 2 years.

- Symptoms:

  - **Emphysema:** progressive dyspnea on exertion; paroxysmal nocturnal dyspnea; pedal edema; weight loss.

  - **Chronic bronchitis:** productive cough with episodes of increased dyspnea with production of discolored sputum; pedal edema.

- Examination:

  - **Emphysema:** decreased level of consciousness and cyanosis during severe exacerbations; increased anterior-posterior chest diameter (barrel chest); use of accessory muscles of breathing: low diaphragms on percussion; decreased breath sounds; prolonged expiratory phase of breathing; expiratory wheezing; clubbing and pedal edema (advanced disease).

  - **Chronic bronchitis:** examination may be relatively normal between acute exacerbations or have low grade scattered expiratory wheezing; acute exacerbations characterized by tachypnea, decreased level of consciousness, fever, increased wheezing, cyanosis, and pedal edema.

DIFFERENTIAL DIAGNOSIS

- Asthma

- Bronchiectasis

- Congestive heart failure

- Acute bronchitis

- Recurrent pulmonary emboli

- Pneumonia

KEYS TO ASSESSMENT

- Acuteness of onset of symptoms and deviation from "baseline"

- New pedal edema may indicate worsening hypoxemia/hypercapnia and cor pulmonale.

- Arterial blood gases (ABG): useful for evaluating the severity of pulmonary dysfunction in both the stable COPD patient (establish baseline values) and during acute exacerbations

  - Look for both hypercapnia and hypoxemia (oximetry is inadequate for these patients in that it does not indicate the $PaCO_2$).

  - Acidosis is a clear indicator of acute hypercapnia.

  - Severe hypoxemia should not be tolerated even in the patient with long-standing advanced COPD; institution of oxygen therapy requires close monitoring of ABG for increasing hypercapnia, and ventilation may be required.

- Chest x-ray: often normal until late-stage disease but is useful for documenting infection

  - Expect flattened diaphragms, increased retrosternal space, enlarged pulmonary arteries, bullae, and scarring in emphysema.

  - Look closely for pneumothorax or acute infiltrates.

- Sputum stain and culture: useful for the diagnosis of chronic bronchitis and for evaluating acute exacerbations of COPD

  - Look for polymorphonucleocytes and bacteria on Gram stain.

  - Most common organisms include *H. influenzae, M. catarrhalis*, and *S. pneumoniae*; in patients with advanced disease, consider *P. aeruginosa*.

- Spirometry

  - Forced expiratory volume in 1 second (FEV_1) is decreased; forced vital capacity (FVC) is also decreased but to a lesser degree such that the FEV_1/FVC ratio is decreased.

  - Total lung capacity (TLC) is normal or increased and residual volume (RV) is increased in emphysema, much less so in chronic bronchitis.

KEYS TO MANAGEMENT

- **Smoking cessation:** many modalities available including hypnosis, nicotine replacements (nasal, oral, dermal), support groups

  - Causes some prompt improvement in pulmonary function.

  - Slows the rate of lung function decline over years.

  - Reduces number of infectious complications and exacerbations.

  - May be associated with an increase in cough and anxiety during first few weeks.

  - Frequent follow-up contacts between the provider and the patient improves the chances for long-term smoking cessation.

- **Oxygen therapy:** in an acute exacerbation with severe hypoxemia, oxygen is vital to sustain life; in patients with sustained hypoxemia and cor pulmonale, home oxygen therapy improves exercise tolerance and survival

  - Supplemental oxygen may depress minute volume (respiratory rate x tidal volume); patient must be monitored for CO_2 retention and ventilated if hypercapnic acidosis develops.

  - Home oxygen therapy should be administered for as many hours a day as the patient will consent to using it, especially at night.

  - Many delivery systems and administration devices are available for maximizing compliance, portability, and overall quality of life.

- **Pharmacotherapy:** COPD will often have some small but potentially symptomatic element of bronchospasm that can be treated with bronchodilators; however, benefits are small, there is little evidence that drugs alter the progression of COPD, and they are often associated with significant side effects

  - **Ipratropium:** Recently recommended to be the first line drug for stable COPD (instead of beta$_2$-agonists due to its more prolonged effectiveness with few side effects); it should be used regularly (2 to 6 inhalations 4 to 6 times per day) rather than prn. Recent studies suggest that it may slow the progression of disease in some patients.

  - **Beta$_2$-agonists:** Now considered second-line drugs that can be used on a prn basis to supplement ipratropium; there is no evidence that continual use is better and the patient must be instructed not to exceed 12 inhalations per day of a short-acting (e.g., albuterol) or twice daily for the long-acting (salmeterol); still the drugs of choice for acute exacerbations due to their rapid onset.

  - **Theophylline:** Controversial benefit:risk ratio; useful at night for sustained relief during sleep; serum levels and potential drug interactions should be monitored carefully if used as continuous therapy.

- **Steroids**: Unlike in asthma, antiinflammatory drugs are not necessary for airway protection in COPD, and only about 20% of patients will improve with steroids; thus a therapeutic trial should be conducted only in severe COPD and the drug discontinued if there is no measurable improvement in FEV_1 in 2 weeks.

- **Antibiotics**: Most studies show no benefit of antibiotics for acute exacerbations unless there is evidence of infection (fever, leukocytosis, purulent sputum, new infiltrate on x-ray); however, recent articles suggest they should be used in all acute exacerbations—more trials pending; empiric choices include amoxicillin (20% of *H. influenza* is resistant to amoxicillin), amoxicillin-clavulanate, a macrolide, tetracycline, trimethoprim-sulfamethoxazole, or ciprofloxacin.

- **Aerosolized surfactant**: Recently studied and found to improve pulmonary function tests and sputum transport by cilia in patients with stable chronic bronchitis.

• **Surgery:** unilateral and bilateral volume reduction improve pulmonary function and symptoms, selection criteria and techniques are still being evaluated. Single or bilateral lung transplantation can be considered in selected patients.

• **Pulmonary rehabilitation:** upper and lower extremity exercise, breathing exercises, nutrition, education, and psychological support have all been shown to improve symptoms

Pathophysiology $\rightarrow$

What is going on in the disease process that influences how the patient presents and how he or she should be managed?

Clinical Link

What should you do now that you understand the underlying pathophysiology?

Pathophysiology	Clinical Link
Cigarette smoke results in irreversible direct damage to bronchial walls as well as indirect damage due to inhibition of protective antielastases in the lung.	Smoking cessation is vital to slow disease progression but will not normalize lung function.
A small minority of patients have a genetic deficiency of the antielastase α_1-antitrypsin as the cause of early-onset emphysema.	A careful examination of family history and genetic testing is indicated in patients with early onset COPD symptoms, especially if there is a minimal smoking history.
Damage to bronchial mucosa and the elastin in bronchial walls results in expiratory airway obstruction due to either loss of airway elasticity, increased mucous production, or both.	Patients with both emphysema and chronic bronchitis present with dyspnea, prolonged expiration and wheezing.
Expiratory obstruction with airtrapping, increased work of breathing, and uneven ventilation result in decreased minute volume and ventilation/perfusion mismatching, especially during late stage disease and acute exacerbations.	Mixed hypercapnia and hypoxemia are common in COPD. Evaluation of arterial blood gases helps determine the severity of disease at "baseline" and contributes to appropriate management decisions during acute exacerbations.
Chronic hypercapnia results in reliance on hypoxic ventilatory drive to maintain adequate ventilation.	Oxygen therapy is vital, but patients must be monitored for decreased minute volume and hypercapnia—some may need mechanical ventilation.
Bronchoconstriction and inflammation are minor components of the disease process in COPD.	Pharmacotherapy is less effective and must be balanced against the risk of side effects.

BIBLIOGRAPHY

American Thoracic Society. (1995). Standards for the care of patients with chronic obstructive pulmonary disease. *American Journal of Respiratory Critical Care, 152*, S78.

Anzueto, A, Jubran, A., Ohar, J., Piquette, C., Renard, S., Colice, G., Pattishall, E., Barrett, J., Engle, M., Perret, K., Rubin, B. (1997) Effects of aerosolized surfactant in patients with stable chronic bronchitis. *Journal of the American Medical Association, 278* (17), 1426-1431.

Ball, P., & Make, B. (1998). Acute exacerbations of chronic bronchitis: An international comparison. *Chest, 113*(3 Suppl), 199S-204S.

Bellone, A., Frisinghelli, A., Pozzi, G., Lapidari, G., & Carnovali, M. (1996). Exercise-induced hypoxaemia in emphysematous type chronic obstructive pulmonary disease. *Monaldi Archives for Chest Disease, 52*(2), 117-119.

Brenner, M., Yusen, R., McKenna, R., Jr., Sciurba, F., Gelb, A. F., Fischel, R., Swain, J., Chen, J. C., Kafie, F., & Lefrak, S. S. (1996). Lung volume reduction surgery for emphysema [review]. *Chest, 110*(1), 205-218.

Celli, B. R. (1996). Current thoughts regarding treatment of chronic obstructive pulmonary disease [review]. *Medical Clinics of North America, 80*(3), 589-609.

Cotton, D. J., Soparkar, G. R., & Grahan, B. L. (1996). Diffusing capacity in the clinical assessment of chronic airflow limitation [review]. *Medical Clinics of North America, 80*(3), 549-564.

Daniel, T. M., Chan, B. B., Bhaskar, V., Parekh, J. S., Walters, P. E., Reeder, J., & Truwit, J. D. (1996). Lung volume reduction surgery. Case selection, operative technique, and clinical results. *Annals of Surgery, 223*(5), 526-531, discussion 532-533.

De Troyer, A. (1997). Effect of hyperinflation on the diaphragm [review, 56 refs]. *European Respiratory Journal, 10*(3), 708-713.

Eda, S., Kubo, K., Fujimoto, K., Matsuzawa, Y., Sekiguchi, M., & Sakai, F. (1997). The relations between expiratory chest CT using helical CT and pulmonary function tests in emphysema. *American Journal of Respiratory and Critical Care Medicine, 155*(4), 1290-1294.

Gelb, A. F., Hogg, J. C., Muller, N. L., Schein, M. J., Kuei, J., Tashkin, D. P., Epstein, J. D., Kollin, J., Green, R. H., Zamel, N., Elliott, W. M., Y Hadjiaghai, L. (1996). Contribution of emphysema and small airways in COPD. *Chest, 109*(2), 353-359.

Grossman, R. F. (1997). Acute exacerbations of chronic bronchitis. *Hospital Practice (Office Edition), 32*, 85-89.

Grossman, R. F. (1997). Guidelines for the treatment of acute exacerbations of chronic bronchitis [review, 29 refs]. *Chest, 112*(6 Suppl), 310S-313S.

Grossman, R. F. (1998). How do we achieve cost-effective options in lower respiratory tract infection therapy? *Chest, 113*(3 Suppl), 205S-210S.

Hanson, M. J. (1997). Caring for the patient with COPD: How to help himn breathe easier once the damage is done [review, 4 refs]. *Nursing, 27*(12), 39-44, quiz 46.

Haraguchi, M., Shimura, S., & Shirato, K. (1996). Morphologic aspects of airways of patients with pulmonary emphysema followed by bronchial asthma-like attack. *American Journal of Respiratory and Critical Care Medicine, 153*(2), 638-643.

Hjalmarson, A., Nilsson,F., Sjostrom, L., & Wiklund, O. (1997) The nicotine inhaler in smoking cessation. *Archives of Internal Medicine 157*, 1721-1728.

Huang, S. L., Su, C. H., & Chang, S. C. (1997). Tumor necrosis factor-alpha gene polymorphism in chronic bronchitis. *American Journal of Respiratory and Critical Care Medicine, 156*(5), 1436-1439.

Keller, C. A., Naunheim, K. S., Osterloh, J., Espiritu, J., McDonald, J. W., & Ramos, R. R. (1997). Histopathologic diagnosis made in lung tissue resected from patients with severe emphysema undergoing lung volume reduction surgery. *Chest, 111*(4), 941-947.

Knight, K. R., Burdon, J., G., Cook, L., Brenton, S., Ayad, M., & Janus, E. D. (1997). The proteinase-antiproteinase theory of emphysema: A speculative analysis of recent advances into the pathogenesis of emphysema [review, 37 refs]. *Respirology, 2*(2), 91-95.

Koyama, H., Nishimura, K., Ikeda, A., Sakai, N., Mishima, M., & Izumi, T. (1996). Influence of baseline airway calibre and pulmonary emphysema on bronchial responsiveness in patients with chronic obstructive pulmonary disease. *Respiratory Medicine, 90*(6), 323-328.

Lefrak, S. S., Yusen, R. D., Trulock, E. P., Pohl, M. S., Patterson, A., & Cooper, J. D. (1997). Recent advances in surgery for emphysema [review, 34 refs]. *Annual Review of Medicine, 48*, 387-398.

Menard-Rothe, K., Sobush, D. C., Bousamra, M., 2nd, Haasler, G. B., & Lipchik, R. J. (1997). Self-selected walking velocity for functional ambulation in patients with end-stage emphysema. *Journal of Cardiopulmonary Rehabilitation, 17*(2), 85-91.

Moody, L. E., Lowry, L., Yarandi, H., & Voss, A. (1997). Psychophysiologic predictors of weaning from mechanical ventilation in chronic bronchitis and emphysema. *Clinical Nursing Research, 6*(4), 311-330, discussion 330-333.

Niven, R. M., Fletcher, A. M., Pickering, C. A., Fishwick, D., Warburton, C. J., Simpson, J. C., Francis, H., & Oldham. L. A. (1997). Chronic bronchitis in textile workers. *Thorax, 52*(1), 22-27.

O'Donnell, D. E., Webb, K. A., Bertley, J. C., Chau, L. K., & Conlan, A. A. (1996). Mechanisms of relief of exertional breathlessness following unilateral bullectomy and lung volume reduction surgery in emphysema. *Chest, 110*(1), 18-27.

Odonohue, W. J. (1996). Home oxygen therapy. *Medical Clinics of North America, 80*(3), 611ff.

Petty, T. L. (1996). Lung cancer and chronic obstructive pulmonary disease. *Medical Clinics of North America, 80*(3), 645ff.

Rogers, R. M., Sciurba, F. C., & Keenan, R. J. (1996). Lung reduction surgery in chronic obstructive lung disease [review]. *Medical Clinics of North America, 80*(3), 623-644.

Schwaiblmair, M., Vogelmeier, C., & Fruhmann, G. (1997). Long-term augmentation therapy in twenty patients with severe alpha-1-antitrypsin deficiency—Three-year follow-up. *Respiration, 64*(1), 10-16.

Sherrill, D. L., Enright, P., Cline, M., Burrows, B., & Lebowitz, M. D. (1996). Rates of decline in lung function among subjects who restart cigarette smoking. *Chest, 111*(4), 1144-1145.

Teramoto, S., Matsuse, T., & Ouchi, Y. (1997). Is the symptomatic improvement after lung volume reduction surgery correlated with FEV1 in patients with diffuse emphysema? [letter]. *Chest, 111*(4), 1144-1145.

Venuta, F., Rendina, E. A., Pescarmona, E. O., De Giacomo, T., Vizza, D., Flaishman, I., & Ricci, C. (1997). Occult lung cancer in patients with bullous emphysema. *Thorax, 52*(3), 289-290.

Voelker, R. (1997). Lung volume reduction surgery puts a new twist on an old technique [news]. *Journal of the American Medical Association, 277*(23), 1830-1831.

Wilcke, J. T., & Dirksen, A. (1997). The effect of inhaled glucocorticosteroids in emphysema due to alpha 1-antitrypsin deficiency. *Respiratory Medicine, 91*(5), 275-279.

Ziering, W., & McElvaine, P. (1998). Randomized comparison of once-daily ceftibuten and twice-daily clarithromycin in the treatment of acute exacerbation of chronic bronchitis. *Infection, 26*(1), 68-75.

Zulueta, J. J., Bloom, S. M., Rozansky, M. I., & White, A. C. (1996). Lung cancer in patients with bullous disease [review]. *American Journal of Respiratory and Critical Care Medicine, 154*(2 Pt 1), 519-522.

CASE STUDY

CHRONIC OBSTRUCTIVE PULMONARY DISEASE

INITIAL HISTORY:
- 58-year-old female presents to the clinic complaining of shortness of breath that has increased slowly for years.
- Worse in recent months; last 2 days much worse with productive cough
- New: ankle swelling

Question 1.
What other questions would you like to ask?

ADDITIONAL HISTORY:
- 60-pack-year smoking history; quit 5 years ago
- Sputum is yellow in color; no blood
- No fever, chills, or chest pain
- Usually brings up only scant white sputum in the A.M.
- No weight loss
- No history of heart disease

Question 2.
What would you like to ask about the past medical history?

PAST MEDICAL HISTORY:
- Has been fairly healthy in the past
- No TB or asbestos exposure; no occupational exposures
- No allergies
- Occasional bronchitis treated as an outpatient with antibiotics
- No history of asthma
- Family history positive for heart disease (brother in 50s)

Question 3.
What is the differential diagnosis at this time?

PHYSICAL EXAMINATION:
- Alert, mild dyspnea with climbing on the exam table
- Afebrile
- P = 95; RR = 28; BP = 135/85, no orthostatic changes
- No cyanosis
- No rashes

HEENT, Neck
- PERRL, fundi without hemorrhages or exudates
- Yellowed teeth
- Nares clear; pharynx clear
- Pursed lip breathing
- Mild jugular venous distension
- Shotty anterior cervical adenopathy

Lungs
- Using accessory muscles at rest
- Barrel chest; decreased diaphragmatic excursion bilaterally
- Percussion hyperresonant; decreased breath sounds throughout
- Prolonged expiration with expiratory wheezes with rhonchi in all lung fields
- No supraclavicular adenopathy

Cardiac
- Regular rate rhythm with occasional premature beat; mild precordial heave
- Normal S_1, loud S_2, no S_3 or S_4

Abdomen, Extremities
- Liver palpable, span 12 cm at the right midclavicular line
- Spleen palpable
- No masses or tenderness
- No cyanosis or clubbing
- 2+ bilateral pitting pedal edema

Neurologic
- Alert, oriented
- Cranial nerves intact
- Strength, sensation, deep tendon reflexes intact and symmetrical
- Gait steady

Question 4.
What are the important positive and negative findings on exam and what might they mean?

Question 5.
What laboratory tests would you order at this time?

LABORATORY:
- SMA 7 normal except bicarbonate = 38
- HCT = 49%; WBC = 9,000, NL DIFF; LFTS = normal; calcium normal
- Sputum = occasional epithelial cell, scattered epithelial cells; PMNs and GM+ diplococci seen

Question 6.
What do these laboratory results tell you?

ARTERIAL BLOOD GAS RESULTS:
- pH = 7.38; $PaCO_2$ = 56; PaO_2 = 54 on room air

Question 7.
What is the A-a gradient?

SPIROMETRY RESULTS:

- Forced expiratory volume in 1 second (FEV_1) = 1.67 L/sec (45% of predicted)
- Forced vital capacity (FVC) = 4.10 L (85% of predicted)
- FEV_1/FVC = 37 (predicted = 72)

Question 8.

What do these spirometry results indicate?

CHEST X-RAY AND READING:

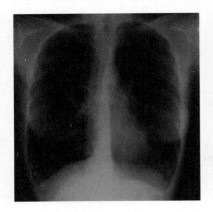 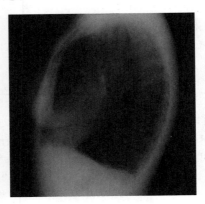

- Hyperinflation with flattened diaphragms
- Increased anterio-posterior diameter and retrosternal space
- Diffuse scarring and bullae especially in the lower lobes
- No acute infiltrates

Question 9.

What is the pathophysiology behind these chest x-ray findings?

Question 10.

What are the key elements of management for this patient?

CHAPTER 7

PNEUMONIA

DEFINITION

- Although the term "pneumonia" can be used to describe a large number of diseases that cause pulmonary parenchymal consolidation, it is most commonly used to refer to infections of the lower respiratory tract.

- Infectious causes may be viral, bacterial, fungal, protozoal, or parasitic.

- May be community-acquired (CAP), nursing home acquired (NHAP), or nosocomial.

EPIDEMIOLOGY

- Advanced age, immunocompromise, reduced forced expiratory volume in 1 second (FEV_1) and high alcohol intake are the greatest risk factors in the general population

- Other risk factors include altered consciousness, smoking, underlying lung disease, endotracheal intubation, malnutrition, airway obstruction, and immobilization.

- Overall incidence of CAP is 3% per year in people >65 years old; mortality ranges from 5% to >30% depending on the etiologic organism. The most common bacterial infections include *S. pneumoniae, H. influenza, M. pneumoniae, C. pneumoniae, L. pneumophila,* and *M. catarrhalis*; influenza is a common viral CAP.

- NHAP has a 13% mortality rate.

- Nosocomial pneumonia the second most common nosocomial infection but has the greatest mortality (60% of deaths attributed to nosocomial infection); it is the most common infection in intensive care units (ICUs), especially in mechanically ventilated patients (42.5% mortality in ICUs).

PATHOPHYSIOLOGY

- Aspiration of oropharyngeal secretions is the most common route of infection. Other routes of inoculation include inhalation, hematogenous spread from remote sites of infection, and direct extension from contiguous sites of infection.

- The upper airway is the first line of defense against infection; however, the clearance of organisms by saliva, mucociliary expulsion, and secretory IgA can be inhibited by many diseases, immunocompromise, smoking, and endotracheal intubation.

- The lower airway defenses include cough, gag reflex, mucociliary expulsion, surfactant, macrophage and polymorphonucleocyte (PMN) phagocytosis, and cellular and humoral immunity. These defenses are inhibited by altered consciousness, smoking, abnormal mucous production (e.g., cystic fibrosis or chronic bronchitis), immunocompromise, intubation and prolonged bedrest.

- The alveolar macrophage is the primary defender against invasion of the lower respiratory tract and it daily clears the airways of aspirated organisms without initiating significant inflammation.

- If the number or virulence of the organisms is too great, the macrophage will recruit PMNs and initiate the inflammatory cascade with release of numerous cytokines including leukotrienes, tumor necrosis factor (TNF), interleukins, oxygen radicals, and proteases.

- This inflammation leads to alveolar filling with ventilation/perfusion mismatching and hypoxemia.

- The infection and inflammation may remain localized to the lung or may cause bacteremia resulting in meningitis or endocarditis, the systemic inflammatory response syndrome (SIRS), and/or sepsis

PATIENT PRESENTATION

- Characteristic presentations and their severity vary with the etiologic organism (Table 7-1) as well as the underlying health of the patient.

- History:

  Age; altered consciousness; immunocompromise; smoking; underlying lung disease; prolonged bedrest; recent hospitalization; intubation.

- Symptoms:

  Upper respiratory prodrome (headache, rhinitis, postnasal drainage); cough; sputum production with discoloration; dyspnea; pleuritic chest pain; hemoptysis; fever; rigors; myalgias.

- Examination:

  Fever; tachypnea; tachycardia; decreased level of consciousness; cyanosis; use of accessory muscles of respiration; splinting; dullness to percussion; inspiratory crackles (rales); egophony; whispered pectoriloquy; increased tactile fremitus; pleural friction rub; tenacious and/or discolored sputum.

DIFFERENTIAL DIAGNOSIS

- Acute or chronic bronchitis

- Upper respiratory infection

- Influenza

- Noninfectious pneumonitis

- Pulmonary embolus

- Asthma

- Congestive heart failure

KEYS TO ASSESSMENT

- Look for source of infection, aspiration.

- Assess for septic shock (hypotension, poor tissue perfusion).

- Arterial blood gases
    - Indicated if the patient is in respiratory distress or has significant underlying lung disease.
    - Expect hypoxemia with respiratory alkalosis in patient without underlying lung disease.
- White blood cell (WBC) count with differential
- Electrolytes and liver function tests may be useful in patients with an atypical presentation or severe symptoms (e.g., patients with *legionella pneumophila*).
- Sputum
    - Gram stain is indicated in all patients: numerous PMNs consistent with bacterial infection (numerous epithelial cells indicate oral contamination of the specimen); organisms may be preliminarily identified by staining characteristics and shape.
    - Sputum culture is indicated in patients who are hospitalized or have been recently discharged, or who present with severe or unusual symptoms.
- Chest x-ray
    - Currently recommended in all patients with a history and physical exam suggestive of pneumonia.
    - Expect lobar or patchy infiltrates; air bronchograms.
- Blood cultures are indicated in hospitalized patients.

KEYS TO MANAGEMENT

- Oxygen and hydration if indicated
- Deep breathing and cough, chest physical therapy (PT) if available
- Antibiotics—for bacterial, parasitic, or fungal pneumonia (not viral)
    - Sputum gram stain may guide therapy but most often empiric coverage is used in outpatients; with inpatients, therapy may need to be altered when cultures with sensitivities become available (48 to 72 hours).
    - Choice of antibiotic varies based on community vs nursing home vs nosocomial acquisition, patient risk factors, and patient presentation.
    - Common empiric antibiotic choices are listed in Table 7-2.
    - Patient presentation and antibiotic choices for selected specific organisms are listed in Table 7-1.
- Hospital admission indicated if:
    - Age over 65, homeless, hospitalized for pneumonia in the past year.
    - Pulse >140/minute, respiratory rate >30/minute, hypotension.
    - Temperature >38.3°C.
    - Altered mental status, cyanosis.
    - Immunosuppression, comorbid condition.
    - High-risk organism (e.g., recent nosocomial pseudomonas infection).

- WBC <4000 or >30,000/μL.

- Partial pressure of oxygen in arterial blood (PaO_2) <60 or $PaCO_2$ >50.

- Chest x-ray with multiple lobes involved or rapid progression.

Table 7-1.
Selected Common Etiologic Organisms:
Important Aspects of Patient Presentation and Suggested Antibiotic Choices

---

COMMUNITY ACQUIRED:

Streptococcus pneumoniae—most common cause of bacterial CAP; patients present with cough productive of "rusty sputum" and dense lobar consolidation; may spread to meninges and endocardium; Rx: penicillin, amoxicillin, erythromycin, doxycycline, cephalosporins.

Haemophilus influenzae—common in children, COPD patients, and alcoholics; patients present with subacute cough and fever progressing to dyspnea and purulent sputum; patchy infiltrates; 30% mortality; Rx: ampicillin + clavulanate, second or third generation cephalosporin, clarithromycin, or trimethoprim-sulfamethoxazole.

Moraxella catarrhalis—common in COPD patients and alcoholics; patients present with fever, pleuritic chest pain, and hemoptysis; lobar pneumonia; Rx: ampicillin + clavulanate, trimethoprim-sulfamethoxazole, or erythromycin.

Anaerobic—aspirated from upper respiratory tract especially in patients with poor dentition; sputum often putrid with lung cavitation and hemoptysis; Rx: clindamycin.

Mycoplasma pneumoniae—common in teenagers and young adults in schools and barracks; patients present with fever, a slow heart rate relative to the degree a pyrexia, pharyngitis, headache and dry cough; Rx: erythromycin, doxycycline, clarithromycin, azithromycin.

Chlamydia pneumoniae—same presentation and Rx as mycoplasma.

Influenza—three major types A, B, and C; occurs in epidemics in winter with sudden onset of prodrome with fever, myalgia, headache, pharyngitis, and dry cough progressing to dyspnea, hypoxia, and significant mortality; may become superinfected with strep or staph; Rx: amantadine if treated in the first 2 days of symptoms; vaccine.

Mycobacterium tuberculosis—immigrants, homeless, alcoholics, immunosuppressed patients; primary infection may be asymptomatic or produce pneumonia and pleurisy; reactivation causes pneumonia with lung cavitation especially of the upper lobes often in the absence of fever; purified protein derivative-negative (PPD-negative) (tuberculin) in up to 25% of patients; sputum cultures sensitive but may take weeks; extrapulmonary disease is common including lymphatic, genitourinary, vertebral, and meningeal; drug resistance is increasingly common, often requires multi-drug regimen (e.g., isoniazid, rifampin, pyrazinamide, ethambutol and/or streptomycin); isolation of patient and prophylaxis of contacts; screening with PPD in at risk populations, Bacillus Calmette-Gúerin (BCG) vaccination in endemic populations.

NURSING HOME ACQUIRED:

Streptococcus, haemophilus, and pseudomonas—common (see above and below).

Klebsiella pneumoniae—diabetics and alcoholics; present with sudden prostration and hemoptysis; significant mortality; requires hospitalization; Rx: third generation cephalosporins, ticarcillin + clavulanate, ciprofloxacin.

Table 7-1 continued:

NOSOCOMIAL:

Pseudomonas aeruginosa—ICU, immunocompromised; patients present with copious purulent sputum, rigors, fever; complicated by abscesses and empyema; 36% to 80% mortality; Rx: aminoglycoside plus imipenem or aztreonam, piperacillin mezlocillin, ceftazidime, ciprofloxacin.

Staphylococcus aureus—may present as superinfection of initial viral pneumonia; fever, dyspnea, chest pain; empyema, cavitation and abscess common; Rx: nafcillin resistance increasingly common, therefore use vancomycin alone or with rifampin .

Enterobacteriaceae—class of organisms including *klebsiella*; patients present with abrupt fever, dyspnea, cough; bibasilar consolidation; mortality 25% to 50%; Rx: aztreonam, floroquinone, aminoglycoside plus cephalosporin, vancomycin.

Acinetobacter—late summer; dry cough, fever; bilateral lower lobe pneumonia; mortality 65%; imipenem plus aminoglycoside.

Table 7-2.
Suggested Empiric Outpatient Antibiotic Therapy for Community and
Nursing Home Acquired Pneumonia (Etiologic Agent Not Identified on Gram Stain)

COMMUNITY ACQUIRED:

Young adult patient (<60 years of age) with typical presentation and no serious underlying disease: erythromycin (clarithromycin or azithromycin in those intolerant of erthromcyin and in smokers) or tetracycline (doxycycline).

Older patient or one with preexisting respiratory disease: second generation cephalopsporin, or sulfamethoxazole - trimethoprim or ampicillin + clavulanate or erythromycin or other macrolide.

NURSING HOME ACQUIRED:

Ampicillin + clavulanate, ciprofloxacin, or ceftriaxone.

Pathophysiology → ## Clinical Link

What is going on in the disease process that influences how the patient presents and how he or she should be managed?

What should you do now that you understand the underlying pathophysiology?

Factors such as smoking, immunocompromise, and recent hospitalization impact the severity of illness, which causative organism is most likely and the potential for antibiotic resistance.	History of risk factors, underlying health of the patient, and where the infection was acquired are keys to assessment and management.
Aspiration of oroparyngeal secretions is the most common route of inoculation of the lower respiratory tract.	Identify patients at risk with compromised protection of the upper airway such as decreased level of consciousness or tracheal intubation.
Infection can spread via the blood to other organs and can lead to widespread inflammation.	Watch for meningitis, endocarditis, or the onset of sepsis, and systemic inflammatory response syndrome (SIRS).
The etiologic organism determines the patient presentation, clinical course, and management, but can be difficult to identify in an outpatient setting.	Sputum stains should be done in all patients with suspected pneumonia, and sputum and blood cultures should be done in hospitalized patients; empiric antibiotic therapy is often necessary.
Inflammation with alveolar filling leads to ventilation/perfusion mismatching and resultant hypoxemia.	Patients with significant respiratory distress or underlying lung disease should have arterial blood gas measurement and may require oxygen.
Although appropriate support and rapid antibiotic therapy are successful in the majority of patients, there remains significant mortality, especially in the elderly.	Patients should be evaluated for admission criteria and be hospitalized if indicated.

BIBLIOGRAPHY

Anonymous. (1997). Guidelines for prevention of nosocomial pneumonia. Centers for Disease Control and Prevention. *Morbidity and Mortality Weekly Report, 46*(RR-1), 1-79.

Astin, G. T., Honig, E., Shipp, C., Moore, B., & McClellan, W. (1997). Initial antibiotic management of community acquired pneumonia. *Journal of the Medical Association of Georgia, 86*(2), 105-108.

Bariffi, F., Sanduzzi, A., & Ponticiello, A. (1995). Epidemiology of lower respiratory tract infections [review]. *Journal of Chemotherapy, 7*(4), 263-276.

Bellemare, J. F., Tepas, J. J., 3rd, Imani, E. R., & Hartland, L. (1996). Complications of trauma care: Risk analysis of pneumonia in 10,001 adult trauma patients. *American Surgeon, 62*(3), 207-211.

Brooks-Brunn, J. A. (1995). Postoperative atelectasis and pneumonia: Risk factors [review]. *American Journal of Critical Care, 4*(5), 340-349, quiz 350-351.

Chastre, J., Trouillet, J. L., & Fagon, J. Y. (1996). Diagnosis of pulmonary infections in mechanically ventilated patients [review]. *Seminars in Respiratory Infections, 11*(2), 65-76.

Chendrasekhar, A. (1996). Are routine blood cultures effective in the evaluation of patients clinically diagnosed to have nosocomial pneumonia? *American Surgeon, 62*(5), 373-376.

Coley, C. M., Li, Y. H., Medsger, A. R., Marrie, T. J., Fine, M. J., Kapoor, W. N., Lave, J. R., Detsky, A. S., Weinstein, M. C., & Singer, D. E. (1996). Preferences for home vs hospital care among low-risk patients with community-acquired pneumonia. *Archives of Internal Medicine, 156*(14), 1565-1571.

Cook, D., De, J. B., Brochard, L., & Brun-Bruisson, C. (1998). Influence of airway management on ventilator-associated pneumonia: Evidence from randomized trials [review, 65 refs]. *Journal of the American Medical Association, 279*(10), 781-787.

Cunnion, K. M., Weber, D. J., Broadhead, W. E., Hanson, L. C., Pieper, C. F., & Rutala, W. A. (1996). Risk factors for nosocomial pneumonia: Comparing adult critical-care populations. *American Journal of Respiratory and Critical Care Medicine, 153*(1), 158-162.

De gelau, J., Guay, D., Straub, K., & Luxenberg, M. G. (1995). Effectiveness of oral antibiotic treatment in nursing home-acquired pneumonia [see comments]. *Journal of the American Geriatrics Society, 43*(3), 245-251.

Doyle, R. (1997). U.S. deaths from pneumonia. *Scientific American, 276*(2), 29.

Ephgrave, K. S., Kleiman-Wexler, R., Pfaller, M., Booth, B. M., Reed, D., Werkmeister, L., & Young, S. (1998). Effects of sucralfate vs antacids on gastric pathogens: Results of a double-blind clinical trial. *Archives of Surgery, 133*(3), 251-257.

Farr, B. M. (1997). Prognosis and decisions in pneumonia [editorial; comment]. *New England Journal of Medicine, 336*(4), 288-289.

Fernandez-Sola, J., Junque, A., Estruch, R., Monforte, R., Torres, A., & Urbano-Marquez, A. (1995). High alcohol intake as a risk and prognostic factor for community-acquired pneumonia. *Archives of Internal Medicine, 155*(15), 1649-1654.

Finch, R. G., & Woodhead, M. A. (1998). Practical considerations and guidelines for the management of community-acquired pneumonia [review, 62 refs]. *Drugs, 55*(1), 31-45.

Fine, M. J., Auble, T. E., Yealy, D. M., Hanusa, B. H., Weissfeld, L. A., Singer, D. E., Coley, C. M., Marrie, T. J., & Kapoor, W. N. (1997). A prediction rule to identify low-risk patients with community-acquired pneumonia [see comments]. *New England Journal of Medicine, 336*(4), 243-250.

Fine, M. J., Smith, M. A., Carson, C. A., Mutha, S. S., Sankey, S. S., Weissfeld, L. A., & Kapoor, W. N. (1996). Prognosis and outcomes of patients with community-acquired pneumonia. A meta-analysis. *Journal of the American Medical Association, 275*(2), 134-141.

Fried, T. R., Gillick, M. R., & Lipsitz, L. A. (1995). Whether to transfer? Factors associated with hospitalization and outcome of elderly long-term care patients with pneumonia. *Journal of General Internal Medicine, 10*(5), 246-250.

Fried, T. R., Gillick, M. R., & Lipsitz, L. A. (1997). Short-term functional outcomes of long-term care residents with pneumonia treated with and without hospital transfer [see comments]. *Journal of the American Geriatrics Society, 43*(3), 302-306.

Garau, J. (1996). Clinical perspectives on the management of community-acquired pneumonia. *Diagnostic Microbiology and Infectious Disease, 25*(4), 205-211.

George, D. L. (1995). Epidemiology of nosocomial pneumonia in intensive care unit patients [review]. *Clinics in Chest Medicine, 16*(1), 29-44.

Gleason, P., Wishwa, N., Stone, R., Lave, J., Obrosky, S., Shulz, R., Singer, D., Coley, C., Marrie, T., Fine, M. (1997) Medical outcomes and antimicrobial costs with the use of the American Thoracic Society Guidelines for outpatients with community-acquired pneumonia. *Journal of the American Medical Association 278*(4), 32-39.

Gilbert, K., Gleason, P. P., Singer, D. E., Marrie, T. J., Coley, C. M., Obrosky, D. S., Lave, J. R., Kapoor, W. N., & Fine, M. J. (1998). Variations in antimicrobial use and cost in more than 2,000 patients with community-acquired pneumonia. *American Journal of Medicine, 104*(1), 17-27.

Granet, K. M., Wallach, S. L., Horvath, K., & Jaeger, J. (1996). Chest radiographs in patients with community-acquired pneumonia. *New Jersey Medicine, 93*(6), 37-41.

Gunter, N., Huang, Y., Moore, L., Eubanks, S., Odom, P., & Gibson, C. (1997). Pneumonia I and Pneumonia II Projects. *Journal of the South Carolina Medical Association, 93*(5), 180-182.

Hand, R., Klemka-Walden, L., & Inczauskis, D. (1997). Mortality and length of stay as performance indicators for pneumonia in the elderly. *Journal of Investigative Medicine, 45*(4), 183-190.

Hauser, C. J., & Poole, G. V. (1996). Ventilator-associated pneumonia. *Critical Care Medicine, 24*(5), 900-901.

Hecht, A., Siple, J., Deitz, S., & Williams, P. (1995). Diagnosis and treatment of pneumonia in the nursing home [review]. *Nurse Practitioner, 20*(5), 24-28.

Hirani, N. A., & Macfarlane, J. T. (1997). Impact of management guidelines on the outcome of severe community-acquired pneumonia. *Thorax, 52*(1), 17-21.

Hixson, S., Sole, M. L., & King, T. (1998). Nursing strategies to prevent ventilator-associated pneumonia [review, 47 refs]. *AACN Clinical Issues, 9*(1), 76-90, quiz 145-146.

Houston, M. S., Silverstein, M. D., & Suman, V. J. (1995). Community-acquired lower respiratory tract infection in the elderly: A community-based study of incidence and outcome. *Journal of the American Board of Family Practice, 8*(5), 347-356.

Iezzoni, L. I., Shwartz, M., Ash, A. S., & Mackiernan, Y. D. (1996). Using severity measures to predict the likelihood of death for pneumonia inpatients. *Journal of General Internal Medicine, 11*(1), 23-31.

Jadavji, T., Law, B., Lebel, M. H., Kennedy, W. A., Gold, R., & Wang, E. E. (1997). A practical guide for the diagnosis and treatment of pediatric pneumonia. *Canadian Medical Association Journal, 156*(5), S703-S711.

Koziel, H., & Koziel, M. J. (1995). Pulmonary complications of diabetes mellitus. Pneumonia [review]. *Infectious Disease Clinics of North America, 9*(1), 65-96.

LaForce, F. M. (1997). Triaging care for patients with pneumonia. Real progress [editorial; comment]. *Archives of Internal Medicine, 157*(1), 15-16.

Leeper, K. V., Jr. (1996). Severe community-acquired pneumonia [review]. *Seminars in Respiratory Infections, 11*(2), 96-108.

Leroy, O., Santre, C., Beuscart, C., Georges, H., Guery, B., Jacquier, J. M., & Beaucaire, G. (1995). A five-year study of severe community-acquired pneumonia with emphasis on prognosis in patients admitted to an intensive care unit. *Intensive Care Medicine, 21*(1), 24-31.

Lipchik, R. J., & Kuzo, R. S. (1996). Nosocomial pneumonia [review]. *Radiologic Clinics of North America, 34*(1), 47-58.

Long, C. O., Ismeurt, R., & Wilson, L. W. (1995). The elderly and pneumonia. Prevention and management [review]. *Home Healthcare Nurse, 13*(5), 43-47.

Mandell, L. A., & Campbell, G. D. J. (1998). Nosocomial pneumonia guidelines: An international perspective. *Chest, 113*(3 suppl), 188S-193S.

Marrie, T. J., & Blanchard, W. (1997). A comparison of nursing home-acquired pneumonia patients with patients with community-acquired pneumonia and nursing home patients without pneumonia. *Journal of the American Geriatrics Society, 45*(1), 50-55.

Mathews, P. (1997). Ventilator-associated infections. Part II. Reducing the risks. *Nursing, 27*(3), 50-51.

Meduri, G. U., & Estes, R. J. (1995). The pathogenesis of ventilator-associated pneumonia: II. The lower respiratory tract [review]. *Intensive Care Medicine, 21*(5), 452-461.

Meeker, D. P., & Longworth, D. L. (1996). Community-acquired pneumonia: An update [review]. *Cleveland Clinic Journal of Medicine, 63*(1), 16-30.

Metlay, J., Kapoor, W., Fine, M. (1997) Does this patient have community-acquired pneumonia: Diagnosing pneumonia by history and physical examination. *Journal of the American Medical Association 278*(17), 1440-1445.

Mokshagundam, S. L., & Minocha, A. (1995). Etiopathogenesis and management of pneumonia [review]. *Comprehensive Therapy, 21*(8), 413-420.

Moroney, C. (1996). Management of pneumonia in elderly people [review]. *Journal of the American Academy of Nurse Practitioners, 8*(5), 237-241.

Mundy, L. M., Auwaerter, P. G., Oldach, D., Warner, M. L., Burton, A., Vance, E., Gaydos, C. A., Joseph, J. M., Gopalan, R., Moore, R. D., et al. (1995). Community-acquired pneumonia: Impact of immune status. *American Journal of Respiratory and Critical Care Medicine, 152*(4 Pt 1), 1309-1315.

Murray, J. F. (1996). Pulmonary complications of HIV infection [review]. *Annual Review of Medicine, 47,* 117-126.

Musher, D. M., & Spindel, S. J. (1996). Community-acquired pneumonia [review]. *Current Clinical Topics in Infectious Diseases, 16,* 102-124.

Nelson, S., Mason, C. M., Kolls, J., & Summer, W. R. (1995). Pathophysiology of pneumonia [review]. *Clinics in Chest Medicine, 16*(1), 1-12.

Niederman, M. S. (1998). Community-acquired pneumonia: A North American perspective. *Chest, 113*(3 Suppl), 179S-182S.

Ortqvist, A., Valtonen, M., Cars, O., Wahl, M., Saikku, P., & Jean, C. (1996). Oral empiric treatment of community-acquired pneumonia. A multicenter, double-blind, randomized study comparing sparfloxacin with roxithromycin. The Scandinavian Sparfloxacin Study Group. *Chest, 110*(6), 1499-1506.

Phillips, K. F., & Crain, H. C. (1998). Effectiveness of a pneumonia clinical pathway: Quality and financial outcomes. *Outcomes Management for Nursing Practice, 2*(1), 16-22, quiz 22-23.

Porath, A., Schlaeffer, F., & Lieberman, D. (1997). The epidemiology of community-acquired pneumonia among hospitalized adults. *Journal of Infection, 34*(1), 41-48.

Schwartz, D. N., Furumoto-Dawson, A., Itokazu, G. S., Chinikamwala, M., Levasseur, S., & Weinstein, R. A. (1998). Preventing mismanagement of community-acquired pneumonia at an urban public hospital: Implications for institution-specific practice guidelines. *Chest, 113*(3 Suppl), 194S-198S.

Stockley, R. A. (1995). Role of inflammation in respiratory tract infections [review]. *American Journal of Medicine, 99*(6B), 8S-13S.

Taylor, D., & Littlewood, S. (1998). Respiratory system: Part I. Pneumonia [review, 5 refs]. *Nursing Times, 94*(7), 48-51.

Trouillet, J. L., Chastre, J., Vuagnat, A., Joly-Guillou, M. L., Combaux, D., Dombret, M. C., & Gibert, C. (1998). Ventilator-assisted pneumonia caused by potentially drug-resistant bacteria. *American Journal of Respiratory and Critical Care Medicine, 157*(2), 531-539.

Vogel, F. (1995). Sequential therapy in the hospital management of lower respiratory infections [review]. *American Journal of Medicine, 99*(6B), 14S-19S.

Wiblin, R. T., & Wenzel, R. P. (1996). Hospital-acquired pneumonia. *Current Clinical Topics in Infectious Diseases, 16*, 194-214.

Woodhead, M. (1998). Community-acquired pneumonia guidelines—an international comparison: A view from Europe. *Chest, 113*(3 Suppl), 183S-187S.

Wunderink, R. G. (1997). Therapy for nosocomial pneumonia [review, 27 refs]. *Current Opinion in Pulmonary Medicine, 3*(2), 120-124.

CASE STUDY

PNEUMONIA

INITIAL HISTORY:
- 63-year-old female bank manager presents in November
- 1-week history of upper respiratory symptoms; 2-day history of increasing fever, malaise, nausea
- Cough productive yellow sputum
- Right-sided pleuritic chest pain

Question 1.
What other questions would you like to ask?

ADDITIONAL HISTORY:
- No rashes, headache, or vomiting; no hemoptysis; some friends recently ill
- Nonsmoker; denies HIV risk (husband died 10 years ago; has not been sexually active since his death)
- Negative past medical history
- No allergies
- Usual childhood immunizations; had a flu shot this year

Question 2.
What is your differential diagnosis based on the history?

PHYSICAL EXAMINATION:
- Alert, flushed, coughing, and using accessory muscles; in moderate respiratory distress
- T = 39.2 orally; P = 100 and regular; RR = 32; BP = 110/80, no orthostatic changes
- Skin warm, moist, and flushed without rashes

HEENT, Neck
- PERRLA, fundi without lesions; nares slightly flared, purulent drainage visible; ears with slight serous fluid seen behind both tympanic membranes
- Pharynx erythematous with purulent postnasal drainage, no tonsillar exudate, mucus membranes moist; neck with mild anterior cervical adenopathy

Lungs
- Normal chest configuration; mild use of accessory muscles; decreased expansion (splinting) over right chest and increased fremitus
- Inspiratory rales, egophony, and whispered pectoriloquy at right anterior axillary line; clear left lung, right upper and right lower lobes

Cardiac, Abdomen, Extremities, Neurological
- Regular rate and rhythm, tachycardiac with I/VI SEM left lower sternal border
- Abdomen soft, nontender, no organomegaly, bowel sounds present
- Extremities warm and flushed without cyanosis or edema, no clubbing
- Alert and oriented; strength, sensation, and deep tendon reflexes 2+ and symmetrical

Question 3.
What are the significant findings on physical exam and what might they mean?

Question 4.
What laboratories should now be obtained?

LABORATORY:

- ABG: pH = 7.56, $PaCO_2$ = 26, PaO_2 = 90 on room air; HCT 42%; WBC 15,000; 5% bands, 83% segs, 10% lymphs, 3% monos, 1% eos; LFT normal.
- Sputum with TNTC (too numerous to count) polymorphonucleocytes and multiple gram + diplococci

Question 5.
What is the A-a gradient?

Question 6.
What do the rest of the laboratories indicate?

CHEST X-RAY:

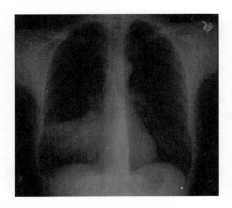 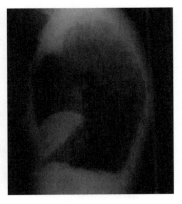

Question 7.
What are the major findings on the chest x-ray?

Question 8.

What are the possible diagnoses now?

Question 9.

How should this patient be managed?

CHAPTER 8

LUNG CANCER

DEFINITION

- Malignant neoplasms arising from the bronchial epithelium
- Classified as non-small cell lung carcinoma (NSCLC) and small cell lung carcinoma (SCLC)
- NSCLC can be further divided:

  - Adenocarcinoma—most common type of lung cancer especially in women.

  - Squamous cell carcinoma—most common type of occult lung cancer.

  - Large cell undifferentiated—relatively uncommon but extremely aggressive tumor.

  - Bronchoalveolar—the only type of lung cancer not associated with smoking

EPIDEMIOLOGY

- Number 1 cancer killer of men and women in the United States (177,000 cases and 158,700 deaths in 1996)
- Number 2 most common cancer in the United States (#1 men = prostate, #1 women = breast)
- There has been a 300% increase in lung cancer deaths in women in the past 20 years; it is estimated that lung cancer will become more common in women than in men in the United States by the year 2010.
- Lung cancer is the #1 cancer killer in the world; women in the United States have the highest incidence of all women in the world.
- Incidence is highest in men >70 years old and women 50 to 60 years old.
- Family history of predisposition; first degree relatives have a 2.5 fold increase in risk
- 80% to 90% caused by smoking; the rest is caused by air pollution, radiation, radon, and industrial exposure (e.g., asbestos, arsenic, sulfur dioxide, formaldehyde, silica, nickel)
- The risk of environmental tobacco smoke (passive smoking) has been estimated to be between 1.4 and 3.0 times the unexposed risk, especially if exposed as children.
- Airflow obstruction as in chronic obstructive pulmonary disease (COPD) is an important indicator of increased risk for lung cancer.
- Overall, smoking rates in the United States have declined and mortality from lung cancer is now leveling off in white males; mortality continues to increase in blacks and women.
- Overall 5 year survival is 14% in whites and 11% in blacks in the United States.

PATHOPHYSIOLOGY

- Initiating events (oxidants and nitrosamines [NNK] from smoking or industrial toxins) plus genetic tendencies (predisposition inherited in a codominant fashion with genotype determining the age of onset of cancer)

- Toxic oxygen radicals and direct injury cause genetic changes.

- "Multiple hit"—many exposures to carcinogens rather than one initiating event; it is estimated that it takes between 10 and 20 genetic mutations to create a lung tumor.

    - Deletion of the short arm of chromosome #3 (86% NSCLC, 100% SCLC)

    - Activation of oncogenes (jun, fos, ras and myc)

    - Inactivation of tumor suppressor genes (p53, RB, DKN2)

    - Overexpression of growth factor producing genes EGFR, ERBB2

    - Mutation of genes that are involved in the metabolism of carcinogens (CYP1A1)

    - Overexpression of genes for multidrug resistance (MDR1)

- Dysplastic cells become carcinoma in situ, then bronchogenic carcinoma.

- Cancer cells produce autocrine growth factors (e.g., epithelial growth factor, tissue growth factor, gastrin-releasing peptide, insulin-like growth factor) that promote tumor growth.

- The type of lung cancer depends on the cell of origin.

    - Non-small cell lung carcinoma (NSCLC)
        1) Adenocarcinoma (arises from glandular cells in bronchial epithelium)
        2) Squamous (from squamous bronchial epithelium)
        3) Large cell (probably either adenocarcinoma or squamous in origin, but the cancer is so anaplastic that the cell of origin cannot be identified)
        4) Bronchiolar-alveolar (from the smallest bronchioles and alveolar septae)

    - Small cell lung carcinoma (SCLC) (arises from neuroendocrine cells in bronchi)

PATIENT PRESENTATION

- 90% are asymptomatic and are discovered incidentally.

- History:

    History of smoking (number of pack years loosely correlated with risk); family history; asbestos exposure; other industrial exposures; pulmonary radiation; history of COPD.

- Symptoms:

    Result from tumor invasion of specific sites or systemic reaction: (1) endobronchial: cough, hemoptysis, dyspnea, atelectasis, postobstructive pneumonia; (2) peripheral (pleura and chest wall): chest pain, pleural effusions; (3) regional spread: dysphagia, stridor, chest pain, syncope, face and arm pain or swelling, hoarseness; (4) metastasis: pain in involved organs, edema, bone pain, seizures, headache; (5) endocrine (paraneoplastic): hyperpigmentation, centripetal obesity, syncope; and (6) constitutional: weight loss, anorexia, weakness, fever.

- <u>Examination</u>:

  Weight loss and cachexia, fever, stridor, vocal cord paralysis, dullness to percussion; localized wheeze, crackles that do not clear with antibiotics, adenopathy (supraclavicular, axillary); decreased strength or sensation in arm, and focal neurologic findings.

DIFFERENTIAL DIAGNOSIS

- Benign lung tumors (hematomas, granulomas)
- Other primary tumor metastatic to the lung (breast, prostate, colon, testicular, etc.)
- COPD)
- Pneumonia
- Tuberculosis
- Pulmonary embolus
- Inhaled foreign body
- Endocrine disorder

KEYS TO MANAGEMENT

- Most cancers remain occult until late stage (only 15% found at stage I, 44% at stage IV).
- Screening is controversial but increasing evidence that high risk (>40 pack years, older, airway obstruction, and symptoms) benefit from yearly x-ray and sputum cytology (Figure 8-1).

Figure 8-1.

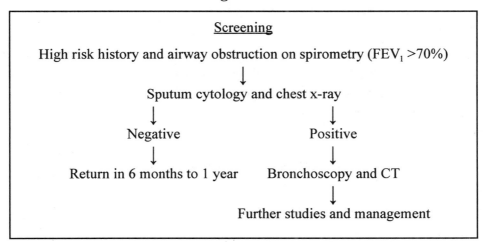

- History of smoking means cancer is always at the top of the list until proven otherwise.
- Hemoptysis in the absence of bronchitis, pneumonia, or sinus infection must be evaluated for possible bronchogenic cancer.

- A history of COPD increases the risk of cancer; pulmonary function testing is important.

- Patient may present with a pneumonia that doesn't clear with antibiotics. Smokers always need follow-up after treatment for pneumonia or bronchitis.

- Patient may present with what appears to be an endocrine disorder (e.g., Cushing syndrome, syndrome of inappropriate antidiuretic hormone [SIADH]); cancer is often found late.

- A supraclavicular node is never normal.

- Chest x-ray is the simplest diagnostic (and screening) modality—solitary pulmonary nodule is common; one may see hilar adenopathy; examine soft tissue, pleura, mediastinum, and bones for regional spread; the appearance of the nodule on the x-ray can help determine whether it is malignant or not—high risk lesions are not densely calcified and have spiculations.

- Sputum cytology may be diagnostic; thoracentesis for pleural effusion.

- Computed tomography (CT) scan or magnetic resonance imagery (MRI) can evaluate for mediastinal involvement and for suspected metastases to abdomen or brain and can guide fine-needle aspiration of the tumor for cytologic diagnosis.

- Bronchoscopy can visualize the tumor and biopsy it under direct visualization unless the lesion is too peripheral in a small bronchus; newest techniques allow for fluorescence bronchoscopy and photodynamic therapy—hematoporphyrin derivative concentrates in tumor cells and fluoresces under light of a certain wavelength such that small lesions can be visualized (also produces toxic oxygen radicals that can kill the tumor cells).

- Endoscopic ultrasound can define the size and depth of the lesion.

- A bone scan is useful for evaluating bone pain if plain films are not diagnostic.

- With SCLC, bone marrow biopsy is usually indicated (high likelihood of bone marrow metastases).

- Serum laboratories results may include pancytopenia from marrow involvement, electrolyte imbalances due to endocrine disorders or hypercalcemia (especially squamous), and hypoglycemia or hyperglycemia.

- Specific hormone markers are becoming increasingly useful for following the cancer once the diagnosis is made, but they are not yet useful for general screening.

  - CYFRA 21-1—cytoskeletal protein sensitive and specific for NSCLC; used to evaluate response to treatment, relapse, and prognosis

  - NSE—neuron specific enolase sensitive and specific for SCLC

  - TPA—tissue polypeptide antigen useful for relapse monitoring in NSCLC

  - SCC—squamous cell carcinoma antigen sensitivity and specificity low

  - CEA—carcinoembryonic antigen sensitivity and specificity low

- The careful assessment is for diagnosis, then for staging.

  - Non-small cell: TNM system for the evaluation of tumor size, nodal involvement, or metastases; determines resectability and prognosis; independent of cell type

  - Small cell: extensive metastatic work up to find the few (<15%) that are "limited disease" and therefore operative candidates

- Performance status testing (eg, Karnofsky scale) is used to assess for operability and prognosis; ventilation/perfusion lung scanning can help to assess viability of tumor-involved lobe

KEYS TO MANAGEMENT

- Prevention

  - Smoking cessation is the only truly effective preventative measure; risk of cancer can return to normal within 5 years.

  - A diet high in fruits and vegetables has been shown to reduce cancer risk.

  - Antioxidants have had mixed results. Some studies have shown that retinoids and vitamin E levels can reduce risk, however, two recent studies have shown a significant increase in risk of cancer in smokers taking beta-carotene (more studies are underway).

  - Other experimental chemoprevention methods include N-acetylcysteine and nonsteroidal antiinflammatory drugs - there are no definitive studies yet available.

- General management

  - A tissue diagnosis is important to planning care: NSCLC and SCLC are treated differently.

  - Once the diagnosis is established, a well-informed patient can best choose if and what kind of therapy is appropriate.

  - Maximizing nutrition and watching for depression and anxiety helps prepare the patient for treatment. Cancer cachexia is a major contributor to morbidity; drugs that may be helpful include metoclopramide, tetrahydrocannabinol, megestrol, and steroids.

- Surgery

  - In all types, lung cancer is a surgical disease if at all possible—complete resection is the only hope for cure.

  - The aggressiveness of the planned surgery is dependent on the patient's operability as well as the tumor's resectability—optimizing strength and stamina preoperatively is important.

  - In NSCLC, relatively healthy patients may be surgical candidates even if they are stage III; in SCLC, very few tumors are found to be resectable.

  - Surgical procedures range from thoracoscopic wedge resection to lobectomy to lung resection with mediastinal dissection.

- Chemotherapy

  - NSCLC does not generally respond dramatically to chemotherapy and it is used primarily as preoperative adjunctive therapy (significantly improves outcome of surgery for stage IIIa) or as palliative care; response rates are 10% to 40% and survival is not greatly affected.

  - SCLC responds dramatically to chemotherapy with tumor responses of 75% to 80% with a marked increase in survival time (an increase from 12 weeks to up to 5 years in some patients).

  - Most commonly used drugs have been cisplatin, adriamycin, cyclophosphamide, vincristine, and etoposide; new drugs are paclitaxel, docetaxel, edatrexate, topotecan, and CPT-11; and the newest of all with exciting response/toxicity ratios are gemcitabine, ifosfamide, and vinorelbine (increased survival with 40% incidence of granulocytopenia but only 8% developed neutropenic fever requiring hospitalization).

- <u>Radiation</u>
  - NSCLC responds fairly well in terms of palliative care, but little hope for cure and considerable lung toxicity is likely.
  - SCLC responds well to radiation, but the extension of survival time is not as good as with chemotherapy.
- <u>Others</u>
  - Laser therapy through the bronchoscope can be palliative especially in patients with significant hemoptysis.
  - Photodynamic therapy (described under Assessment above)
  - Endobronchial brachytherapy—palliative
  - Biologic response modifiers (monoclonal antibodies to growth factors, interleukins)
  - Cranial radiation in SCLC to prevent the high incidence of brain metastases

Pathophysiology   →

What is going on in the disease process that influences how the patient presents and how he or she should be managed?

Clinical Link

What should you do now that you understand the underlying pathophysiology?

Pathophysiology	Clinical Link
Most lung cancer arises from bronchial epithelial cells that have been exposed to cigarette smoke.	Smoking cessation is the most important step toward prevention; the risk increases with pack-years of smoking and returns to normal 5 years after cessation.
Multiple genetic mutations have been found in cancerous lung cells including oncogenes, loss of tumor-suppressor genes, chromosomal deletions, and other tumor growth and drug resistance-inducing gene abnormalities.	The ability to detect early genetic changes may lead to early detection of susceptible high-risk individuals, and may lead to gene therapies. Current work is around transplanting "wild" p53 genes and monoclonal antibodies to growth factor receptors.
Many of the genetic mutation seen in lung cancer are felt to be the result of toxic oxygen radicals from smoke and industrial toxins.	Antioxidants are being researched as prevention and treatment for lung cancer; current results are mixed, and there is even some evidence they may be harmful. Studies are ongoing.
Lung tumors cause symptoms by endobronchial obstructions, pleural disease, metastases, endocrine abnormalities, and constitutional abnormalities, but most are asymptomatic until late stage.	Screening remains controversial, but according to recent data, high-risk individuals (>40 pack years, airway obstruction, symptoms of COPD) should receive yearly chest x-rays and sputum cytology.
Lung tumors produce a large number of tumor markers such as CYFRA 21-1, NSE, and TPA.	Although current methods of identifying tumor markers are not adequate for general screening, they are useful for following response to treatment, relapse, and prognosis.
NSCLC cells are resistant to chemotherapy; complete tumor removal is the only hope for cure; SCLC is rarely adequately localized for surgery but responds dramatically to chemotherapy prolonging life even though it rarely cures.	Patients with NSCLC should be nutritionally, physically, educationally, and emotionally optimized to increase operability—a decision to add chemotherapy should take into account the likelihood of minimal gain vs toxicity; those with SCLC should receive the same supportive care to minimize toxicity to chemotherapeutic agents.

BIBLIOGRAPHY

Arriagada, R. (1997). Optimizing chemotherapy and radiotherapy in locally advanced non-small cell lung cancer [review, 37 refs]. *Hematology/Oncology Clinics of North America, 11*(3), 461-472.

Baldwin, P. D. (1996). Vinorelbine tartrate: A promising new chemotherapeutic agent [review, 36 refs]. *Journal of Intravenous Nursing, 19*(1), 16-27.

Beith, J. M., Clarke, S. J., Woods, R. L., Bell, D. R., & Levi, J. A. (1996). Long-term follow-up of a randomized trial of combined chemoradiotherapy induction treatment, with and without maintenance chemotherapy in patients with small cell carcinoma of the lung [review, 21 refs]. *European Journal of Cancer, 32A*(3), 438-443.

Broderick, L. S., Tarver, R. D., & Conces, D. J. J. (1997). Imaging of lung cancer: Old and new [review, 53 refs]. *Seminars in Oncology, 24*(4), 411-418.

Bunn, P. A. J. (1996). The North American experience with paclitaxel combined with cisplatin or carboplatin in lung cancer [review, 34 refs]. *Seminars in Oncology, 23*(6 Suppl 16), 18-25.

Bunn, P. A. J., & Carney, D. N. (1997). Overview of chemotherapy for small cell lung cancer [review, 44 refs]. *Seminars in Oncology, 24*(2 Suppl 7), S7-69-S7-74.

Carbone, D. P. (1997). The biology of lung cancer [review, 181 refs]. *Seminars in Oncology, 24*(4), 388-401.

Carney, D. N. (1996). Chemotherapy in the management of patients with inoperable non-small cell lung cancer [review, 59 refs]. *Seminars in Oncology, 23*(6 Suppl 16), 71-75.

Charloux, A., Quoix, E., Wolkove, N., Small, D., Pauli, G., & Kreisman, H. (1997). The increasing incidence of lung adenocarcinoma: Reality or artifact? A review of the epidemiology of lung adenocarcinoma [review, 100 refs]. *International Journal of Epidemiology, 26*(1), 14-23.

Chlebowski, R. T., Palomares, M. R., Lillington, L., & Grosvenor, M. (1996). Recent implications of weight loss in lung cancer management [review, 61 refs]. *Nutrition, 12*(1 Suppl), S43-S47.

Dancey, J., & Le, C. T. (1997). Non-small cell lung cancer: An overview of current management [review, 88 refs]. *European Journal of Cancer, 33*(Suppl 1), S2-S7.

De, L. L. M., & Ross, S. A. (1996). Beta-carotene increases lung cancer incidence in cigarette smokers [review, 17 refs]. *Nutrition Reviews, 54*(6), 178-180.

Desch, C. E., Hillner, B. E., & Smith, T. J. (1996). Economic considerations in the care of lung cancer patients [review, 39 refs]. *Current Opinion in Oncology, 8*(2), 126-132.

Devereux, T. R., Taylor, J. A., & Barrett, J. C. (1996). Molecular mechanisms of lung cancer. Interaction of environmental and genetic factors. Giles F. Filley Lecture [review, 80 refs]. *Chest, 109*(3 Suppl), 14S-19S.

Dholakia, S., & Rappaport, D. C. (1996). The solitary pulmonary nodule. Is it malignant or benign? [review, 4 refs]. *Postgraduate Medicine, 99*(2), 246-250.

Ebert, W., Muley, T., & Drings, P. (1996). Does the assessment of serum markers in patients with lung cancer aid in the clinical decision making process? [review, 27 refs]. *Anticancer Research, 16*(4B), 2161-2168.

Edelman, M. J., & Gandara, D. R. (1996). Promising new agents in the treatment of non-small cell lung cancer [review, 96 refs]. *Cancer Chemotherapy and Pharmacology, 37*(5), 385-393.

Edelman, M. J., Gandara, D. R., Roach, M., & Benfield, J. R. (1996). Multimodality therapy in stage III non-small cell lung cancer [review, 60 refs]. *Annals of Thoracic Surgery, 61*(5), 1564-1572.

Elias, A. D. (1997). Small cell lung cancer: State-of-the-art therapy in 1996 [review, 51 refs]. *Chest, 112*(4 Suppl), 251S-258S.

Elias, A. D. (1997). Future directions in lung cancer research and therapeutics [review, 8 refs]. *Hematology/Oncology Clinics of North America, 11*(3), 519-527.

Ettinger, D. S. (1996). Ifosfamide in the treatment of small cell lung cancer [review, 20 refs]. *Seminars in Oncology, 23*(3 Suppl 6), 2-6.

Fossella, F. V., Lee, J. S., & Hong, W. K. (1997). Management strategies for recurrent non-small cell lung cancer [review, 54 refs]. *Seminars in Oncology, 24*(4), 455-462.

Fossella, F. V., Rivera, E., & Roth, J. A. (1996). Preoperative chemotherapy for stage IIIa non-small cell lung cancer [review, 41 refs]. *Current Opinion in Oncology, 8*(2), 106-111.

Frei, E. (1997). Non-small cell lung cancer: Novel treatment strategies [review, 8 *refs]. Chest, 112*(4 Suppl), 266S-268S.

Giaccone, G. (1996). New drugs for the management of lung cancer [review, 45 refs]. *British Journal of Hospital Medicine, 55*(10), 634-638.

Giaccone, G. (1996). Oncogenes and antioncogenes in lung tumorigenesis [review, 46 refs]. *Chest, 109*(5 Suppl), 130S-134S.

Ginsberg, R. J. (1997). Resection of non-small cell lung cancer: How much and by what route [review, 36 refs]. *Chest, 112*(4 Suppl), 203S-205S.

Govindan, R., & Ihde, D. C. (1997). Practical issues in the management of the patient with small cell lung cancer [published erratum appears in Chest Surg Clin N Am 1997 Aug;7(3):447] [review, 74 refs]. *Chest Surgery Clinics of North America, 7*(1), 167-181.

Groeger, A. M., Esposito, V., Mueller, M. R., Caputi, M., Kaiser, H. E., & Giordano, A. (1997). Advances in the understanding of lung cancer [review, 57 refs]. *Anticancer Research, 17*(4A), 2519-2522.

Hainsworth, J. D. (1997). Chemotherapy in the treatment of non-small cell lung cancer [review, 31 refs]. *American Family Physician, 55*(6), 2265-2272.

Herbst, R. S., Dang, N. H., & Skarin, A. T. (1997). Chemotherapy for advanced non-small cell lung cancer [review, 204 refs]. *Hematology/Oncology Clinics of North America, 11*(3), 473-517.

Jassem, J. (1996). Biological treatment of NSCLC. The need for conclusive studies [review, 61 refs]. *Chest, 109*(5 Suppl), 119S-124S.

Johnson, D. H. (1996). Ifosfamide in non-small cell lung cancer [review, 27 refs]. *Seminars in Oncology, 23*(3 Suppl 6), 7-10.

Johnson, D. H. (1997). Small cell lung cancer in the elderly patient [review, 65 refs]. *Seminars in Oncology, 24*(4), 484-491.

Jones, S. F., & Burris, H. A. (1996). Vinorelbine: A new antineoplastic drug for the treatment of non-small-cell lung cancer [see comments] [review, 29 refs]. *Annals of Pharmacotherapy, 30*(5), 501-506.

Kelly, K. (1997). Overview of the randomized phase III trials in non-small cell lung cancer in North America [review, 10 refs]. *Seminars in Oncology, 24*(3 Suppl 8), S8-2-S8-5.

Khuri, F. R., Kurie, J. M., & Hong, W. K. (1997). Chemoprevention of respiratory tract cancer [review, 72 refs]. *Hematology/Oncology Clinics of North America, 11*(3), 387-408.

Koo, L. C. (1997). Diet and lung cancer 20+ years later: More questions than answers? [review, 82 refs]. *International Journal of Cancer,* (Suppl 10), 22-29.

Langer, C. J., & Rosvold, E. (1996). Newer aspects in the diagnosis, treatment, and prevention of non-small cell lung cancer. Part II [review, 380 refs]. *Current Problems in Cancer, 20*(4), 217-279.

Lillington, G. A. (1997). Management of solitary pulmonary nodules. How to decide when resection is required [review, 10 refs]. *Postgraduate Medicine, 101*(3), 145-150.

Marchioli, C. C., & Graziano, S. L. (1997). Paraneoplastic syndromes associated with small cell lung cancer [review, 99 refs]. *Chest Surgery Clinics of North America, 7*(1), 65-80.

Mentzer, S. J. (1997). Mediastinoscopy, thoracoscopy, and video-assisted thoracic surgery in the diagnosis and staging of lung cancer [review, 21 refs]. *Hematology/Oncology Clinics of North America, 11*(3), 435-447.

Mentzer, S. J., Swanson, S. J., DeCamp, M. M., Bueno, R., & Sugarbaker, D. J. (1997). Mediastinoscopy, thoracoscopy, and video-assisted thoracic surgery in the diagnosis and staging of lung cancer [review, 10 refs]. *Chest, 112*(4 Suppl), 239S-241S.

Midthun, D. E., & Jett, J. R. (1997). Chemotherapy for advanced lung cancer. When to expect a response [review, 20 refs]. *Postgraduate Medicine, 101*(3), 187-188.

Mooney, L. A., & Perera, F. P. (1996). Application of molecular epidemiology to lung cancer chemoprevention [review, 33 refs]. *Journal of Cellular Biochemistry,* (Suppl 25), 63-68.

Mossman, B. T., Kamp, D. W., & Weitzman, S. A. (1996). Mechanisms of carcinogenesis and clinical features of asbestos-associated cancers [review, 126 refs]. *Cancer Investigation, 14*(5), 466-480.

Muers, M. F., & Haward, R. A. (1996). Management of lung cancer [editorial; comment] [see comments] [review, 40 refs]. *Thorax, 51*(6), 557-560.

Nally, A. T. (1996). Critical care of the patient with lung cancer [review, 55 refs]. *AACN Clinical Issues, 7*(1), 79-94, quiz 177-178.

Naruke, T., Tsuchiya, R., Kondo, H., Asamura, H., & Nakayama, H. (1997). Implications of staging in lung cancer [review, 35 refs]. *Chest, 112*(4 Suppl), 242S-248S.

Perry, M. C. (1997). Future directions in the therapy of small cell lung cancer [review, 56 refs]. *Chest Surgery Clinics of North America, 7*(1), 183-194.

Petty, T. L. (1996). Lung cancer and chronic obstructive pulmonary disease [review, 19 refs]. *Medical Clinics of North America, 80*(3), 645-655.

Petty, T. L. (1997). Lung cancer and chronic obstructive pulmonary disease [review, 19 refs]. *Hematology/Oncology Clinics of North America, 11*(3), 531-541.

Petty, T. L. (1997). The predictive value of spirometry. Identifying patients at risk for lung cancer in the primary care setting [review, 14 refs]. *Postgraduate Medicine, 101*(3), 128-130.

Ramanathan, R. K., & Belani, C. P. (1997). Chemotherapy for advanced non-small cell lung cancer: Past, present, and future [review, 132 refs]. *Seminars in Oncology, 24*(4), 440-454.

Reilly, J. J. (1997). Preoperative and postoperative care of standard and high-risk surgical patients [review, 42 refs]. *Hematology/Oncology Clinics of North America, 11*(3), 449-459.

Reilly, J. J. (1997). Preparing for pulmonary resection: Preoperative evaluation of patients [review, 15 refs]. *Chest, 112*(4 Suppl), 206S-208S.

Risser, N. L. (1996). Prevention of lung cancer: The key is to stop smoking [review, 69 refs]. *Seminars in Oncology Nursing, 12*(4), 260-269.\

Rozenberg, S., Liebens, F., Kroll, M., & Vandromme, J. (1996). Principal cancers among women: Breast, lung and colorectal [review, 33 refs]. *International Journal of Fertility and Menopausal Studies, 41*(2), 166-171.

Ruckdeschel, J. C. (1997). Combined modality therapy of non-small cell lung cancer [review, 110 refs]. *Seminars in Oncology, 24*(4), 429-439.

Sabichi, A. L., & Birrer, M. J. (1996). Regulation of nuclear oncogenes expressed in lung cancer cell lines [review, 31 refs]. *Journal of Cellular Biochemistry,* (Suppl 24), 218-227.

Saka, H., & Shimokata, K. (1997). Chemotherapy for small-cell lung cancer: More is not better [review, 21 refs]. *Cancer Chemotherapy and Pharmacology, 40*(Suppl), S107-S109.

Sandler, A. B. (1997). Current management of small cell lung cancer [review, 71 refs]. *Seminars in Oncology, 24*(4), 463-476.

Scott, C. L., Zalcberg, J. R., & Irving, L. B. (1996). Treatment principles in advanced non-small-cell lung cancer [review, 44 refs]. *Australian and New Zealand Journal of Surgery, 66*(10), 688-693.

Shepherd, F. A. (1997). The role of chemotherapy in the treatment of small cell lung cancer [review, 82 refs]. *Chest Surgery Clinics of North America, 7*(1), 113-133.

Sing, A., Freudenberg, N., Kortsik, C., Wertzel, H., Klosa, B., & Hasse, J. (1997). Comparison of the sensitivity of sputum and brush cytology in the diagnosis of lung carcinomas [review, 67 refs]. *Acta Cytologica, 41*(2), 399-408.

Splinter, T. A. (1997). Introduction to the treatment of lung cancer [review, 44 refs]. *Seminars in Oncology, 24*(4 Suppl 12), S12-1-S12-5.

Strauss, G. M. (1997). Measuring effectiveness of lung cancer screening: From consensus to controversy and back [review, 88 refs]. *Chest, 112*(4 Suppl), 216S-228S.

Strauss, G. M., Gleason, R. E., & Sugarbaker, D. J. (1997). Screening for lung cancer. Another look; a different view [see comments] [review, 93 refs]. *Chest, 111*(3), 754-768.

Thatcher, N., Hopwood, P., & Anderson, H. (1997). Improving quality of life in patients with non-small cell lung cancer: Research experience with gemcitabine [review, 33 refs]. European Journal of Cancer, 33(Suppl 1), S8-S13.

Thatcher, N., Niven, R. M., & Anderson, H. (1996). Aggressive vs nonaggressive therapy for metastatic NSCLC [review, 52 refs]. *Chest, 109*(5 Suppl), 87S-92S.

Todd, T. R. (1997). The surgical treatment of pulmonary metastases [review, 57 refs]. *Chest, 112*(4 Suppl), 287S-290S.

Turrisi, A. T. (1997). Concurrent chemoradiotherapy for limited small-cell lung cancer [review, 25 refs]. *Oncology, 11*(9 Suppl 9), 31-37.

Urschel, J. D., Antkowiak, J. G., & Takita, H. (1997). Is there a role for surgery in small-cell lung cancer? [review, 53 refs]. *Journal of the Royal Society of Medicine, 90*(7), 387-390.

Valanis, B. G. (1996). Epidemiology of lung cancer: A worldwide epidemic [review, 51 refs]. *Seminars in Oncology Nursing, 12*(4), 251-259.

Vansteenkiste, J. F., Simons, J. P., Wouters, E. F., & Demedts, M. G. (1996). Hormonal treatment in advanced non-small cell lung cancer: Fact or fiction? [review, 48 refs]. *European Respiratory Journal, 9*(8), 1707-1712.

Wagner, H. J. (1997). Combined-modality therapy of locally advanced non-small-cell lung cancer [review, 34 refs]. *Oncology, 11*(9 Suppl 9), 43-50.

Weintraub, S. J. (1996). Inactivation of tumor suppressor proteins in lung cancer [review, 39 refs]. *American Journal of Respiratory Cell and Molecular Biology, 15*(2), 150-155.

Weynants, P., Marchandise, F. X., & Sibille, Y. (1997). Pulmonary perspective: Immunology in diagnosis and treatment of lung cancer [review, 212 refs]. *European Respiratory Journal, 10*(8), 1703-1719.

Williams, C. L. (1997). Basic science of small cell lung cancer [review, 140 refs]. *Chest Surgery Clinics of North America, 7*(1), 1-19.

Wolpaw, D. R. (1996). Early detection in lung cancer. Case finding and screening [review, 74 refs]. *Medical Clinics of North America, 80*(1), 63-82.

Works, C. R., & Gallucci, B. B. (1996). Biology of lung cancer [review, 90 refs]. *Seminars in Oncology Nursing, 12*(4), 276-284.

Zulueta, J. J., Bloom, S. M., Rozansky, M. I., & White, A. C. (1996). Lung cancer in patients with bullous disease [review, 28 refs]. *American Journal of Respiratory and Critical Care Medicine, 154*(2 Pt 1), 519-522.

CASE STUDY

LUNG CANCER

INITIAL HISTORY:
- 52-year-old female smoker with a history of emphysema comes in for routine yearly check-up.
- Over the past year, she has had a mild increase in her chronic dyspnea, with a dramatic worsening over the past 4 months.
- She has begun coughing more frequently.

Question 1.
Based on this limited history, what is your differential diagnosis?

Question 2.
What questions about her symptoms would you like to ask this patient?

ADDITIONAL HISTORY:
- She is now dyspneic on walking to her bathroom and back.
- She denies change in her chronic production of scant white sputum.
- She denies fever.
- She denies hemoptysis.
- She has had increasing discomfort in her left chest with deep breathing and cough.
- She denies substernal chest pain, palpitations, or edema.
- She admits to a 10 pound weight loss over the past year.

Question 3.

What questions about her past medical history would you like to ask?

PAST MEDICAL HISTORY:

- 60 pack/year smoker
- Emphysema diagnosed 5 years ago managed with inhaled beta agonist and ipratropium
- Last pulmonary function testing was at the time of emphysema diagnosis; she doesn't know results
- Had pneumonia 3 years ago treated at home
- Seen in the emergency room with bronchitic exacerbation of her emphysema last year
- Has never had angina or congestive heart failure (CHF) symptoms
- Has no allergies
- Is on no other medications
- Had influenza vaccine last year and pneumococcal vaccine 2 years ago

PHYSICAL EXAMINATION:

- Alert thin woman looking older than stated age in mild respiratory distress, became dyspneic moving from chair to exam table
- T = 37 orally; P = 90 and regular; RR = 22 and mildly labored; BP = 124/74
- Pursed-lip breathing, no cyanosis

HEENT, Skin, Neck

- PERRLA, pharynx clear, pursed-lip breathing
- No rashes
- No thyromegaly or bruits

Lungs

- Increase in anteroposterior (AP) diameter
- Use of accessory muscles of respiration
- Chest tympanic without dullness
- Diaphragms low with decreased excursion bilaterally
- Scattered wheezes without crackles or rhonchi
- No rubs

Cardiac

- Apical pulse felt at 5th intercostal space at the midclavicular line
- Regular rate and rhythm; no murmurs or gallops

Abdomen, Extremities, Neurological

- Bowel sounds present, no masses, tenderness, or organomegaly
- No edema, pulses full, no bruits
- Cognition intact; strength, sensation, and reflexes normal and symmetrical; gait steady

Question 4.
What are the pertinent positives and negatives on the exam and what might they mean?

Question 5.
How has your differential diagnosis changed?

Question 6.
What tests would be indicated now?

INITIAL DIAGNOSTICS:
- Arterial blood gases: pH = 7.42, $PaCO_2$ = 48, PaO_2 = 68 on room air
- Electrocardiogram (ECG) reveals sinus tachycardia without evidence of ischemia
- Pulmonary function testing reveals forced expiratory volume in 1 second (FEV_1) = 55% of predicted

CHEST X-RAY AND READING:

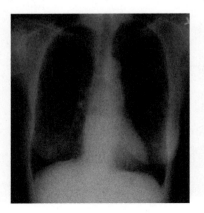
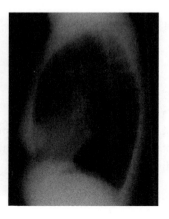

- Small, peripheral, noncalcified, and spicuated lesion in the upper left lobe
- No evidence of hilar adenopathy
- No evidence of soft tissue or bone disease
- Lungs otherwise reveal hyperexpansion, bullae, and scarring consistent with emphysema

SPUTUM CYTOLOGY:
- Atypical cells suspicious for carcinoma but not diagnostic

Question 7.
What is your interpretation of these findings?

Question 8.
What other studies might be indicated?

ADDITIONAL EVALUATION:
- She is referred to a pulmonologist.
- CT scan reveals the lesion seen on x-ray, no mediastinal disease
- Bronchoscopy cannot visualize the lesion, CT-guided fine needle aspiration reveals adenocarcinoma
- Stage is 1, V/Q scanning and functional status testing indicates operability
- There is no evidence of another primary tumor

Question 9.
The patient returns for advice prior to surgery, what should she be told?

POSTOPERATIVE FOLLOW-UP:
- 3 weeks after left lower lobectomy, the patient returns feeling weak and still having pain at the incision.
- Her dyspnea is gradually improving after getting much worse immediately post-OP.
- She reports that she was told that the operation was a success; there were no complications.
- She is concerned about whether she will need chemotherapy and about her prognosis.

Question 10.
What can you tell the patient now?

CHAPTER 9

BREAST CANCER

DEFINITION

- Neoplastic proliferation of breast cells

- Classification of breast tumor types include the following:

    - Ductal—arises from duct epithelium
        1) Carcinoma in situ (DCIS)—50% of cases will progress to invasive carcinoma
        2) Infiltrating ductal—most common breast cancer
        3) Others include medullary, tubular, mucinous, papillary, adenocystic, carcinosarcoma

    - Lobular
        1) Carcinoma in situ (LCIS)
        2) Infiltrating lobular

    - Other
        1) Pagets disease—oozing and itching of the nipple
        2) Inflammatory breast cancer—skin edema, redness and warmth, automatic stage IV

EPIDEMIOLOGY

- It is the most common cancer affecting women in the United States (184,000 cases in 1996).

- One in every 8 women in the United States develops breast cancer in her lifetime.

- There has been a dramatic increase in incidence in the past decade.

- The peak age is 75 to 79; it is the major cause of death for women aged 35 to 54.

- Risk factors:

    - **Genetics**—overall, family history increases risk 9-fold
        1) Hereditary (approximately 10% of cases)
            - Mutation of BRCA1 gene—located on the long arm of chromosome 17; autosomal dominant transmission; 54% risk of breast cancer by age 60, 30% risk of ovarian cancer
            - Mutation of BRCA2 gene—located on chromosome 13; 85% lifetime risk for breast cancer; 10% to 20% risk of ovarian cancer; 6% lifetime risk of male breast cancer (100-fold increase in risk over the general population)
            - Li Fraumeni syndrome—germline deletion of p53 (p53 is a tumor-suppressor gene that normally induces apoptosis in mutated cells); increase in breast, brain, and adrenal tumors, as well as sarcomas and leukemias
            - Others—rare syndrome such as Cowden, androgen receptor mutation, HRAS1

2) Sporadic (approximately 90% of cases)
- Multiple mutations have been identified including oncogenes Her2/neu (ERBB2), MYC, CPY17, and CCND1 and tumor-suppressor genes p53, RB1, and CDKN2.
- Acquired mutations in BRCA1 and BRCA2 are rare in sporadic tumors, but there may be some depression in these tumor-suppressor gene products.

- **Reproductive/hormonal**—overall, parity and breastfeeding decrease risk
  1) Early menarch (<age 12) or late menopause (>age 55)
  2) Nulliparity or late first pregnancy
  3) Termination of pregnancy remains controversial; recent studies suggest no risk
  4) Postmenopausal estrogen replacement—controversy remains over magnitude of risk and the amount, timing, and type of hormones associated with the greatest risk; overall estimated increase in risk is 1.4 for all ages and 1.7 for women aged 60 to 64 who are current users for more than 5 years
  5) Oral contraceptives do not increase risk

- **Environmental**—Incidence of breast cancer cannot be fully explained by genetic and reproductive/ hormonal risks but direct links to environmental toxins have been difficult.
  1) Dietary fats—still controversial but recent data suggest an increase in risk due to fat-induced increases in endogenous estrogens and the production of tumor-promoting eicosanoids
  2) Smoking—new data suggests that nicotine and N-nitrosamines (carcinogens in cigarette smoke) are concentrated in breast tissue, and that postmenopausal women smokers with a polymorphism of the gene responsible for detoxifying these carcinogens (slow acetylators) have about a 4-fold increased risk for breast cancer
  3) Alcohol—mixed studies, but there is an overall increase in breast cancer with alcohol consumption
  4) Polycyclic aromatic hydrocarbons (fossil fuel pollution)
  5) Heterocyclic amines (overcooked meat)
  6) Ionizing radiation—risk is greatest if exposed before age 19; questionable risk of radon

- **Proliferative breast disease** (including fibrocysts)
  1) Affects 1.2 million women in the United States.
  2) It complicates screening, but there is no increased risk unless atypical hyperplasia occurs (approximately 20% of benign breast biopsies), then the risk increases by 1.6.

- **Past history of breast cancer** in contralateral breast—48% of cases will develop carcinoma in situ, with 1% per year developing invasive carcinoma

PATHOPHYSIOLOGY

- The period between menarche and first pregnancy is believed to be the most vulnerable time for mutagenesis of breast cells.

- **Lob 1**

  - Mammary cancer originates in areas of the breast called Lob 1, which are undifferentiated terminal structures of the mammary gland.

  - Lob 1 contains many undifferentiated cells with high proliferation rates and is particularly sensitive to carcinogens.

- Pregnancy, especially with breastfeeding, reduces the amount of Lob 1 in the breast. Most of Lob 1 matures to what are called Lob 2 or Lob 3 that are more differentiated and less vulnerable to mutagenesis.

- **BRCA1**

    - Breast tissue taken from prophylactic mastectomy from patients with mutated BRCA1 gene reveals high amounts of Lob 1, even if the patient was parous.

    - The normal BRCA1 gene product is a growth inhibitor that controls proliferation of breast cells; this gene product is lost when the gene is mutated.

- **Estrogen receptors (ER)**

    - ER are cystol proteins present on the cell surface of normal breast cells and on primary breast tumors or their metastases.

    - Estrogens stimulate growth factor production. In normal cells, this causes breast maturation and proliferation, but the effect is balanced by growth inhibitors.

    - In neoplastic cells, ER stimulation results in an overexpression of growth factor production and an uncontrolled cell proliferation.

    - 60% of primary tumors are considered ER positive. Many tumors also have progesterone receptors (PR). These tumors have slower growth rates, better prognoses, and better responses to hormone manipulation therapy than ER/PR negative tumors.

- **Cell adhesion molecules**

    - Normal mammary epithelial cells are arranged in 2 layers—a luminal and a basal layer. The basal layer is highly proliferative and is closest to the basement membrane that separates the mammary tissue from the surrounding structures.

    - Tumor cells must escape normal cell-cell and cell-basement membrane adhesion molecules in order to invade.

    - One of the most important adhesion molecules in breast tissue is E-cadherin, which is downregulated in breast cancer.

- **Multidrug resistance gene (MDR1)**—produces a glycoprotein "efflux pump" and decreases intracellular concentration of anticancer agents

- **Matrix metalloproteinases and cathepsins**

    - Extracellular proteinases modulate cell-basement membrane interactions and can degrade the membrane to allow for invasion and metastasis.

    - Breast cancer is characterized by high levels of these enzymes.

- **Immunologic tumor markers**—oncogene peptide products that can be recognized by the immune system, including mucin (MUC1), HER2/neu (ERBB2), and epithelial-derived growth factor (EDGF)

PATIENT PRESENTATION

- History:

    Medical history of breast disease; reproductive history (age of onset of menses, number of pregnancies and age at first pregnancy, age of onset of menopause); history of hormone use; family history of breast cancer.

- Symptoms:

    Breast and axillary symptoms (mass, pain, nipple discharge or retraction, skin changes, arm swelling); symptoms of metastases (headache, seizure, bone pain, dyspnea); fatigue; weight loss.

- Examination:

    Breast mass (size, location, consistency, fixation to skin); skin changes (erythema, dimpling, edema); nipple changes (retraction, thickening, discharge); nodal status (axillary—size, location fixation, supraclavicular nodes).

DIFFERENTIAL DIAGNOSIS

- Fibroademona

- Mastitis

- Metastases from another primary tumor

KEYS TO ASSESSMENT

- Screening for breast cancer in the general public

    - Screening for cancer—monthly self-exam plus yearly clinical exam and mammography

    - Recommendations for mammography are controversial; it is unclear whether to do screening before age 50, but 25% to 33% of breast cancers occur in women younger than 59, and evidence is mounting that screening can reduce mortality by 23% to 44% in this age group

- Screening of women with an inherited predisposition (BRCA1, BRCA2, Li Fraumeni) for breast cancer

    - Monthly self-exam beginning at age 18; semiannual clinical exam beginning at age 25.

    - Mammography beginning at age 25 (every other year until age 35, then every year thereafter).

    - Ovarian cancer surveillance with yearly transvaginal ultrasound and serum CA-125.

- Assessment once a breast mass is discovered

    - Careful history of risk factors and family history.

    - An examination consistent with a breast mass must be followed with diagnostics to determine if it likely to be benign or malignant.
        1) Mammography—digital mammography is more sensitive
        2) Ultrasound—cystic vs solid
        3) MRI—3D RODEO MRI—detected 85% of carcinomas versus 31% with mammogram
        4) Tc99m sestamibi scan

- Tissue diagnosis
    1) Fine needle aspiration (FNA)—98% accuracy if combined with exam and mammogram
    2) Core biopsy, excisional biopsy (lumpectomy)

- Assessing nodal status
    1) Sentinel node biopsy—if sentinel node is negative, then, in 98% of the cases, the rest of the axillary nodes are negative It may eliminate the need for more extensive axillary biopsies
    2) Axillary dissection

- Chest x-ray, bone scan for metastases

- Staging—"TNM" system (Tumor size, Nodal status, Metastases)

KEYS TO MANAGEMENT

- Prevention of breast cancer

    - Smoking cessation

    - Exercise—clearly decreases risk

    - Decrease fat intake; increase percentage of unsaturated fats

    - Decrease alcohol intake

    - Vitamin E (α-tocopherol)—antioxidant—studies are mixed, but there is a strong trend toward decreased risk with supplementation, especially in postmenopausal women

    - Retinoids (4-HPR, 9-cis-RA)—induce transforming growth factor B (TGF-B) to promote differentiation of breast cells and depress proliferation

    - Flavonoids—contained in soybeans; questionable epidemiologic support for these in cancer prevention

    - Antiestrogens—tamoxifen decreases the incidence of cancer in the contralateral breast by as much as 50%; large scale trials of this and other antiestrogens are underway in high risk patients. There is a concern over an increased risk for endometrial cancer.

- Surgical

    - Lumpectomy—used when the tumor is small and there is no obvious axillary involvement; results clearly show survival similar to mastectomy, even if axillary nodes are positive

    - Modified radical mastectomy—preserves pectoralis muscle with improved cosmesis over radical mastectomy; it is used most often for stage II to stage III if there is no fixation to muscle

    - Total mastectomy (simple mastectomy)—no axillary dissection; it is used for CIS, prophylactic removal of a contralateral breast, local recurrence after lumpectomy, and palliation of bulky tumor

    - Radical mastectomy—breast is removed en bloc, along with all axillary nodes and both pectoralis muscles. It is used if the tumor is fixed to the pectoralis muscle or if there is bulky axillary involvement.

- Endocrine therapy (hormone manipulation)

    - It is used as adjuvant therapy after surgery for both pre- and postmenopausal women; use with cytotoxic therapy in node-positive disease.

- It increases survival and disease-free survival, and decreases the risk for the contralateral breast.

- Tamoxifen—there is a 25% decrease in recurrence and a 17% decrease in mortality for both ER-positive and ER-negative tumors; it works best if it is used for 2 to 5 years and if the patient is over 50 years old

- Newer antiestrogens (toremifene, droloxifene, raloxifene) may have equal antitumor effects with less risk of endometrial cancer; studies are ongoing

- Other hormonal manipulations—ovarian ablation; progestins (megestrol); aromatase inhibitors (anastrazole, 4 hydroxyandrostenedione); androgens

- Chemotherapy

  - Use chemotherapy when nodes are positive in all; consider it as adjunct in premenopausal node (-).

  - It clearly works best in premenopausal women; the toxicity profile is high in older women.

  - It clearly improves survival in the early stage of the disease.

  - The overall response rates in metastatic disease is 20% to 80%; the duration is 7 to 13 months.

  - Chemotherapy is often used with tamoxifen in the advanced stage of the disease.

Conventional	New/experimental
Methotrexate	Losoxantrone, telosantrone
Cyclophosphamide	Edatrexate
Doxorubicin	Gemcitabine
Vinblastine	Mitefosine
5-FU	Docetaxel, paclitaxel
Etoposide	Vinrelobine

  - A high dose of cyclophosphamide with either doxorubicin or cisplatin plus supporting granulocyte-colony stimulating factor (G-CSF) and blood stem cells has been found to be a highly effective and safe outpatient regimen for many patients.

  - Cyclophosphamide plus doxorubicin that is given preoperatively shrinks tumors and makes lumpectomy a surgical option in some patients with a relatively large primary tumor prior to chemotherapy.

  - High dose of chemotherapy and an autologous bone marrow transplant provide dramatic results in some patients, but it is associated with high morbidity.

- Trastuzumab (herceptin) —Monoclonal antibody to Her2/neu growth factor receptor. In phase III trials for advanced disease, used alone or with chemotherapy improves response rates and survival time with minimal toxicity. There is a significant risk for cardiac dysfunction but this is usually manageable.

- Psychological support—improves survival and slows disease progression

Pathophysiology →

What is going on in the disease process that influences how the patient presents and how he or she should be managed?

Clinical Link

What should you do now that you understand the underlying pathophysiology?

Strong genetic component to risk.	The family history is important, and genetic screening should be considered.
Numerous environmental toxins accumulate in breast tissue and are associated with carcinogenesis.	Women should be counseled to avoid smoking and should consider dietary modification including reduced fat and alcohol intake and increased antioxidant intake.
Breast cancer is associated with high amounts of Lob 1 in the breast.	Nulliparous women are at greater risk; pregnancy, especially with lactation, reduces risk.
BRCA1 is associated with high amounts of Lob 1; this mutation leads to loss of an important growth inhibitor.	Patients with BRCA1 gene require careful screening beginning at age 25.
When estrogen receptors are stimulated, they cause the production of growth factors that induce cell division.	Tamoxifen is an antiestrogen that blocks estrogen receptors and can be used in both prevention and treatment.
Positive axillary nodes indicate spread of the primary tumor.	Axillary sentinel node biopsy or full axillary dissection is crucial to proper staging for treatment.
When the tumor is small, there is less likelihood of tumor spread.	Early stage tumors should be treated with lumpectomy; individual consideration should be given to adjuvant endocrine or chemotherapy.

BIBLIOGRAPHY

Anonymous. (1997). National Institutes of Health Consensus Development Conference Statement: Breast cancer screening for women ages 40-49, January 21-23, 1997. National Institutes of Health Consensus Development Panel [review, 94 refs]. *Journal of the National Cancer Institute, 89*(14), 1015-1026.

Antman, K. H., Rowlings, P. A., Vaughan, W. P., Pelz, C. J., Fay, J. W., Fields, K. K., Freytes, C. O., Gale, R. P., Hillner, B. E., Holland, H. K., Kennedy, M. J., Klein, J. P., Lazarus, H. M., McCarthy, P. L. J., Saez, R., Spitzer, G., Stadtmauer, E. A., Williams, S. F., Wolff, S., Sobocinski, K. A., Armitage, J. O., & Horowitz, M. M. (1997). High-dose chemotherapy with autologous hematopoietic stem-cell support for breast cancer in North America. *Journal of Clinical Oncology, 15*(5), 1870-1879.

Apostolopoulos, V., McKenzie, I. F., & Pietersz, G. A. (1996). Breast cancer immunotherapy: Current status and future prospects [review, 41 refs]. *Immunology and Cell Biology, 74*(5), 457-464.

Biesecker, B. B., & Brody, L. C. (1997). Genetic susceptibility testing for breast and ovarian cancer: A progress report [review, 82 refs]. *Journal of the American Medical Womens Association, 52*(1), 22-27.

Blackwood, M. A., & Weber, B. L. (1996). Recent advances in breast cancer biology [review, 49 refs]. *Current Opinion in Oncology, 8*(6), 449-454.

Bonadonna, G., & Valagussa, P. (1996). Primary chemotherapy in operable breast cancer [review, 36 refs]. *Seminars in Oncology, 23*(4), 464-474.

Braga, C., La Vecchia, C., Negri, E., Franceschi, S., & Parpinel, M. (1997). Intake of selected foods and nutrients and breast cancer risk: An age- and menopause-specific analysis. *Nutrition and Cancer, 28*(3), 258-263.

Brodie, A. M., & Njar, V. C. (1996). Aromatase inhibitors and breast cancer [review, 118 refs]. *Seminars in Oncology, 23*(4 Suppl 9), 10-20.

Brody, J. G., Rudel, R., Maxwell, N. I., & Swedis, S. R. (1996). Mapping out a search for environmental causes of breast cancer [review, 44 refs]. *Public Health Reports, 111*(6), 494-507.

Bryla, C. M. (1996). The relationship between stress and the development of breast cancer: A literature review [review, 50 refs]. *Oncology Nursing Forum, 23*(3), 441-448.

Burke, W., Daly, M., Garber, J., Botkin, J., Kahn, M. J., Lynch, P., McTiernan, A., Offit, K., Perlman, J., Petersen, G., Thomson, E., & Varricchio, C. (1997). Recommendations for follow-up care of individuals with an inherited predisposition to cancer. II. BRCA1 and BRCA2. Cancer Genetics Studies Consortium [review, 120 refs]. *Journal of the American Medical Association, 277*(12), 997-1003.

Cady, B. (1997). Traditional and future management of nonpalpable breast cancer [review, 24 refs]. *American Surgeon, 63*(1), 55-58.

Cagnoni, P. J., & Shpall, E. J. (1997). High-dose chemotherapy for the treatment of breast and ovarian cancer [see comments] [review, 32 refs]. *Current Opinion in Oncology, 9*(2), 122-125.

Cahn, M. D., Tran, T., Theur, C. P., & Butler, J. A. (1997). Hormone replacement therapy and the risk of breast lesions that predispose to cancer. *American Surgeon, 63*(10), 858-860.

Cameron, D. A., Anderson, E. D., Levack, P., Hawkins, R. A., Anderson, T. J., Leonard, R. C., Forrest, A. P., & Chetty, U. (1997). Primary systemic therapy for operable breast cancer—10-year survival data after chemotherapy and hormone therapy. *British Journal of Cancer, 76*(8), 1099-1105.

Carlson, R. W. (1997). Scientific review of tamoxifen. Overview from a medical oncologist [review, 19 refs]. *Seminars in Oncology, 24*(1 Suppl 1), S1-151-S1-7.

Clarke, R., Hilakivi-Clarke, L., Cho, E., James, M. R., & Leonessa, F. (1996). Estrogens, phytoestrogens, and breast cancer [review, 141 refs]. *Advances in Experimental Medicine and Biology, 401*, 63-85.

Cleary, M. P., & Maihle, N. J. (1997). The role of body mass index in the relative risk of developing premenopausal versus postmenopausal breast cancer [review, 215 refs]. *Proceedings of the Society for Experimental Biology and Medicine, 216*(1), 28-43.

Cohen, C. J. (1997). Tamoxifen and endometrial cancer: Tamoxifen effects on the human female genital tract [review, 61 refs]. *Seminars in Oncology, 24*(1 Suppl 1), S1-55-S1-64.

Conte, P. F., Baldini, E., Michelotti, A., Salvadori, B., Gennari, A., Da Prato, M., Tibaldi, C., Giannessi, P. G., & Gentile, A. (1996). Paclitaxel combinations as front-line and salvage chemotherapy regimens in advanced breast cancer [review, 10 refs]. *Seminars in Oncology, 23*(6 Suppl 15), 39-42.

Cornelisse, C. J., Cornelis, R. S., & Devilee, P. (1996). Genes responsible for familial breast cancer [review, 77 refs]. *Pathology, Research and Practice, 192*(7), 684-693.

Crabbe, W. W. (1996). The tamoxifen controversy [review, 32 refs]. *Oncology Nursing Forum, 23*(5), 761-766.

de Vries, E. G., Mastenbroek, C. C., & Rodenhuis, S. (1997). High-dose chemotherapy for breast cancer [letter; comment]. *Annals of Internal Medicine, 126*(11), 917-918.

Donegan, W. L. (1997). Tumor-related prognostic factors for breast cancer [review, 174 refs]. *CA: A Cancer Journal for Clinicians, 47*(1), 28-51.

Dorssers, L. C., & van Agthoven, T. (1996). Genetic mechanisms of estrogen-independence in breast cancer [review, 117 refs]. *Pathology, Research and Practice, 192*(7), 743-751.

Earnshaw, J. J., & Stephenson, Y. (1997). First two years of a follow-up breast clinic led by a nurse practitioner. *Journal of the Royal Society of Medicine, 90*(5), 258-259.

Feigelson, H. S., Ross, R. K., Yu, M. C., Coetzee, G. A., Reichardt, J. K., & Henderson, B. E. (1996). Genetic susceptibility to cancer from exogenous and endogenous exposures [review, 48 refs]. *Journal of Cellular Biochemistry—Supplement, 25*, 15-22.

Fisher, B., Brown, A., Mamounas, E., Wieand, S., Robidoux, A., Margolese, RG., Cruz, AB., Fisher, ER., Wickerham, D., Wolmark, N., DeCillis, A., Hoehn, J., Lees, A., & Dimitrov, N. (1997) The effect of preoperative chemotherapy on local-regional disease in women with operable breast cancer: Findings from National Surgical Adjuvant Breast and Bowel Project B-18. *Journal of Clinical Oncology 15*,(7), 2483-2493

Forbes, J. F. (1997). The incidence of breast cancer: The global burden, public health considerations [review, 15 refs]. *Seminars in Oncology, 24*(1 Suppl 1), S1-20-S1-35.

Forbes, J. F. (1997). The control of breast cancer: The role of tamoxifen [review, 33 refs]. *Seminars in Oncology, 24*(1 Suppl 1), S1-5-S1-19.

Galloway, S., Graydon, J., Harrison, D., Evans-Boyden, B., Palmer-Wickham, S., Burlein-Hall, S., Rich-van der Bij, L., West, P., & Blair, A. (1997). Informational needs of women with a recent diagnosis of breast cancer: Development and initial testing of a tool. *Journal of Advanced Nursing, 25*(6), 1175-1183.

Garrett, T. J., Vahdat, L. T., & Kinne, D. W. (1997). Systemic adjuvant therapy of breast cancer [review, 35 refs]. *Journal of Surgical Oncology, 64*(2), 167-172.

Gluck, S., des Rochers, C., Cano, C., Dorreen, M., Germond, C., Gill, K., Lopez, P., & Sinoff, C. (1997). High-dose chemotherapy followed by autologous blood cell transplantation: A safe and effective outpatient approach. *Bone Marrow Transplantation, 20*(6), 431-434.

Goldhirsch, A., & Gelber, R. D. (1996). Endocrine therapies of breast cancer [review, 105 refs]. *Seminars in Oncology, 23*(4), 494-505.

Greene, M. H. (1997). Genetics of breast cancer [review, 99 refs]. *Mayo Clinic Proceedings, 72*(1), 54-65.

Greenwald, P., Sherwood, K., & McDonald, S. S. (1997). Fat, caloric intake, and obesity: Lifestyle risk factors for breast cancer [review, 76 refs]. *Journal of the American Dietetic Association, 97*(7 Suppl), S24-30.

Haffty, B. G., Ward, B., Pathare, P., Salem, R., McKhann, C., Beinfield, M., Fischer, D., & Reiss, M. (1997). Reappraisal of the role of axillary lymph node dissection in the conservative treatment of breast cancer [see comments]. *Journal of Clinical Oncology, 15*(2), 691-700.

Hargreaves, M. K., Buchowski, M. S., Hardy, R. E., Rossi, S. R., & Rossi, J. S. (1997). Dietary factors and cancers of breast, endometrium, and ovary: Strategies for modifying fat intake in African American women [review, 134 refs]. *American Journal of Obstetrics and Gynecology, 176*(6), S255-S264.

Harms, S. E. (1996). MRI in breast cancer diagnosis and treatment [review, 111 refs]. *Current Problems in Diagnostic Radiology, 25*(6), 193-215.

Hayes, D. F. (1996). Serum (circulating) tumor markers for breast cancer [review, 52 refs]. *Recent Results in Cancer Research, 140*, 101-113.

Holmes, F. A. (1996). Paclitaxel combination therapy in the treatment of metastatic breast cancer: A review [review, 55 refs]. *Seminars in Oncology, 23*(5 Suppl 11), 46-56.

Hortobagyi, G. N., & Piccart-Gebhart, M. J. (1996). Current management of advanced breast cancer [review, 21 refs]. *Seminars in Oncology, 23*(5 Suppl 11), 1-5.

Howell, T. (1997). New endocrine agents [review, 28 refs]. *Cancer Treatment Reviews, 23*(Suppl 1), S49-S57.

Huang, Z., Hankinson, S. E., Colditz, G. A., Stampfer, M. J., Hunter, D. J., Manson, J. E., Hennekens, C. H., Rosner, B., Speizer, F. E., & Willett, W. C. (1997). Dual effects of weight and weight gain on breast cancer risk [see comments]. *Journal of the American Medical Association, 278*(17), 1407-1411.

Hudis, C. A., & Norton, L. (1996). Adjuvant drug therapy for operable breast cancer [review, 99 refs]. *Seminars in Oncology, 23*(4), 475-493.

Hulka, B. S. (1996). Epidemiology of susceptibility to breast cancer [review, 52 refs]. *Progress in Clinical and Biological Research, 395*, 159-174.

Ingram, D., Sanders, K., Kolybaba, M., & Lopez, D. (1997). Case-control study of phyto-estrogens and breast cancer [see comments]. *Lancet, 350*(9083), 990-994.

Joensuu, H. (1996). Autologous stem cell transplantation in breast cancer [review, 35 refs]. *Annals of Medicine, 28*(2), 145-149.

Khandekar, J. D. (1996). Recommendations on follow-up of breast cancer patients following primary therapy [review, 37 refs]. *Seminars in Surgical Oncology, 12*(5), 346-351.

Kimmick, G. G., Bell, R. A., & Bostick, R. M. (1997). Vitamin E and breast cancer: A review [review, 60 refs]. *Nutrition and Cancer, 27*(2), 109-117.

Kramer, M. M., & Wells, C. L. (1996). Does physical activity reduce risk of estrogen-dependent cancer in women? [review, 117 refs]. *Medicine and Science in Sports and Exercise, 28*(3), 322-334.

La, V. C., Ferraroni, M., Franceschi, S., Mezzetti, M., Decarli, A., & Negri, E. (1997). Fibers and breast cancer risk. *Nutrition and Cancer, 28*(3), 264-269.

Lopez, M. J., & Porter, K. A. (1996). The current role of prophylactic mastectomy [review, 51 refs]. *Surgical Clinics of North America, 76*(2), 231-242.

Love, R. R., & Vogel, V. G. (1997). Breast cancer prevention strategies. *Oncology, 11*(2), 161-168, discussion 168-173.

Lynch, H. T., & Lynch, J. F. (1996). Breast cancer genetics: Family history, heterogeneity, molecular genetic diagnosis, and genetic counseling [review, 67 refs]. *Current Problems in Cancer, 20*(6), 329-365.

McKeon, V. A. (1997). The Breast Cancer Prevention Trial: Evaluating tamoxifen's efficacy in preventing breast cancer [review, 62 refs]. *Journal of Obstetric, Gynecologic, and Neonatal Nursing, 26*(1), 79-90.

Melbye, M., Wohlfahrt, J., Olsen, J. H., Frisch, M., Westergaard, T., Helweg-Larsen, K., & Andersen, P. K. (1997). Induced abortion and the risk of breast cancer [see comments]. *New England Journal of Medicine, 336*(2), 81-85.

Merkel, D. E. (1996). Pregnancy and breast cancer [review, 43 refs]. *Seminars in Surgical Oncology, 12*(5), 370-375.

Pharoah, P. D., Day, N. E., Duffy, S., Easton, D. F., & Ponder, B. A. (1997). Family history and the risk of breast cancer: A systematic review and meta-analysis. *International Journal of Cancer, 71*(5), 800-809.

Piccart, M. (1997). New cytotoxic agents [review, 28 refs]. *Cancer Treatment Reviews, 23*(Suppl 1), S59-S67.

Piccart, M. J., & Hortobagyi, G. N. (1997). Conclusions: Future strategies in the treatment of breast cancer [review, 71 refs]. *Seminars in Oncology, 24*(1 Suppl 3), S34-S40.

Powles, T. J. (1997). Efficacy of tamoxifen as treatment of breast cancer [review, 50 refs]. *Seminars in Oncology, 24*(1 Suppl 1), S1-48-S1-54.

Ranson, M. R., Carmichael, J., O'Byrne, K., Stewart, S., Smith, D., & Howell, A. (1997). Treatment of advanced breast cancer with sterically stabilized liposomal doxorubicin: Results of a multicenter phase II trial. *Journal of Clinical Oncology, 15*(10), 3185-3191.

Reid, S. E., Murthy, M. S., Kaufman, M., & Scanlon, E. F. (1996). Endocrine and paracrine hormones in the promotion, progression and recurrence of breast cancer [review, 126 refs]. *British Journal of Surgery, 83*(8), 1037-1046.

Richardson, M. A., Post-White, J., Grimm, E. A., Moye, L. A., Singletary, S. E., & Justice, B. (1997). Coping, life attitudes, and immune responses to imagery and group support after breast cancer treatment. *Alternative Therapies in Health and Medicine, 3*(5), 62-70.

Rose, D. P. (1997). Dietary fatty acids and cancer [review, 56 refs]. *American Journal of Clinical Nutrition, 66*(4 Suppl), 998S-1003S.

Simon, M. S., Heilbrun, L. K., Boomer, A., Kresge, C., Depper, J., Kim, P. N., Valeriote, F., & Martino, S. (1997). A randomized trial of a low-fat dietary intervention in women at high risk for breast cancer. *Nutrition and Cancer, 27*(2), 136-142.

Smith, G., & Henderson, I. C. (1996). New treatments for breast cancer [review, 161 refs]. *Seminars in Oncology, 23*(4), 506-528.

Stoll, B. A. (1997). Eating to beat breast cancer: Potential role for soy supplements. *Annals of Oncology, 8*(3), 223-225.

Thune, I., Brenn, T., Lund, E., & Gaard, M. (1997). Physical activity and the risk of breast cancer [see comments]. *New England Journal of Medicine, 336*(18), 1269-1275.

Ursin, G., Henderson, B. E., Haile, R. W., Pike, M. C., Zhou, N., Diep, A., & Bernstein, L. (1997). Does oral contraceptive use increase the risk of breast cancer in women with BRCA1/BRCA2 mutations more than in other women? *Cancer Research, 57*(17), 3678-3681.

van der Pompe, G., Antoni, M., Visser, A., & Garssen, B. (1996). Adjustment to breast cancer: The psychobiological effects of psychosocial interventions [review, 77 refs]. *Patient Education and Counseling, 28*(2), 209-219.

Vogel, C. L. (1996). Hormonal approaches to breast cancer treatment and prevention: An overview [review, 41 refs]. *Seminars in Oncology, 23*(4 Suppl 9), 2-9.

Wolff, M. S., Collman, G. W., Barrett, J. C., & Huff, J. (1996). Breast cancer and environmental risk factors: Epidemiological and experimental findings [review, 116 refs]. *Annual Review of Pharmacology and Toxicology, 36*, 573-596.

CASE STUDY*

BREAST CANCER

INITIAL HISTORY:
- 44-year-old white premenopausal woman
- Presents for annual GYN examination
- States her breasts are "cystic"
- Concerned about a "lump" in her left breast
- History of 7 to 8 year use of birth control pills
- Denies pain, nipple discharge, or skin changes of her breasts

Question 1.
What is your differential diagnosis based on the information you now have?

Question 2.
What other questions would like to ask this patient?

ADDITIONAL HISTORY:
- The patient does practice breast self-exam, but not routinely.
- She never had a mammogram.
- She noticed the lump approximately 8 weeks ago.
- Maternal grandmother was diagnosed with breast cancer at age 78.
- No previous breast biopsies.
- One child, age 10; has never breast fed.
- No significant health history, no medications, exercises 3 times a week.
- Menarche age 12, first child at age 34.

* Kathleen R. Haden, RN, CS, MSN, ANP, OCN, contributed this case study.

Question 3.

What are the major risk factors of breast cancer?

Question 4.

What are the controversial risk factors associated with breast cancer?

PHYSICAL EXAMINATION:
- Well appearing 44-year-old white female in no acute distress
- Afebrile, vital signs stable
- Weight stable at 125 lbs
- Height 5' 4"

HEENT
- Head exam normal
- Neck supple, no JVD
- No palpable cervical, supraclavicular, infraclavicular or axillary adenopathy
- Thyroid nonpalpable

Breast Exam
- Symmetrical breasts
- No dimpling, puckering, or nipple discharge
- Normal skin appearance
- Diffuse small mobile cystic nodules palpable in the upper outer quadrants of both breasts
- One is approximately 1 cm, firm, nonmobile nodule palpable in the left upper outer quadrant of the left breast.

Chest, Cardiac, Abdomen, Gynecologic
- Exam unremarkable

Question 5.
What do you think of her exam findings?

Question 6.
What would you do at this point?

Question 7.
What would you tell the patient about her examination and the scheduled testing?

ADDITIONAL FINDINGS:

- Mammogram reveals an approximately 2 cm noncystic dominant mass with irregular borders within the left upper outer quadrant of the left breast.
- During her exam, the radiologist informs you about the findings, and the patient agrees to undergo a core biopsy of the lesion.
- Results reveal an infiltrating ductal carcinoma.

Question 8.
What do you do now?

ADDITIONAL INFORMATION:
- All laboratory tests and chest x-ray are normal.
- Breast surgeon educates patient about two surgical options including:
  - Lumpectomy with axillary dissection followed by local irradiation.
  - Mastectomy with axillary lymph node dissection with or without reconstruction surgery.

PATIENT ALSO MET WITH RADIATION ONCOLOGIST TO DISCUSS THE POTENTIAL SIDE EFFECTS OF RADIATION THERAPY:
- Acute changes such as skin changes (erythema and desquamation), lymphadema of the breast, and fatigue
- Chronic problems such as rib fracture, breast retraction, scarring of lumpectomy incision, and the potential of pneumonitis

Question 9.
On what basis is breast conservation therapy (lumpectomy) based?

MORE INFORMATION:
- The patient elects breast conservation therapy (lumpectomy) and axillary dissection with RT.
- The pathology reveals a 1.8 cm infiltrating ductal carcinoma.
- Graded III/III
  - None of the 12 lymph nodes are positive.
  - All surgical margins are clear.
  - Estrogen receptors/progesterone receptors are negative.
- Stage I

Question 10.
Would you refer her to a medical oncologist at this time?

Question 11.
What therapy would be recommended?

Question 12.
What side effects would be discussed with the patient?

ADDITIONAL INFORMATION:
- Patient elects CMF chemotherapy for 6 months, followed by 6 weeks of radiation treatment since she had breast-conserving therapy.
- Following therapy, the patient will be followed every 3 to 4 months for the first 2 years, then every 6 months until 5 years, and then annually.
- Only routine yearly chest x-ray, routine chemistries, and mammography are ordered for follow-up, unless clinical suspicion for recurrence.

Question 13.
Where are the most common sites of breast cancer recurrence that would be important to ask during routine review of system history taken during follow-up visits?

CHAPTER 10

CUTANEOUS MALIGNANT MELANOMA

DEFINITION

- Intraepidermal proliferation of malignant melanocytes with or without extension into the subcutaneous layers

- Melanoma types include the following:

    - Superficial spreading melanoma

    - Acral lentiginous melanoma

    - Nodular melanoma

EPIDEMIOLOGY

- It is the 7th most common cancer in the United States.

- Incidence has increased dramatically over the past 2 decades (approximately 4% per year).

- The lifetime risk for developing melanoma is 1.2% for whites, and 0.1% for blacks in the United States; incidence increases with age.

- Worldwide, Australia has the highest incidence; in the United States, California has the highest incidence.

- Overall 5-year survival has increased to 85%.

- Risk factors

    - Sun exposure—strongest risk factor known; intermittent intense sun exposures, especially repeated sunburns as children, have the highest risk; occupational exposure and residing in a sunny part of the world also increases risk

    - Pigment traits—blue eyes, fair complexion, red hair, freckling, sunburns easily

    - Nevi—the total number of benign melanocytic nevi has been related to up to a 10-fold increased melanoma risk; dysplastic nevi are the precursor lesion to melanoma; the dysplastic nevus syndrome is an inherited entity associated with 25 to 75 such nevi per individual and a high risk for melanoma

    - Family history—one relative = 2 times the risk; 2 relatives = 14 times the risk

    - Genetics—melanoma susceptibility loci have been identified on chromosomes 9 (p16 or CDKN2), 12 (CDK4), 1, and 6

    - Immunosuppression—risk is increased by 4- to 8-fold

PATHOPHYSIOLOGY

- Ultraviolet radiation can act as an initiator, a promoter, a cocarcinogen, and an immunosuppressive agent.

- UVA and UVB radiation are absorbed by the deoxyribonucleic acid (DNA) and by melanin with released toxic oxygen radicals; both stimulate proliferation of melanocytes, increased deposition of melanin in keratinocytes, and skin thickening.

- The basic fibrinogen growth factor (bFGF) stimulates autonomous melanocyte proliferation; an increased activity of bFGF is associated with a p53 mutation.

- Mutation of CDK4 locus results in inactivation of inhibitors of melanocyte division.

- 30% of melanoma arises from a dysplastic nevi that occur in about 10% of the Caucasian population; there is stepwise progression from a symmetrical, uniformly pigmented macule to an increasingly asymmetrical, variegated, elevated lesion with atypia and patchy lymphocyte invasion.

- Intraepidermal proliferation of malignant melanocytes (radial growth phase) are followed by malignant cell nests and single cells spreading outward and down through the dermis and into the subcutaneous fat.

- The untraepidermal phase is not associated with metastasis; once growth is vertical (nodular with penetration through the dermis), then metastasis is likely.

PATIENT PRESENTATION

- History:

   Fair skinned with a history of frequent sunburns as a child; multiple "moles;" outdoor occupation; residence in sunny location; family history; immunosuppression.

- Symptoms:

   Enlarging pigmented lesion on trunk, legs, neck, head or arms, occasionally on palms, soles, or nail plate; may present with dyspnea from pulmonary involvement.

- Examination:

   Superficial spreading—lesions on the back or the legs with irregular, asymmetric borders and color variegation; size is generally >6 mm to 8 mm.

   Acral lentiginous—soles, palms, and beneath the nail plate with irregular pigmentation and large size (≥3 cm); pigmentation of the proximal or lateral nail folds (Hutchinson sign) is diagnostic of subungual melanoma.

   Lentigo maligna—elderly with lesions on head, neck, and arms occurring in a previously benign lesion (often present for numerous years); tan on brown patch with hypopigmented areas and nodular areas.

   Nodular melanoma—the back and the trunk with rapid growth and the presence of a raised dark nodule with frequent bleeding and ulceration.

DIFFERENTIAL DIAGNOSIS

- Seborrheic keratoses
- Common acquired melanocytic nevi
- Traumatized benign nevi (bleeding mole)
- Blue nevus
- Spitz nevus
- Congenital melanocytic nevi
- Dysplastic nevi

KEYS TO ASSESSMENT

- Visually recognize suspicious nevi—recent change, asymmetry, variegated color, nodularity, location in unusual areas (palms, soles, under breasts)
- Punch biopsy; excisional biopsy
- Determination of prognostic indicators include the following:
    - Anatomic level of invasion (Clark): 5 levels of invasion based on anatomic landmarks (e.g., I is intraepidermal only, V is infiltration of the subcutaneous fat)
    - Linear depth of invasion (Breslow)—millimeters from the top to the deepest tumor cell
    - Histiogenic type (superficial spreading, acral lentiginous)
    - Evidence of regression or ulceration
- Lymphoscintigraphy—identify lymphatic basins draining the primary melanoma
- Sentinel node biopsy—if positive, do complete regional lymph node dissection (LND)
- Polymerase chain reaction (PCR) detection of melanoma markers detect nodal micrometastases (can also use PCR to detect circulating melanoma cells in the blood)
- Chest x-ray; chest computerized tomography (CT) or magnetic resonance imaging (MRI); abdominal CT/MRI
- Tumor/Nodes/Metastasis (TNM) staging

KEYS TO MANAGEMENT

- Surgical
    - Wide excision of primary lesion (2 to 4 cm margins).
    - Sentinel node biopsy after lymphatic mapping—if negative, there is a 99% assurance that the remaining nodes are negative and the procedure is terminated; if positive, then complete lymph node dissection is performed.
    - Complications include postoperative lymphedema.
    - Local recurrences are widely excised.

- Intransit lesions (lesions >2 cm from the primary site) receive hyperthermic perfusion and/or intraarterial infusion chemotherapy before excision.

- Resection of distant metastases is indicated if there is a small number of lesions (<4) and a disease-free interval after primary resection of 1 to 2 years—subcutaneous, pulmonary, and gastrointestinal.

- Stereotactic radiosurgery for palliation of brain metastases.

- Chemotherapy

  - Isolated hyperthermic chemotherapy for limb recurrence or intransit melanoma, or as an adjunct to primary excision, improves survival and decreases the need for major amputation.

  - Chemotherapy for metastatic disease consists of single agent or combinations of decarbazine, nitrosureas, interleukin-2 and interferon alpha with response rates of 10% to 50% and improved survival in responders.

- Immunotherapy

  - Interferon alpha-2b is used as adjuvant therapy in patients at high risk for recurrence. It increases 5-year survival, but has a high toxicity.

  - Interferons are also used for metastatic disease, alone or in combination with other chemotherapy agents; there are response rates of approximately 50%, with complete remission in 10%.

  - Interleukin-2, given alone or in combination with lymphokine activated killer cells, have provided response rates of 15% to 25% but with high toxicity.

  - Nonspecific immunotherapy with bacille Calmette-Guerin (BCG) via intralesional injection controls local disease but does not improve the ultimate outcome.

  - Tumor vaccines made from tumor cells or antigens cause induction of cytotoxic T cells and antibodies with some clinical response.

  - Passive immunotherapy with human antimelanoma monoclonal antibodies has shown partial remissions.

  - Adaptive cellular therapy in which tumor infiltrating leukocytes are extracted from the primary tumor, activated with interleukin-2, and reinfused show response rates of 20% to 35%.

- Radiation

  - It is used as primary therapy for inoperable tumors with response rates of 30% to 70%.

  - It is used as adjuvant therapy for mucosal and uveal melanomas.

  - It is used as palliation for unresectable loco-regional disease and brain metastases.

- Prevention

  - Avoidance of excessive sun exposure.

  - Use of sunscreens that block UVA and UVB radiation.

  - Careful self-exam for suspicious moles.

  - Prompt evaluation by healthcare provider of suspicious moles.

Pathophysiology →

What is going on in the disease process that influences how the patient presents and how he or she should be managed?

Clinical Link

What should you do now that you understand the underlying pathophysiology?

UVA and UVB radiation, especially when associated with recurrent childhood sunburns, cause changes in melanocyte DNA and increase melanoma risk.	Protection from excessive sun exposure, especially in children, is essential for the prevention of melanoma.
Many melanomas arise from dysplastic nevi, especially in inherited dysplastic nevus syndrome.	Patients with multiple nevi require frequent examinations to screen for malignancy.
There are four melanoma types, each with somewhat different likely locations and appearances.	Patients must be examined carefully for suspicious lesions.
Malignant lesions initially spread within the epidermis and have little risk of metastasis, but once intradermal invasion occurs with formation of a nodular lesion, there is significant risk for distant spread.	Careful biopsy to evaluate for Clark level and depth of invasion is essential to staging and prognostic evaluation.
Melanoma spread first through the lympahtics, and outcomes can be improved with lymph node removal if positive nodes are found on biopsy.	Lymphoscintigraphy and sentinel node biopsy are essential to determining the appropriate extent of surgical removal.
Melanoma cells are relatively responsive to immunologic intervention.	Interferons, interleukins, monoclonal antibodies, tumor vaccines, and passive immunotherapy are all being used to treat malignant melanoma.

BIBLIOGRAPHY

Agarwala, S. S., & Kirkwood, J. M. (1996). Interferons in melanoma [review, 57 refs]. *Current Opinion in Oncology, 8*(2), 167-174.

Ahmed, I. (1997). Malignant melanoma: Prognostic indicators [review, 40 refs]. *Mayo Clinic Proceedings, 72*(4), 356-361.

Alexander, H. R. J., Fraker, D. L., & Bartlett, D. L. (1996). Isolated limb perfusion for malignant melanoma [review, 85 refs]. *Seminars in Surgical Oncology, 12*(6), 416-428.

Baran, R., & Kechijian, P. (1996). Hutchinson's sign: A reappraisal [review, 21 refs]. *Journal of the American Academy of Dermatology, 34*(1), 87-90.

Berg, P., & Lindelof, B. (1997). Differences in malignant melanoma between children and adolescents. A 35-year epidemiological study [review, 20 refs]. *Archives of Dermatology, 133*(3), 295-297.

Berwick, M., & Halpern, A. (1997). Melanoma epidemiology [see comments] [review, 55 refs]. *Current Opinion in Oncology, 9*(2), 178-182.

Bezwoda, W. R. (1997). The treatment of disseminated malignant melanoma with special reference to the role of interferons, vinca alkaloids and tamoxifen [review, 144 refs]. *Cancer Treatment Reviews, 23*(1), 17-34.

Cannon-Albright, L. A., Kamb, A., & Skolnick, M. (1996). A review of inherited predisposition to melanoma [review, 66 refs]. *Seminars in Oncology, 23*(6), 667-672.

Donawho, C., & Wolf, P. (1996). Sunburn, sunscreen, and melanoma [review, 57 refs]. *Current Opinion in Oncology, 8*(2), 159-166.

Elwood, J. M. (1996). Melanoma and sun exposure [review, 69 refs]. *Seminars in Oncology, 23*(6), 650-666.

Fraser, M. C., Goldstein, A. M., & Tucker, M. A. (1997). The genetics of melanoma [review, 72 refs]. *Seminars in Oncology Nursing, 13*(2), 108-114.

Gattoni-Celli, S., & Cole, D. J. (1996). Melanoma-associated tumor antigens and their clinical relevance to immunotherapy [review, 39 refs]. *Seminars in Oncology, 23*(6), 754-758.

Greene, M. H. (1997). Genetics of cutaneous melanoma and nevi [review, 75 refs]. *Mayo Clinic Proceedings, 72*(5), 467-474.

Halaban, R. (1996). Growth factors and melanomas [review, 145 refs]. *Seminars in Oncology, 23*(6), 673-681.

Hayward, N. K. (1996). The current situation with regard to human melanoma and genetic inferences [review, 69 refs]. *Current Opinion in Oncology, 8*(2), 136-142.

Houghton, A. N., Meyers, M. L., & Chapman, P. B. (1996). Medical treatment of metastatic melanoma [review, 113 refs]. *Surgical Clinics of North America, 76*(6), 1343-1354.

Katsambas, A., & Nicolaidou, E. (1996). Cutaneous malignant melanoma and sun exposure. Recent developments in epidemiology [review, 62 refs]. *Archives of Dermatology, 132*(4), 444-450.

Kawakami, Y., Robbins, P. F., & Rosenberg, S. A. (1996a). Human melanoma antigens recognized by T lymphocytes [review, 78 refs]. *Keio Journal of Medicine, 45*(2), 100-108.

Kawakami, Y., Robbins, P. F., Wang, R. F., & Rosenberg, S. A. (1996b). Identification of tumor-regression antigens in melanoma [review, 140 refs]. *Important Advances in Oncology*, 3-21.

Koh, H. K., Geller, A. C., Miller, D. R., Grossbart, T. A., & Lew, R. A. (1996). Prevention and early detection strategies for melanoma and skin cancer. Current status [editorial] [review, 88 refs]. *Archives of Dermatology, 132*(4), 436-443.

Le, A. D., Fenske, N. A., Glass, L. F., & Messina, J. L. (1997). Malignant melanoma: Differential diagnosis of pigmented lesions [review, 45 refs]. *Journal of the Florida Medical Association, 84*(3), 166-174.

Legha, S. S. (1997). Durable complete responses in metastatic melanoma treated with interleukin-2 in combination with interferon alpha and chemotherapy [review, 25 refs]. *Seminars in Oncology, 24*(1 Suppl 4), S39-S43.

Legha, S. S. (1997). The role of interferon alfa in the treatment of metastatic melanoma [review, 35 refs]. *Seminars in Oncology, 24*(1 Suppl 4), S24-S31.

Liu, T., & Soong, S. J. (1996). Epidemiology of malignant melanoma [review, 66 refs]. *Surgical Clinics of North America, 76*(6), 1205-1222.

Marks, R. (1996). Prevention and control of melanoma: The public health approach [review, 46 refs]. *CA: A Cancer Journal for Clinicians, 46*(4), 199-216.

Mc Clay, E. F., & Mc Clay, M. E. (1996). Systemic chemotherapy for the treatment of metastatic melanoma [review, 91 refs]. *Seminars in Oncology, 23*(6), 744-753.

Neifeld, J. P. (1996). Endocrinology of melanoma [review, 37 refs]. *Seminars in Surgical Oncology, 12*(6), 402-406.

Nelson, M. A., Thompson, F. H., Emerson, J., Aickin, M., Adair, L., Trent, J. M., Leong, S. P., & Taetle, R. (1996). Clinical implications of cytogenetic abnormalities in melanoma [review, 65 refs]. *Surgical Clinics of North America, 76*(6), 1257-1271.

Parmiani, G., Arienti, F., Sule-Suso, J., Melani, C., Colombo, M. P., Ramakrishna, V., Belli, F., Mascheroni, L., Rivoltini, L., & Cascinelli, N. (1996). Cytokine-based gene therapy of human tumors. An overview [review, 21 refs]. *Folia Biologica, 42*(6), 305-309.

Peck, G. L. (1997). Diagnosis of pigmented skin lesions aided by epiluminescence microscopy [review, 5 refs]. *Maryland Medical Journal, 46*(5), 247-250.

Philip, P. A., & Flaherty, L. (1997). Treatment of malignant melanoma with interleukin-2 [review, 64 refs]. *Seminars in Oncology, 24*(1 Suppl 4), S32-S38.

Prehn, R. T. (1996). The paradoxical association of regression with a poor prognosis in melanoma contrasted with a good prognosis in keratoacanthoma [review, 43 refs]. *Cancer Research, 56*(5), 937-940.

Rees, J. L., & Healy, E. (1996). Molecular genetic approaches to non-melanoma and melanoma skin cancer [review, 141 refs]. *Clinical and Experimental Dermatology, 21*(4), 253-262.

Rigel, D. S. (1996). Malignant melanoma: Perspectives on incidence and its effects on awareness, diagnosis, and treatment [editorial] [review, 21 refs]. *CA: A Cancer Journal for Clinicians, 46*(4), 195-198.

Rigel, D. S. (1997). Malignant melanoma: Incidence issues and their effect on diagnosis and treatment in the 1990s [review, 35 refs]. *Mayo Clinic Proceedings, 72*(4), 367-371.

Rogers, R. S., & Gibson, L. E. (1997). Mucosal, genital, and unusual clinical variants of melanoma [review, 15 refs]. *Mayo Clinic Proceedings, 72*(4), 362-366.

Seykora, J., & Elder, D. (1996). Dysplastic nevi and other risk markers for melanoma [review, 52 refs]. *Seminars in Oncology, 23*(6), 682-687.

Shields, J. A., Shields, C. L., De Potter, P., & Singh, A. D. (1996). Diagnosis and treatment of uveal melanoma [review, 23 refs]. *Seminars in Oncology, 23*(6), 763-767.

Slingluff, C. L. J. (1996). Tumor antigens and tumor vaccines: Peptides as immunogens [review, 89 refs]. *Seminars in Surgical Oncology, 12*(6), 446-453.

Villikka, K., & Pyrhonen, S. (1996). Cytokine therapy of malignant melanoma [review, 63 refs]. *Annals of Medicine, 28*(3), 227-233.

Vrouenraets, B. C., Nieweg, O. E., & Kroon, B. B. (1996). Thirty-five years of isolated limb perfusion for melanoma: Indications and results [review, 131 refs]. *British Journal of Surgery, 83*(10), 1319-1328.

CASE STUDY*

MELANOMA

INITIAL HISTORY:
- 39-year-old white, red-haired, green-eyed male with light, freckled skin
- History of numerous nevi since childhood
- Now with a larger dark, irregular-shaped skin lesion on his midback
- Physical education teacher
- Positive family history of dysplastic nevus syndrome

Question 1.
What of this patient's history are considered risk factors for melanoma, and what are other warning signs?

Question 2.
Is there a relationship between dysplastic nevus syndrome and melanoma?

Question 3.
What would be the relationship between sunlight and melanoma for this patient?

---

* **Patrice Y. Neese, RN, MSN, CS, ANP, contributed this case study.**

PHYSICAL EXAMINATION:

HEENT, Neck, Lungs, Cardiac, Abdomen, Neurological
- Conjunctival and fundoscopic exam without lesions
- No supraclavicular or cervical adenopathy
- Clear to auscultation and percussion, no axillary adenopathy
- Regular rate and rhythm (RRR) without murmurs
- Soft, nontender, no liver enlargement
- Strength and reflex +2 and equal bilaterally

Integument
- Numerous nevi and freckles
- 5 mm, irregularly-shaped, darker lesion, midback
- Moderate sun damage to face, neck, chest, and back

Question 4.
What are the pertinent positive and negative findings of this patient's physical exam?

Question 5.
Does melanoma always appear on the skin?

Question 6.
What are the most common sites of metastases?

Question 7.
What type of biopsy should be done for this patient?

BIOPSY RESULTS:
- Clark level IV
- Breslow 2.2 mm
- Superficial spreading melanoma

Question 8.
What does this tell you about his prognosis?

Question 9.
What is the significance of this histologic subgroup of melanoma?

Question 10.
What tests should be ordered for staging?

MANAGEMENT:
- Patient proceeds with wide local excision and sentinel lymph node biopsy.

Question 11.
What is the role of sentinel lymph node mapping and biopsy in melanoma for this patient?

RESULTS OF SURGERY:
- Lymphoscintigraphy results: one hot spot identified in right axilla
- Lymph node biopsy: negative
- Scar and inflammatory changes in remainder of wide local excision

Question 12.
Should interferon therapy be considered as adjuvant treatment for this patient?

Question 13.
What is the pertinent patient education the practitioner should convey?

Question 14.
What is the appropriate follow-up for this patient?

CHAPTER 11

TYPE 2 (Noninsulin-Dependent) DIABETES MELLITUS*

DEFINITION

- In 1997, the Expert Committee on the Diagnosis and Classification of Diabetes Mellitus in the United States recommended replacing the term noninsulin-dependent diabetes mellitus (NIDDM) with type 2 diabetes, although both terms are still used throughout the world literature.

- As defined by the National Diabetes Data Group and the World Health Organization, type 2 diabetes is diabetes with resistance to ketoacidosis in the absence of exogenous insulin.

- It can further be defined as a metabolic disorder of carbohydrate metabolism characterized by hyperglycemia and glucose underutilization with peripheral and hepatic insulin resistance and absolute or relative insulin deficiency.

EPIDEMIOLOGY

- It is the most common endocrine disease.

- Prevalence in the United States is 6% to 7% in persons 45 to 65 years old, and 10% to 12% in persons over 65 years old; 8 million people in the United States have been diagnosed with diabetes of whom 90% have type 2 diabetes.

- A large percentage of all Medicare patients have diabetes or glucose intolerance.

- It has been estimated that the average time from onset of type 2 diabetes to diagnosis is 10 to 12 years; ¼ of patients have long-term complications at the time of diagnosis.

- It is the 7th leading cause of death in the United States, causing 17% of all deaths in persons over 25 years old; it is responsible for 300,000 deaths annually.

- It is the leading cause of blindness, end-stage renal disease, and lower extremity amputations.

- It increases risk of coronary disease and stroke 2 to 5 times.

- By the year 2000, many primary care practitioners will have 15% to 20% of their practice made up of patients with diabetes.

---

* Lucy R. Deivert, RN, BA, BSN, coauthored this chapter.

PATHOPHYSIOLOGY

- Genetics

    - It is a heterogenous disorder with its various expressions linked only by glucose intolerance.

    - It is genetically complex with multiple genetic factors that interact with exogenous influences to produce the phenotype.

    - Defects occur at a minimum of two loci (insulin action and insulin secretion).

    - It is hypothesized that there are primary diabetogenes (analogous to oncogenes) and secondary or diabetes-related genes (such as those predisposing one to obesity).

- Insulin resistance

    - The major causes of insulin resistance in skeletal muscle include a genetic deficiency of glycogen synthase activation, metabolic disorders, receptor down regulation, and glucose transporter abnormalities.

    - It results in a reduced insulin-induced glucose uptake.

    - The liver is also resistant to insulin; insulin fails to decrease glucose production despite ambient hyperglycemia. This leads to an inappropriately raised basal hepatic glucose output.

    - Abdominal obesity with an increase in omental fat and a high intake of free fatty acids are strongly correlated with peripheral insulin resistance.

- Beta-cell dysfunction

    - Peripheral and hepatic insulin resistance increases beta-cell demand.

    - Beta-cell dysfunction results in the inability of the pancreas to produce sufficient insulin to compensate for insulin resistance.

    - It is theorized that hyperglycemia may render the beta-cells increasingly unresponsive to glucose due to glucose toxicity.

    - Insulin secretion normally occurs in two phases. The first phase occurs within 5 minutes of glucose loading and represents release of the insulin stored in the beta-cells; the second phase represents the release of newly synthesized insulin. In type 2 diabetes the acute first phase of insulin release is completely lost.

    - The "thrifty phenotype" hypothesis suggests that people with low birth weight and poor nutrition early in life have pancreatic underdevelopment and therefore have an inability to adequately compensate for insulin resistance later in life.

    - Patients with type 2 diabetes have deposits of islet amyloid polypeptide that cause extensive beta-cell damage, but it is unknown whether amyloid deposits impair insulin secretion or occur secondary to impaired insulin secretion.

PATIENT PRESENTATION

- History:

    Positive family history of diabetes mellitus; associated cardiovascular risk factors (hypertension, dyslipidemia, smoking); physical inactivity; obesity of long duration; personal history of impaired glucose tolerance or gestational diabetes.

- Symptoms:

  Frequently asymptomatic, a patient may have severe hyperglycemia without losing sense of well-being; classical symptoms of hyperglycemia—polyuria, polydipsia, fatigue, abnormalities of healing, polyphagia, weight loss, and increasing occurrence of certain infections such as yeasts; first presentation may be symptom of diabetic late complications—sensory loss and pain secondary to diabetic neuropathy, or visual changes such as blurry vision due to diabetic retinopathy.

- Examination:

  Truncal obesity with increased waist to hip ratio; sensory neuropathy; skin rashes or ulcers; retinopathy; evidence of cardiovascular disease or hypertension.

DIFFERENTIAL DIAGNOSIS

- Type 1 diabetes (insulin-dependent diabetes mellitus)

- Latent autoimmune diabetes in adults

- Maturity onset diabetes of youth

- Gestational diabetes mellitus

- Secondary diabetes mellitus—pancreatic disorder (hemochromatosis, chronic pancreatitis, pancreatectomy), hormonal disorder (Cushing syndrome, thyrotoxicosis, acromegaly), and others (cystic fibrosis, congenital rubella syndrome, Down's syndrome)

- Several rare clinical syndromes associated with insulin resistance—type A insulin resistance syndrome and a variant, Rabson-Mendenhall syndrome

KEYS TO ASSESSMENT

- Screening for diabetes

  - All patients at age 45 and every 3 years thereafter

  - Begin younger in patients who
    1) Are obese
    2) Have first-degree relative with diabetes
    3) Are members of a high-risk ethnic population (African American or Native American)
    4) Have a history of gestational diabetes
    5) Are hypertensive and/or have dyslipidemia

- General evaluation

  - Review of systems strategically focused on: heart disease, eye disease, renal disease, and major vascular disease

  - Weight, pulse, and blood pressure measurements

  - Eye fundus exam (or referral to ophthalmologist)

  - Visual inspection of patient's feet

  - Neuro exam—testing of vibration or proprioception in feet

  - Electrocardiogram

- Urine dipstick for albuminuria

- Serum electrolytes, total cholesterol and serum lipoproteins, blood urea nitrogen, and creatinine

- Establishing the diagnosis

    - New criteria for the diagnosis of diabetes have been proposed by the 1997 Expert Committee on the Diagnosis and Classification of Diabetes Mellitus in the United States. Diabetes is diagnosed by one of three criteria:
        1) Fasting plasma glucose (FPG) $\geq$7 mmol/L (126 mg/dL)
        2) Symptoms of diabetes plus a casual plasma glucose concentration $\geq$11.1 mmol/L (200 mg/dl)
        3) A 2-hour plasma glucose level of $\geq$11.1 mmol/L during an oral glucose tolerance test (OGTT); if abnormal the OGTT should be confirmed on another day; this test has poor reproducibility and is inconvenient and unpleasant for patients and is no longer routinely recommended

    - Glycosylated hemoglobin (HbA1c) is an average indication of overall glycemic control over a 2 to 3 month period.

    - **Current diagnostic recommendations** suggest a combination of the FPG and the more expensive HbA1c.
        1) Patients with a FPG <6.4 mmol/L (115 mg/dL) probably have normal glucose tolerance and have no need for further testing, unless they have risk factors in which an annual check is suggested.
        2) Patients with intermediate FPG concentrations 6.4 to 7 mmol/L (115 to 126 mg/dL) most likely have impaired glucose tolerance or diabetes mellitus. Follow up by measuring their HbA1c; if it is >7.0%, they have diabetes.
        3) Patients with a FPG >7 mmol/L (126 mg/dL) have diabetes and should have follow-up by repeat FPG and HbA1c level for management planning.

    - Serum concentration of des 31, 32 split proinsulin measures the degree of exposure of the beta-cells to glucose. Elevated concentrations may provide an early indication of the pathogenic events leading to type 2 diabetes; they are not routinely measured at this time.

    - Urinary microalbuminuria has been correlated with a marked increase in renal disease and cardiovascular risk; testing for urine protein is recommended annually.

KEYS TO MANAGEMENT

- **Therapeutic goals** include optimizing blood glucose control, reducing obesity, normalizing lipid disturbances, and reducing hypertension, thus improving the patient's sense of well-being and decreasing the risk for diabetic late complications.

- **Goals for glycemic control** are a preprandial serum glucose of 80 to 120 mg/dL and a bedtime glucose of 100 to 140 mg/dL.

- **Self-monitoring of blood glucose** is desirable in patients with type 2 diabetes, but the optimal frequency of testing is not known.

- **Exercise:** After screening for cardiovascular risk factors, patients should begin an individualized and realistic exercise regime emphasizing aerobic low-impact exercise at least 4 days per week for 20 to 45 minutes; they should begin gradually and build up as tolerated; exercise reduces insulin resistance by increasing insulin sensitivity in skeletal muscle and adipose tissue.

- **The diabetic diet** aims to normalize blood glucose and lipid levels, as well as maintain optimal body weight; again there is great emphasis on an individualized approach based on the patient's metabolic profile.

  - Caloric restriction decreases hepatic glucose production via glycogen depletion.

  - Current dietary recommendations advocate:
    1) High carbohydrate diet with a decreased caloric intake; carbohydrates should be complex and rich in fiber and make-up 55% to 60% of the total energy intake.
    2) Total fat should be reduced to 30% to 35% of total energy intake; animal fats should be replaced with monounsaturated or polyunsaturated fats.
    3) Protein should be reduced to 10% of total caloric intake.
    4) Cholesterol intake should be limited.
    5) Alcohol consumption should be curtailed.

  - Recent studies have reported a more favorable lipid, glucose, and insulin profile following the ingestion of a diet high in monounsaturated fats compared to the traditional high-carb, low-fat diet; substituting monounsaturated fat for carbohydrates improves plasma glucose, triglyceride, and insulin concentrations, while not adversely affecting low density lipoprotein (LDL) or high density lipoprotein (HDL) levels.

- Oral hypoglycemics and insulin

  - In the face of poor glycemic control due to failure of diet and exercise intervention, the use of oral hypoglycemic agents is warranted to achieve tight glycemic control.

  - The use of home glucose monitoring is essential when striving for intensive glycemic control as these programs increase the risk of hypoglycemia.

  - There are four main categories of oral hypoglucemics:
    1) **Sulfonylureas** (tolbutamide, acetohexamide, chlorpropamide, glyburide, glipizide, glimepiride)
       - They stimulate insulin release from the beta-cells enhancing the second phase of secretion, and enhance the ability of insulin to turn off hepatic glucose output.
       - When used alone, they will reduce fasting plasma glucose 40%.
       - Side effects include weight gain and hypoglycemia.
       - Drug interactions—alcohol, aspirin, and sulfonamides—may lead to hypoglycemia.
       - They are contraindicated in severe insulin deficiency, pregnancy, intercurrent illness, and the perioperative patient.
    2) **Biguanides** (metformin)
       - They lower blood glucose by decreasing intestinal glucose absorption, enhancing peripheral glucose uptake, and inhibiting hepatic glucose production; they also reduce plasma insulin levels.
       - Other benefits include decreased total cholesterol, triglyceride, and LDL levels, and an increase in the HDL level.
       - Due to the side effects of reduced appetite and weight loss, this drug is preferred in the treatment of the obese patient.
       - Side effects include minor gastrointestinal (GI) effects that can be modulated by dosage. A rare serious consequence is lactic acidosis; this usually occurs when a contraindication such as renal insufficiency has been overlooked.
       - They are contraindicated in renal impairment, pregnancy, and severe insulin deficiency, and should be used with caution in patients with liver, heart, or lung disease; cimetidine increases metformin serum levels.

3) **Alpha-glucosidase inhibitors** (acarbose, voglibose, miglitol)
   - They slow the rate at which polysaccharides and sucrose are digested, resulting in a subsequent delay in the absorption of glucose and increased control of the postprandial blood glucose levels.
   - Other benefits include a decrease in the serum triglyceride and very low density lipoprotein (VLDL).
   - They decrease hyperinsulinemia and hyperglycemia, and have a protective beta-cell effect.
   - They do not cause changes in body weight and are associated with minimal risk of hypoglycemia.
   - Side effects are primarily GI irritability.
   - They are especially useful in the elderly for whom use of sulfonylureas, metformin, and insulin are contraindicated.

4) **Thiazolidinediones** (troglitazone)
   - They enhance hepatic sensitivity to the suppressive effects of insulin on hepatic glucose production, improve peripheral insulin sensitivity, and reduce hyperinsulinism.
   - Other benefits include: lower triglycerides and increased HDL; increased LDL but reduced LDL oxidation and incorporation into vessel walls; powerful antioxidants; and lower blood pressure.
   - Side effects are minimal and include mild reversible reductions in hematocrit (HCT) and transient increases in liver function enzymes.
   - They have been only recently approved for use in the United States, but early results are positive.

- **Insulin**

  - Exogenous insulin substitutes for the beta-cell defect by reducing glucose toxicity, suppressing overproduction of glucose by the liver, and increasing glucose uptake into peripheral tissues after meals.

  - Other benefits include a slight improvement in plasma lipids.

  - Insulin treatment is initiated after insufficient metabolic control is obtained with maximal doses of oral hypoglycemic agents; large doses (200 to 300 units daily) may be required to overcome the insulin resistance.

  - Side effects of an intensive insulin regime include weight gain and a three-fold increase of hypoglycemic episodes.

  - Insulin may be useful during acute medical or surgical events, when oral hypoglycemics are contraindicated.

- **For general management** begin treatment with one of the oral hypoglycemic agents (preferably metformin or troglitazone); if ineffective add another drug from another class of oral agents (usually a sulfonylurea); if still ineffective add insulin at bedtime.

- **Monitoring and management of diabetic complications**

  - Macrovascular disease is atherosclerosis of the large vessels, which can be reduced by similar strategies of exercise and diet.

- Microvascular disease, including retinopathy, nephropathy, and neuropathy, may all be delayed or prevented by tight glycemic control (HbA1c averaging 7% or less) and aggressive treatment of hypertension.

    1) Retinopathy includes microaneurysms, dot and flame hemorrhages, hard exudates, infarcts, and proliferative retinopathy; yearly eye exams are recommended and, in cases of severe proliferative retinopathy, laser photocoagulation may be beneficial.

    2) Nephropathy results in urinary albumin excretion of 30+ mg in 24 hours due to glomerulosclerosis; eating a low protein diet and using angiotensin converting enzyme inhibitors as antihypertensives may slow the anticipated decline in glomerular filtration rate.

    3) Neuropathy is the primary factor in the pathogenesis of diabetic foot ulcers; restricting alcohol consumption, maintaining adequate nutrition, practicing good foot care, and avoiding physical injury to the feet will all decrease the risk of foot ulcers and, potentially, amputations.

    4) Skin involvement results in an increased risk for bacterial or fungal infections, itching, diabetic dermopathy, and eruptive xanthomatosis; diabetic patients with skin lesions should see a dermatologist every 6 months.

    5) Diabetic foot infections account for nearly half of all nontraumatic lower-extremity amputations in the United States. Patients should examine their feet daily and wear appropriate shoes; foot examination including vascular, neurologic, and dermatologic should be done every 3 to 6 months with immediate evaluation of ingrown toenails and ulcers.

Pathophysiology

What is going on in the disease process that influences how the patient presents and how he or she should be managed?

→

Clinical Link

What should you do now that you understand the underlying pathophysiology?

There is increasing evidence that there are specific diabetogenes as well as diabetes-related genes that predispose an individual to the development of type 2 diabetes.	Type 2 diabetes is a familial disorder; patients with a family history (especially a first-degree relative) should be screened regularly.
Insulin resistance results from a variety of mechanisms including genetic enzyme deficiency, metabolic disorders, receptor down regulation, and glucose transporter abnormalities.	Diabetes is heterogenous in its pathogenesis and management techniques must be multifaceted in their effects; the newer oral hypoglycemic drugs target several of these mechanisms.
Abdominal obesity is strongly correlated with insulin resistance.	Weight loss is one of the most effective management modalities.
Caloric restriction decreases hepatic glucose production.	Diet modification is a key component of management.
End-organ effects from diabetes occur frequently in patients prior to their diagnosis and may begin early in the course of the disease.	At-risk patients should be screened regularly. The criteria for diagnosis have been modified to identify patients with the earliest indications of increased fasting blood sugar.
Diabetes affects many organ systems including skin, eyes, kidneys, nerves, and blood vessels.	Patients with diabetes require careful screening for skin infections, foot ulcers, retinopathy, microalbuminuria, neuropathy, and atherosclerosis (ischemic heart disease, cerebrovascular disease, and peripheral vascular disease).

BIBLIOGRAPHY

Anonymous. (1997). Type II diabetes mellitus clinical guidelines at primary health care level. A SEMDSA Consensus Document, 1997, in association with DESSA, ADSA [review, 13 refs]. *South African Medical Journal, 87*(4 Pt 3), 493-512.

Bailey, C. J., & Turner, R. C. (1996). Metformin [review]. *New England Journal of Medicine, 334*(9), 574-579, Feb. 29.

Baliga, B. S., & Fonseca, V. A. (1997). Recent advances in the treatment of type II diabetes mellitus [review, 20 refs]. *American Family Physician, 55*(3), 817-824.

Bell, P. M., & Hadden, D. R. (1997). Metformin. *Endocrinology and Metabolism Clinics of North America, 26*(3), 523-537.

Boden, G. (1997). Role of fatty acids in the pathogenesis of insulin resistance and NIDDM [published erratum appears in *Diabetes*, 1997 Mar, 46(3), 536] [review, 74 refs]. *Diabetes, 46*(1), 3-10.

Bodzin, B. J. (1997). Type II (noninsulin-dependent) diabetes: New treatment options [review, 11 refs]. *Home Healthcare Nurse, 15*(1), 41-47.

Boel, E., Selmer, J., Flodgaard, H. J., & Jensen, T. (1995). Diabetic late complications: Will aldose reductase inhibitors or inhibitors of advanced glycosylation endproduct formation hold promise? [review]. *Journal of Diabetes Complications, 9*(2), 104-129.

Bosello, O., Armellini, F., Zamboni, M., & Fitchet, M. (1997). The benefits of modest weight loss in type II diabetes [review, 44 refs]. *International Journal of Obesity and Related Metabolic Disorders, 21*(Suppl 1), S10-13.

Bourn, D. M. (1996). The potential for lifestyle change to influence the progression of impaired glucose tolerance to non-insulin-dependent diabetes mellitus [review, 55 refs]. *Diabetic Medicine, 13*(11), 938-945.

Bressler, R., & Johnson, D. G. (1997). Pharmacological regulation of blood glucose levels in non-insulin-dependent diabetes mellitus [review, 234 refs]. *Archives of Internal Medicine, 157*(8), 836-848.

Burge, M. R., & Schade, D. S. (1997) Insulins. *Endocrinology and Metabolism Clinics of North America, 26*(3), 575-598.

Campbell, L. K., White, J. R., & Campbell, R. K. (1996). Acarbose: Its role in the treatment of diabetes mellitus [see comments] [review, 33 refs]. *Annals of Pharmacotherapy, 30*(11), 1255-1262.

Capriotti, T. (1997). Beyond sulfonylureas: New oral medications in the treatment of NIDDM (type II DM), [review, 25 refs]. *MEDSURG Nursing, 6*(3), 166-169.

Cirone, N. (1996). Diabetes in the elderly, Part I. Unmasking a hidden disorder [review, 4 refs]. *Nursing, 26*(3), 34-39, quiz 46-47.

Cirone, N., & Schwartz, N. (1996). Diabetes in the elderly, Part II. Finding the balance for drug therapy [review, 4 refs]. *Nursing, 26*(3), 40-45, quiz 46-47.

Cooper, M. E. (1996). Renal protection and angiotensin converting enzyme inhibition in microalbuminuric type I and type II diabetic patients [review, 47 refs]. *Journal of Hypertension, 14*(Suppl 6), S11-S14.

Csorba, T. R.., & Edwards, A. L. (1995).The genetics and pathophsiology of type II and gestational diabetes. *Critical Reviews in Clinical Laboratory Sciences, 32*(5-6), 509-550.

Dagogo-Jack, S., & Santiago, J. V. (1997). Pathophysiology of type 2 diabetes and modes of action of therapeutic interventions [review, 181 refs]. *Archives of Internal Medicine, 157*(16), 1802-1817.

Davidson, M. B., & Peters, A. L. (1997). An overview of metformin in the treatment of type 2 diabetes mellitus [review, 87 refs]. *American Journal of Medicine, 102*(1), 99-110.

Dinneen, S. F., & Gerstein, H. C. (1997). The association of microalbuminuria and mortality in non-insulin-dependent diabetes mellitus. A systematic overview of the literature [review, 33 refs]. *Archives of Internal Medicine, 157*(13), 1413-1418.

Drass, J. A., & Peterson, A. (1996). Type II diabetes: Exploring treatment options [review, 8 refs]. *American Journal of Nursing, 96*(11), 45-49, quiz 50.

Eastman, R. C., & Keen, H. (1997). The impact of cardiovascular disease on people with diabetes: The potential for prevention [review, 29 refs]. *Lancet, 350*(Suppl 1), SI29-SI32.

Feener, E. P., & King, G. L. (1997). Vascular dysfunction in diabetes mellitus [review, 35 refs]. *Lancet, 350*(Suppl 1), SI9-S13.

Flick, M., & Schumann, L. (1997). Non-insulin-dependent diabetes mellitus [review, 41 refs]. *Journal of the American Academy of Nurse Practitioners, 9*(7), 337-344, quiz 346-347.

Folsch, U.R. (1995) Clinical experience as first line therapy in NIDDM [review]. *Clinical and Investigative Medicine, 18*(4), 312-317.

Fore, W. W. (1995). Noninsulin-dependent diabetes mellitus. The prevention of complications. *Medical Clinics of North America, 79*(2), 287-298.

Franz, M. J. (1997). Lifestyle modification for diabetes management. *Endocrinology and Metabolism Clinics of North America, 26*(3), 499-510.

Garg, A., et al. (1994). Effects of varying carbohydrate content of diet in patients with non-insulin-dependent diabetes mellitus. *Journal of the American Medical Association, 271*(18), 1421-1428.

Gautier, J. F., Scheen, A., & Lefebvre, P. J. (1995). Exercise in the management of non-insulin-dependent (type 2) diabetes mellitus [review]. *International Journal of Obesity and Related Metabolic Disorders, 19*(Suppl 4), S58-S61.

Gerich, J. E. (1996). Pathogenesis and treatment of type 2 (noninsulin-dependent) diabetes mellitus (NIDDM) [review, 53 refs]. *Hormone and Metabolic Research, 28*(9), 404-412.

Goldstein, D. E., & Little, R. R. (1997). Monitoring glycemia in diabetes. *Endocrinology and Metabolism Clinics of North America, 26*(3), 475-486.

Groop, L. C., & Tuomi, T. (1997). Non-insulin-dependent diabetes mellitus--a collision between thrifty genes and an affluent society [review, 179 refs]. *Annals of Medicine, 29*(1), 37-53.

Guthrie, R. (1997). Treatment of non-insulin-dependent diabetes mellitus with metformin [review, 57 refs]. *Journal of the American Board of Family Practice, 10*(3), 213-221.

Haffner, S. M. (1995). Risk Factors for non-insulin-dependent diabetes mellitus [review]. *Journal of Hypertension, 13*(Suppl 3), S73-S76.

Haffner, S. M., & Miettinen, H. (1997). Insulin resistance implications for type II diabetes mellitus and coronary heart disease [review, 106 refs]. *American Journal of Medicine, 103*(2), 152-162.

Hales, C, N. (1994). The pathogenesis of NIDDM. *Diabetologia, 37*(Suppl 2), S162-168.

Hales, C. N., Desai, M., & Ozanne, S. E. (1997). The Thrifty Phenotype hypothesis: How does it look after 5 years? [review, 53 refs]. *Diabetic Medicine, 14*(3), 189-195.

Harris, M. I. (1995). Epidemiologic studies on the pathogenesis of non-insulin-dependent diabetes mellitus (NIDDM) [review]. *Clinical and Investigative Medicine, 18*(4), 231-239.

Harris, M. I., & Eastman, R. C. (1996). Early detection of undiagnosed non-insulin-dependent diabetes mellitus. *Journal of the American Medical Association, 276*(15), 1261-1262.

Harrower, A. D. (1994). Comparison of efficacy, secondary failure rate, and complications of sulfonylureas [review]. *Journal of Diabetes and Its Complications, 8*(4), 201-203.

Henry, H. R. (1996). Glucose control and insulin resistance in non-insulin-dependent diabetes mellitus. *Annals of Internal Medicine, 124*(1 Pt 2), 97-103.

Henry, H. R. (1997). Thiazolidinediones. *Endocrinology and Metabolism Clinics of North America, 26*(3), 553-573.

Henry, H. R., & Genuth, S. (1996). Forum one: Current recommendations about intensification of metabolic control in non-insulin-dependent diabetes mellitus. *Annals of Internal Medicine, 124*(1 Pt 2), 175-177.

Henry, R. R. (1996). Effects of troglitazone on insulin sensitivity [review, 9 refs]. *Diabetic Medicine, 13*(9 Suppl 6), S148-S150.

Hirsch, I. B., Paauw, D. S., & Brunzell, J. (1995). Inpatient management of adults with diabetes [review]. *Diabetes Care 18*(6), 870-878.

Ilarde, A., & Tuck, M. (1994). Treatment of non-insulin-dependent diabetes mellitus and its complications. A state-of-the-art review [review]. *Drugs Aging, 4*(6), 470-491.

Kahn, C. R., Vicent, D., & Doria, A. (1996). Genetics of non-insulin-dependent (type-II) diabetes mellitus [review, 157 refs]. *Annual Review of Medicine, 47,* 509-531.

Keen, H. (1996). Management of non-insulin-dependent diabetes mellitus. The United Kingdom experience, [review]. *Annals of Internal Medicine, 124*(1 Pt 2),156-159.

Kerr, C. P. (1995). Improving outcomes in diabetes: A review of outpatient care of NIDDM patients, [review]. *Journal of Family Practice, 40*(1), 63-75.

Knowler, W. C., Narayan, K. M., Hanson, R. L., et al. (1995). Preventing non-insulin-dependent diabetes, [review]. *Diabetes, 44*(5), 483-488.

Kopelman, P. G., & Albon, L. (1997). Obesity, non-insulin-dependent diabetes mellitus and the metabolic syndrome [review, 95 refs]. *British Medical Bulletin, 53*(2), 322-340.

Laakso, M. (1996). Lipids and lipoproteins as risk factors for coronary heart disease in non-insulin-dependent diabetes mellitus, [review, 53 refs]. *Annals of Medicine, 28*(4), 341-345.

Laakso, M., & Kuusisto, J. (1996). Epidemiological evidence for the association of hyperglycaemia and atherosclerotic vascular disease in non-insulin-dependent diabetes mellitus [review, 23 refs]. *Annals of Medicine, 28*(5), 415-418.

Liebovitz, H. E. (1997). Alpha-glucosidase inhibitors. *Endocrinology and Metabolism Clinics of North America, 26*(3), 539-551.

Manson, J. E., & Spelsberg, A. (1994). Primary prevention of non-insulin-dependent diabetes mellitus [review]. *American Journal of Preventive Medicine, 10*(3), 172-184.

Mazze, R. S., Bergenstal, R., & Ginsberg, B. (1995). Intensified diabetes management: Lessons from the diabetes control and complications trial [review]. *International Journal of Clinical Pharmacology and Therapeutics, 33*(1), 43-51.

Melchior, W. R., & Jaber, L. A. (1996). Metformin: An antihyperglycemic agent for treatment of type II diabetes [review, 48 refs]. *Annals of Pharmacotherapy, 30*(2), 158-164.

Moller, D. E., Bjorbaek, C., & Vidal-Puig, A. (1996). Candidate genes for insulin resistance [review, 45 refs]. *Diabetes Care, 19*(4), 396-400.

Nathan, D. M. (1995). Prevention of long-term complications of non-insulin-dependent diabetes mellitus, [review]. *Clinical Investigative Medicine, 18*(4), 332-339.

Peters, A. L., Davidson, M. B., Schriger, D. L. , & Hasselblad. V. (1996). A Clinical approach for the diagnosis of diabetes mellitus [review]. *Journal of the American Medical Association, 276*(15), 1246-1252

Pontiroli, A.E., Caldera, A., & Pozza, G. (1994). Secondary failure of oral hypoglycaemic agents: Frequency, possible causes, and management [review]. *Diabetes/Metabolism Reviews, 10*(1), 31-43.

Porte, D., Jr., & Kahn, S. E. (1995). The key role of islet dysfunction in type II diabetes mellitus [review]. *Investigative Medical Clinics, 18*(4), 247-254.

Reaven, G. M. (1995). Pathophysiology of insulin resistance in human disease [review]. *Physiology Reviews, 75*(3), 473-486.

Riddle, M. C. (1996). Combined therapy with a sulfonylurea plus evening insulin: Safe, reliable, and becoming routine [review, 30 refs]. *Hormone and Metabolic Research, 28*(9), 430-433.

Roman, S. H., & Harris, M. I. (1997). Management of diabetes mellitus from a public health perspective. *Endocrinology and Metabolism Clinics of North America, 26*(3), 443-474.

Sacks, D. B., & McDonald, J. M. (1996). The pathogenesis of type II diabetes mellitus. A polygenic disease [review, 44 refs]. *American Journal of Clinical Pathology, 105*(2), 149-156.

Saltiel, A. R., & Olefsky, J. M. (1996). Thiazolidinediones in the treatment of insulin resistance and type II diabetes [review, 53 refs]. *Diabetes, 45*(12), 1661-1669.

Saudek, C. D. (1997). Novel forms of insulin delivery. *Endocrinology and Metabolism Clinics of North America, 26*(3), 599-610.

Sheard, N. F. (1995). The diabetic diet: Evidence for a new approach [review]. *Nutrition Review, 53*(1), 16-18.

Susman, J. L., & Helseth, L. D. (1997). Reducing the complications of type II diabetes: A patient-centered approach [review, 51 refs]. *American Family Physician, 56*(2), 471-480.

Tan, G. H., & Nelson, R. L. (1996). Pharmacologic treatment options for non-insulin-dependent diabetes mellitus [see comments] [review, 26 refs]. *Mayo Clinic Proceedings, 71*(8), 763-768.

Vidt, D. G., Speerhas, R. A., & Reddy, S. S. (1997). Troglitazone: A new antihyperglycemic agent [review, 8 refs]. *Cleveland Clinic Journal of Medicine, 64*(5), 238-240.

Virtanen, S. M., & Aro, A. (1994). Dietary factors in the etiology of diabetes [review]. *Annals of Medicine, 26*(6), 469-478.

Wildasin, E. M., Skaar, D. J., Kirchain, W. R., & Hulse, M. (1997). Metformin, a promising oral antihyperglycemic for the treatment of noninsulin-dependent diabetes mellitus [review, 51 refs]. *Pharmacotherapy, 17*(1), 62-73.

Williams, G. (1994). Management of non-insulin-dependent diabetes mellitus [review] *Lancet 343*(8889), 95-100.

Wolffenbuttel, B. H., & van Haeften, T. W. (1995), Prevention of complications in non-insulin-dependent diabetes mellitus (NIDDM) [review]. *Drugs 50*(2), 263-288.

Yki-Jarvinen, H. (1994). Pathogenesis of non-insulin-dependent diabetes mellitus [review]. *Lancet, 343*(8999), 91-95.

Zimmerman, B. R. (1997). Sulfonylureas. *Endocrinology and Metabolism Clinics of North America, 26*(3), 511-522.

Zimmet, P. Z. (1995). The pathogenesis and prevention of diabetes in adults. Genes, autoimmunity, and demography [review]. *Diabetes Care 18*(7), 1050-1064.

Zimmet, P. Z., & Alberti, K. G. (1997). The changing face of macrovascular disease in non-insulin-dependent diabetes mellitus: An epidemic in progress [review, 37 refs]. *Lancet, 350*(Suppl 1), SI1-SI4.

CASE STUDY

TYPE 2 DIABETES MELLITUS

INITIAL HISTORY:
- 52-year-old African American female
- Diagnosed with type 2 diabetes 6 years ago but did not follow-up with recommendations for care
- Now complaining of weakness in her right foot and an itching rash in her groin area

Question 1.
What questions would you like to ask her about her symptoms?

ADDITIONAL HISTORY:
- She says her foot has been weak for about a month and is difficult to dorsiflex; it also feels numb.
- She denies any other weakness, numbness, difficulty speaking or walking, change in vision, syncope, or seizures.
- She has had some increased thirst and gets up more often at night to urinate.
- She says she has had the rash on and off for many years. It is worst when the weather is warm. She gets some relief from "salt baths."
- She denies any chest pain, shortness of breath, edema, change in bowel or bladder habits, or skin ulcers.

Question 2.
What other questions would you like to ask her about her diabetes?

DIABETES HISTORY:

- She remembers being told her blood sugar "was around 200" when she was diagnosed—she had gone for a work physical and felt fine at the time and saw no need for "expensive drugs."
- Her mother and her sister have diabetes. Both of them were diagnosed in their 40s and are on "both pills and shots."
- She has been completely asymptomatic, except for the rash, until the foot weakness.
- She has gained 18 pounds over the past year and eats a diet high in fats and refined sugars.
- She works as a banking executive and gets little exercise.

Question 3.
What would you like to ask about her past medical history?

PHYSICAL EXAMINATION:

- Obese female in no acute distress
- T = 37 orally; P = 80 and regular; RR = 15 and unlabored; BP = 162/98 right arm sitting

Skin
- Erythematous scaling rash in both inguinal areas and in the axillae
- No petechia or ecchymoses

HEENT, Neck
- PERRL, fundi with mild vascular narrowing
- Nares and tympanic membranes clear
- Pharynx clear
- Neck without bruits or thyromegaly

Lungs, Cardiac
- Lungs clear to auscultation and percussion
- Cardiac exam with a regular rate and rhythm without murmurs or gallops

Abdomen, Extremities
- Abdomen moderately obese with bowel sounds heard in all four quadrants; no abdominal bruits, tenderness, masses, or organomegaly
- Extremities without edema; pulses diminished to 1+ in both feet

Neurological
- Alert and oriented
- Cranial nerves II-XII intact (including good visual acuity)
- Strength 5/5 throughout except 2/5 on dorsiflexion of the right foot
- Sensory to light touch, proprioception, and vibration slightly diminished in both feet
- Deep tendon reflexes 1+ and symmetrical throughout
- Gait normal except for right foot drop, negative Romberg

Question 4.

What are the pertinent positives and negatives on exam?

Question 5:

What laboratory tests would you order now?

LABORATORY RESULTS:
- Serum electrolytes, including BUN and creatinine, calcium, and magnesium all within normal limits
- Random glucose = 253 mg/dL
- HbA1c = 9.1%
- Urine dipstick positive for glucose, negative for protein; microscopic without significant cellular or infectious findings
- Wet prep of smear from rash consistent with candida albicans
- ECG with evidence of early left ventricular hypertrophy (LVH) by voltage

BLOOD PRESSURE AND FOLLOW-UP LABORATORY RESULTS THE FOLLOWING WEEK:
- BP = 150/100 both arms sitting
- Fasting glucose = 168 mg/dL.
- Fasting total cholesterol = 246 mg/dL with HDL = 28 mg/dL and triglucerides = 458 mg/dL
- 24-hour urine for protein = 100 mg/24 hrs
- Electromyography consistent with peripheral neuropathy

Question 6.
How would you interpret these laboratory findings?

Question 7:
What would you recommend at this time?

CHAPTER 12

ANEMIA

DEFINITION

- A decrease in red blood cells (RBC)—often reported as a decrease in hematocrit (HCT) or a decrease in hemoglobin concentration (HgB).

- Results in decreased oxygen carrying capacity of the blood.

- Anemia can be divided into 2 major categories:

    - insufficient production of RBC or

    - increased destruction of RBC.

- Selected causes of anemia:

    - Insufficient production
        1) Microcytic anemia (iron deficiency, anemia of chronic disease [ACD])
        2) Macrocytic anemia (vitamin B_{12} or folate deficiency, alcoholism)
        3) Marrow disease (leukemia, aplastic anemia, other myelodysplastic diseases)
        4) Renal disease with decreased erythropoietin

    - Increased destruction
        1) Immune hemolytic anemia
        2) Inherited hemolytic anemia
            - Hereditary spherocytosis
            - Sickle cell disease
            - Thalassemias

PATHOPHYSIOLOGY

- Microcytic anemia

    - 9% of toddlers aged 1 to 2 years and 9% to 11% of adolescent girls and women of childbearing age are iron deficient; less than 1% of older male children and men are iron deficient.
        1) Normally, approximately 1 mg of iron is absorbed and lost per day; an imbalance between intake, requirements, and loss of iron leads to iron deficiency.
        2) Dietary iron deficiency is common in states of increased iron requirements such as infancy and pregnancy; inadequate iron absorption can occur after partial gastrectomy and in diseases of the small intestine such as celiac disease.
        3) Increased iron loss occurs in menstruation (up to 20 mg with each period) and with chronic blood loss (e.g., peptic ulcer disease, colon cancer, repetitive phlebotomy).
        4) Iron deficiency leads to diminished iron stores (decreased ferritin, decreased bone marrow iron stores).

    5) Lack of iron leads to abnormal RBC production.
    6) RBCs are small (microcytic—decreased mean corpuscular volume [MCV]) and pale (hypochromic—decreased mean corpuscular hemoglobin concentration [MCHC]).

- Anemia of chronic disease is the most common anemia in hospitalized patients.
    1) Anemia is associated with underlying inflammatory and neoplastic conditions.
    2) Mechanisms of the anemia are not well understood but include impaired erythropoiesis, relative erythropoietin deficiency, and decreased utilization of iron.
    3) Abnormal hemoglobin synthesis and decreased RBC survival.

- **Macrocytic anemia**

  - Alcoholism is the most common cause of macrocytic anemia, followed by vitamin B_{12} and folate deficiency, liver disease, certain drugs, and hypothyroidism.

  - RBCs have abnormal deoxyribonucleic acid (DNA) synthesis in their precursor marrow stem cells (megaloblastic) with inadequate and abnormal RBC production.

  - Alcohol interferes with RBC maturation and is also associated with vitamin B_{12} and folate deficiency, thus is a common cause of macrocytic anemia.

  - Some patients are unable to absorb vitamin B_{12} due to autoimmune destruction of intrinsic factor, which is made in the stomach and is necessary for normal B_{12} absorption in the ileum (pernicious anemia).

  - Postgastrectomy patients also may have low levels of intrinsic factor and decreased B_{12} absorption.

- **Marrow disease**

  - Marrow disease can result in:
    1) Displacement of the normal erythropoietic stem cells by leukemic blasts or metastatic tumor cells.
    2) Aplasia of the marrow (aplastic anemia).
    3) Abnormal differentiation of the hematopoietic stem cells seen in myelodysplastic syndromes. These abnormalities result in decreased marrow production of RBC.

- **Renal disease**

  - Patients with chronic renal disease have inadequate erythropoietin and diminished RBC production. Treatment with recombinant erythropoietin is highly effective but can result in a state of relative iron deficiency requiring iron supplementation.

- **Immune hemolytic anemia**

  - Binding of antibodies and/or complement to RBC

  - May be mediated by IgG antibody that reacts with RBC at body temperature (warm antibody) or by IgM that reacts with RBC at colder temperatures (cold antibody)

  - 50% are idiopathic; secondary causes
    1) Neoplasia (chronic leukemia, lymphoma)
    2) Collagen vascular disorders (systemic lupus erythematosus, rheumatoid arthritis)
    3) Drugs (α-methyldopa, penicillin)
    4) Infections (mycoplasma, infectious mononucleosis)

  - RBCs may be lysed or are removed from the circulation by the spleen.

- Inherited hemolytic anemia

    - Hereditary spherocytosis
        1) Autosomal dominant inheritance; common in northern Europeans
        2) Defect in the proteins of the red cell cytoskeleton results in spherocytes that have reduced membrane surface area compared with cell volume
        3) RBCs are fragile and are removed by the spleen

- Sickle cell anemia

    - Sickle cell trait occurs in about 8% of African Americans, with the disease present in 0.15%; autosomal recessive inheritance with several degrees of penetrance.

    - Substitution of an amino acid results in intracellular polymerization of the hemoglobin molecule in response to deoxygenation, low temperature, and acidosis.

    - Sickled cells adhere to the endothelium and cause microvascular obstruction with organ infarcts. They are removed by the spleen, which can result in sickle cell crisis with severe pain and profound anemia.

    - Complications include susceptibility to infection and sepsis (splenic dysfunction), delayed growth and development, lung and kidney dysfunction, stroke, skin ulcers, bone necrosis, pulmonary failure, retinal hemorrhage, and narcotic addiction.

- Thalassemias

    - α-thalassemia and β-thalassemia occur in people from Asia, Africa, and the Mediterranean.

    - Hereditary defects in hemoglobin synthesis: α-thalassemia results from decreased production of alpha globin; β-thalassemia is from abnormal beta globin synthesis.

    - Three major clinical categories include carrier, trait, and disease, with varying degrees of microcytic hypochromic anemia with hemolysis and splenic destruction.

PATIENT PRESENTATION

- History:

    - Pregnancy; menorrhagia; unusual diet (e.g., strict vegetarian); alcohol abuse; chronic underlying illness; gastric surgery; drugs; family history; history of pain crises or sepsis.

- Symptoms:

    - Mild cases are often asymptomatic; fatigue; dyspnea on exertion; weakness; palpitations; edema; symptoms of underlying disease; more severe cases may present with congestive heart failure, transient ischemic attacks, syncope, or angina.

    - Iron deficiency is associated with menometrorrhagia or other blood loss (melena, hematochezia, hematemesis, hemoptysis, hematuria); patients may complain of pica for starch, ice, or clay.

    - Sickle cell disease is characterized by pain crises, skin ulcers, and organ infarcts that may be manifested by acute pain, neurologic deficits, or symptoms of other specific organ dysfunction.

- Examination:

    - Pallor; tachycardia; systolic murmurs; edema; splenomegaly; severe anemia may be manifested with evidence of congestive heart failure; signs of alcohol abuse; signs of specific underlying illnesses.

- Iron deficiency is associated with glossitis, angular cheilitis, and brittle nails.

- Sickle cell disease is associated with evidence of organ infarction including focal neurologic deficits, skin ulcers, evidence of infection or kidney disease, and pulmonary congestion (acute chest syndrome).

KEYS TO ASSESSMENT

- Mild anemia may be asymptomatic and should be suspected in infants, women of menstruation age, and pregnant women.

- Alcohol abuse can be associated with direct marrow toxicity, vitamin deficiency, and upper gastrointestinal (GI) blood loss and is a common cause of a mixed microcytic and macrocytic anemia.

- A family history of anemia is common, especially in certain racial and ethnic groups.

- A logical progression of investigative studies should be undertaken (Figure 12-1):

Figure 12-1.

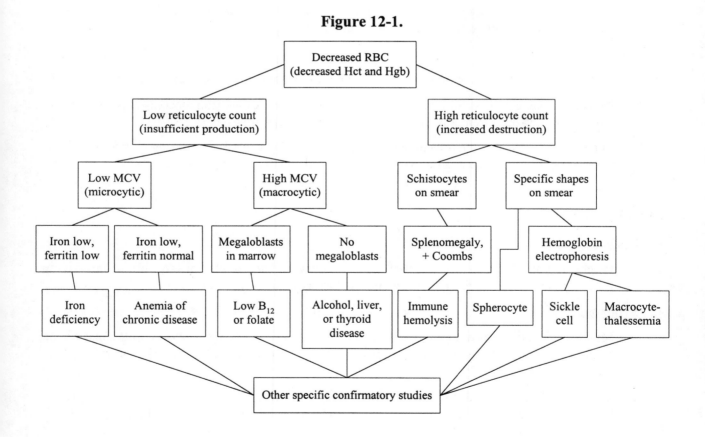

- Specific tests

    - Iron deficiency: serum iron, iron binding capacity, ferritin

    - Megaloblastic anemia: serum and RBC folate, serum B_{12}, and Schilling test

    - Nonmegaloblastic macrocytic anemia: liver function testing, thyroid function tests

    - Immune hemolysis: measurement of specific warm and cold antibodies

- Immune hemolysis: measurement of specific warm and cold antibodies
- Hereditary hemolytic anemias: specific hemoglobin and genetic profiles

KEYS TO MANAGEMENT

- Treating any underlying systemic disease is vital.

- Discontinuation of alcohol intake should be recommended for most patients.

- Transfusion should be limited to those patients with severe anemia and symptoms such as chest pain, dyspnea at rest, congestive heart failure, or neurologic complaints.

- Unexplained iron deficiency in adult males and postmenopausal women must be evaluated thoroughly, including a complete GI work-up.

- Specific therapies

  - Iron deficiency
    1) Oral iron (60 mg three times a day)—GI side effects such as dyspepsia and constipation are common and may require a decrease in dosage.
    2) Normalization of RBC count should occur in 6 to 8 weeks.
    3) Malabsorption or iron losses exceeding the maximal oral replacement are indications for parenteral iron replacement with iron dextran; toxicity is high including anaphylaxis and patients should receive a test dose with epinephrine at the bedside.

  - Anemia of chronic disease (ACD)
    1) Successful treatment of the underlying disease will result in normalization of the HCT.
    2) Erythropoietin therapy has been used in rheumatoid arthritis and is being tested in other causes of ACD.

  - B_{12} and folate deficiency
    1) Oral replacement is indicated in dietary insufficiency without malabsorption; in patients with B12 malabsorption (pernicious anemia, postgastrectomy), B_{12} should be given monthly via intramuscular injection.

  - Bone marrow disease
    1) Treatment of the underlying disease is the only way to improve anemia; however, many of the indicated treatments (e.g., chemotherapy, bone marrow transplant) may result in a transient worsening of the RBC count and may necessitate transfusion.
    2) Myelodysplastic syndromes may respond to androgens, differentiating agents (retinoic acid), or growth factors (erythropoietin).

  - Chronic renal disease
    1) Recombinant erythropoietin with iron supplementation when indicated.

  - Immune hemolysis
    1) Removal of causative drugs and treatment of underlying disease.
    2) Splenectomy may be necessary in some chronic diseases.
    3) Plasmapheresis has been used in cold antibody immune hemolysis.
    4) Steroids and cytotoxic agents (e.g., cyclosporin) may be indicated in severe cases.

  - Hereditary spherocytosis
    1) Splenectomy
    2) Vaccination to reduce the risk of infection after splenectomy

- Sickle cell disease
    1) Pain crises—oxygen, hydration, pain control (patient-controlled analgesia has been effective in emergency room and clinic settings)
    2) Severe anemia (aplastic crisis)—oxygen, transfusion
    3) Chronic therapy—hydroxyurea or 5-azacitidine (increase HgB F) decreases symptoms and extends time between transfusions
    4) Clotrimazole and magnesium help retain RBC water content by reducing potassium and water efflux; early trials have documented decreased sickling when these are used.
    5) Bone marrow transplant has been successful in selected extreme cases.
    6) Monitor and treat the many potential complications.

- Thalassemia
    1) Many patients require no treatment.
    2) Plasmapheresis with transfusions followed by iron chelation therapy are indicated in severe anemia.
    3) Bone marrow transplant has been successful in selected extreme cases.
    4) Successful cord blood transplantation if diagnosed in utero has been reported.

Pathophysiology →

What is going on in the disease process that influences how the patient presents and how he or she should be managed?

Clinical Link

What should you do now that you understand the underlying pathophysiology?

Iron deficiency can result from increased requirement for iron, decreased intake of iron, or increased loss of iron.	Patients at risk for iron deficiency anemia include infants, women of menstrual age, pregnant women, postgastrectomy patients, and patients with chronic blood loss.
Normally, iron is recycled in the body after RBC destruction and is reused to make new RBCs such that only 1 gm of iron is lost and needs to be replaced per day.	Men and postmenstrual women who become iron deficient should be evaluated for sites of blood loss, especially from the GI tract (ulcers, cancers).
Macrocytosis can result form direct toxicity from alcohol, or from abnormal RBC maturation due to B_{12} and/or folate deficiency, which are common in alcoholism.	A patient with macrocytic anemia should be questioned about alcohol use and have B_{12} and folate levels measured in the blood.
Intrinsic factor is produced in the stomach and is necessary for adequate B_{12} absorption in the ileum. Some patients have autoimmune antibodies to intrinsic factor (pernicious anemia); other patients are postgastrectomy and have low levels of intrinsic factor.	Patients with pernicious anemia can be diagnosed by measuring intrinsic factor antibodies. Treatment for these patients and patients who are postgastrectomy require intramuscular injection of B_{12}.
Immune hemolytic anemias are associated with a variety of underlying conditions and the intake of certain drugs; patients will demonstrate autoimmune antibodies in their own RBCs.	Patients with lymphoma, chronic leukemia, rheumatoid arthritis, systemic lupus erythematosus, mycoplasma, or Epstein Barr virus infections, or who are on penicillin or α-methyldopa who develop anemia should be evaluated with a Coombs test for autoantibodies.
Inherited hemolytic anemias can result in significant clinical disease and require specific therapy.	A thorough family history is important in evaluating childhood anemia with testing to identify specific etiologies.

BIBLIOGRAPHY

Abernathy, K. A., & Meuleman, J. R. (1996). Appropriateness of iron prescribing: A retrospective study. *Pharmacotherapy, 16*(3), 473-476.

Allen, L. H. (1997). Pregnancy and iron deficiency: Unresolved issues [review, 93 refs]. *Nutrition Reviews, 55*(4), 91-101.

Anonymous. (1997). Case records of the Massachusetts General Hospital. Weekly clinicopathological exercises. Case 13-1997. A 32-year-old man with IgG antibody and Coombs'-positive hemolytic anemia resistant to corticosteroid therapy [clinical conference]. *New England Journal of Medicine, 336*(17), 1235-1241.

Bampton, P. A., & Holloway, R. H. (1996). A prospective study of the gastroenterological causes of iron deficiency anaemia in a general hospital. *Australian and New Zealand Journal of Medicine, 26*(6), 793-799.

Blaylock, B. (1996). Sickle cell leg ulcers [review, 16 refs]. *MEDSURG Nursing, 5*(1), 41-43.

Bookchin, R. M., & Lew, V. L. (1996). Pathophysiology of sickle cell anemia [review, 61 refs]. *Hematology Oncology Clinics of North America, 10*(6), 1241-1253.

Booth, I. W., & Aukett, M. A. (1997). Iron deficiency anaemia in infancy and early childhood [review, 42 refs]. *Archives of Disease in Childhood, 76*(6), 549-553, discussion 553-554.

Boutry, M., & Needlman, R. (1996). Use of diet history in the screening of iron deficiency. *Pediatrics, 98*(6 Pt 1), 1138-1142.

Bunn, H. F. (1997). Pathogenesis and treatment of sickle cell disease [review, 73 refs]. *New England Journal of Medicine, 337*(11), 762-769.

Burns, D. L., Mascioli, E. A., & Bistrian, B. R. (1996). Effect of iron-supplemented total parenteral nutrition in patients with iron deficiency anemia. *Nutrition, 12*(6), 411-415.

Childs, F., Aukett, A., Darbyshire, P., Ilett, S., & Livera, L. N. (1997). Dietary education and iron deficiency anaemia in the inner city. *Archives of Disease in Childhood, 76*(2), 144-147.

Davenport, J. (1996). Macrocytic anemia [see comments] [review, 30 refs]. *American Family Physician, 53*(1), 155-162.

Dickey, W., Kenny, B. D., McMillan, S. A., Porter, K. G., & McConnell, J. B. (1997). Gastric as well as duodenal biopsies may be useful in the investigation of iron deficiency anaemia. *Scandinavian Journal of Gastroenterology, 32*(5), 469-472.

Drueke, T. B., Barany, P., Cazzola, M., Eschbach, J. W., Grutzmacher, P., Kaltwasser, J. P., Macdougall, I. C., Pippard, M. J., Shaldon, S., & van, W. D. (1997). Management of iron deficiency in renal anemia: Guidelines for the optimal therapeutic approach in erythropoietin-treated patients [review, 69 refs]. *Clinical Nephrology, 48*(1), 1-8.

Eckman, J. R. (1996). Leg ulcers in sickle cell disease [review, 74 refs]. *Hematology Oncology Clinics of North America, 10*(6), 1333-1344.

Eliason, B. C. (1996). RDW to detect iron deficiency [letter; comment]. *Journal of Family Practice, 43*(3), 223-224.

Frewin, R., Henson, A., & Provan, D. (1997). ABC of clinical haematology. Iron deficiency anaemia [see comments] [review, 0 refs]. *British Medical Journal, 314*(7077), 360-363.

Govaker, D. (1996). Low MCV anemia. *Journal of Family Practice, 43*(3), 307.

Gupte, S. C. (1996). Autoimmune haemolytic anaemia: Laboratory aspects. *Indian Journal of Medical Sciences, 50*(5), 155-161.

Harris, L. H., & Gore, S. (1996). Sickle cell disease: Care throughout the life span [review, 30 refs]. *Journal of National Black Nurses Association, 8*(1), 33-44.

Hash, R. B., Sargent, M. A., & Katner, H. (1996). Anemia secondary to combined deficiencies of iron and cobalamin [review, 25 refs]. *Archives of Family Medicine, 5*(10), 585-588.

Hoffbrand, V., & Provan, D. (1997). ABC of clinical haematology. Macrocytic anaemias [see comments] [review, 0 refs]. *British Medical Journal, 314*(7078), 430-433.

Howard, R. J. (1996). Management of sickling conditions in pregnancy [review, 20 refs]. *British Journal of Hospital Medicine, #19-Jul 9;56*(1), 7-10.

Hoyt, R. E. (1997). Popcorn, pica, and impaction. *American Journal of Medicine, 103*(1), 70

Jolobe, O. M. (1997). Iron deficiency in benign duodenal ulcer [letter; comment]. *Lancet, 349*(9054), 809-810.

Kattamis, C. A., & Kattamis, A. C. (1995). Management of thalassemias: Growth and development, hormone substitution, vitamin supplementation, and vaccination [review, 46 refs]. *Seminars in Hematology, 32*(4), 269-279.

Kaul, D. K., Fabry, M. E., & Nagel, R. L. (1996). The pathophysiology of vascular obstruction in the sickle syndromes [review, 153 refs]. *Blood Reviews, 10*(1), 29-44.

King, K. E., & Ness, P. M. (1996). Treating anemia [review, 71 refs]. *Hematology Oncology Clinics of North America, 10*(6), 1305-1320.

Lane, P. A. (1996). Sickle cell disease [review, 108 refs]. *Pediatric Clinics of North America, 43*(3), 639-664.

Looker, A. C., Dallman, P. R., Carroll, M. D., Gunter, E. W., & Johnson, C. L. (1997). Prevalence of iron deficiency in the United States. *Journal of the American Medical Association, 277*(12), 973-976.

Marchiondo, K., & Thompson, A. (1996). Pain management in sickle cell disease [review, 30 refs]. *MEDSURG Nursing, 5*(1), 29-33.

Marignani, M., Angeletti, S., Bordi, C., Malagnino, F., Mancino, C., Delle, F. G., & Annibale, B. (1997). Reversal of long-standing iron deficiency anaemia after eradication of Helicobacter pylori infection. *Scandinavian Journal of Gastroenterology, 32*(6), 617-622.

Pathare, A. V. (1996). Management of autoimmune hemolytic anemia. *Indian Journal of Medical Sciences, 50*(5), 162-167.

Pearson, H. A. (1996). Pharmacologic manipulation of fetal hemoglobin levels in sickle cell diseases and thalassemia: Promise and reality [57 refs]. *Advances in Pediatrics, 43*, 309-334.

Pollitt, E. (1997). Iron deficiency and educational deficiency [review, 12 refs]. *Nutrition Reviews, 55*(4), 133-141.

Richer, S. (1997). A practical guide for differentiating between iron deficiency anemia and anemia of chronic disease in children and adults [29 refs]. *Nurse Practitioner, 22*(4), 82-86.

Robbins, K. C., Senger, J. M., Kerhulas, S., & Fishbane, S. (1997). Iron management in ESRD and the role of the nephrology nurse [review, 23 refs]. *Anna Journal, 24*(2), 265-272, quiz 273-274.

Sanchez-Medal, L., & Loria, A. (1996). Erythrocyte production in iron deficiency anemia. *Acta Haematologica, 96*(3), 146-149.

Seppa, K., Heinila, K., Sillanaukee, P., & Saarni, M. (1996). Evaluation of macrocytosis by general practitioners. *Journal of Studies on Alcohol, 57*(1), 97-100.

Smieja, M. J., Cook, D. J., Hunt, D. L., Ali, M. A., & Guyatt, G. H. (1996). Recognizing and investigating iron-deficiency anemia in hospitalized elderly people. *Canadian Medical Association Journal, 155*(6), 691-696.

Steensma, D. P., & Matteson, E. L. (1997). 80-year-old woman with dizziness. *Mayo Clinic Proceedings, 72*(8), 781-784.

Steinberg, M. H. (1996). Review: Sickle cell disease: Present and future treatment [review, 103 refs]. *American Journal of the Medical Sciences, 312*(4), 166-174.

Stellon, A. J., & Kenwright, S. E. (1997). Iron deficiency anaemia in general practice: presentations and investigations. *British Journal of Clinical Practice, 51*(2), 78-80.

Swain, R. A., & St, C. L. (1997). The role of folic acid in deficiency states and prevention of disease [review, 53 refs]. *Journal of Family Practice, 44*(2), 138-144.

Thomas, V. N., & Westerdale, N. (1997). Sickle cell disease [review, 30 refs]. *Nursing Standard, 11*(25), 40-45, quiz 46-47.

Tibble, J. A., Ireland, A., & Duncan, J. R. (1997). Acute auto immune haemolytic anaemia secondary to hepatitis A infection. *Clinical and Laboratory Haematology, 19*(1), 73-75.

Till, S. H., & Grundman, M. J. (1997). Prevalence of concomitant disease in patients with iron deficiency anaemia. *British Medical Journal, 314*(7075), 206-208.

Tucker, K. L., Mahnken, B., Wilson, P. W., Jacques, P., & Selhub, J. (1996). Folic acid fortification of the food supply. Potential benefits and risks for the elderly population [see comments] [published erratum appears in JAMA 1997 Mar 5;277(9):714]. *Journal fo the American Medical Association, 276*(23), 1879-1885.

Walter, T., Olivares, M., Pizarro, F., & Munoz, C. (1997). Iron, anemia, and infection [review, 89 refs]. *Nutrition Reviews, 55*(4), 111-124.

Wong, W. Y., Elliott-Mills, D., & Powars, D. (1996). Renal failure in sickle cell anemia [review, 69 refs]. *Hematology Oncology Clinics of North America, 10*(6), 1321-1331.

CASE STUDY

ANEMIA

INITIAL HISTORY:
- 47-year-old male presents with the gradual onset of dyspnea on exertion and fatigue.
- Also complaints of frequent dyspepsia with nausea and occasional epigastric pain.
- Has a history of alcohol abuse.

Question 1.
What questions would you like to ask this patient about his symptoms?

ADDITIONAL HISTORY:
- He says he has not had his usual energy levels for several months; the dyspnea has become much worse in the past few weeks.
- He denies chest pain, orthopnea, edema, cough, wheezing, or recent infections.
- He states he has had occasional episodes of hematemesis after drinking heavily, and subsequently had several days of dark stools.
- He drinks up to a 2 six-packs of beer a day for the past 8 years since losing his job.
- Nothing seems to make his breathing any better, but antacids help his epigastric discomfort and dyspepsia.

Question 2.
What questions would you like to ask about his past medical history?

PAST MEDICAL HISTORY:
- He denies any history of cardiac or pulmonary disease.
- He has been diagnosed with a duodenal ulcer in the past and was on "three drugs at once" for a while 2 years ago, but stopped them due to expense.
- His only surgery was a childhood tonsillectomy.
- He does not smoke.
- He is on no medications except over-the-counter antacids.
- He has no known allergies.

PHYSICAL EXAMINATION:
- Thin, pale, white male looking older than stated age in no acute distress
- T = 37 orally; P = 95 and regular; RR = 16 and unlabored; BP = 128/72 sitting, right arm

Skin, HEENT, Neck
- Skin pale without rash; no spider angiomata
- Sclera pale
- PERRL, fundi without lesions
- Pharynx clear without postnasal drainage
- No thyromegaly or adenopathy
- No bruits

Lungs, Cardiac
- Good lung expansion; lungs clear to auscultation and percussion
- PMI at the 5th ICS at the midclavicular line
- RRR with a II/VI systolic ejection murmur at the left sternal border
- No gallops, heaves, or thrills

Abdomen, Rectal
- Abdomen nondistended; bowel sounds present
- Liver 8 cm at the midclavicular line
- Moderate epigastric tenderness without rebound or guarding
- Prostate not enlarged and nontender
- Stool heme positive

Extremities, Neurological
- No joint deformity or muscle tenderness
- No edema
- Alert and oriented x3
- Strength 5/5 throughout and sensation intact
- Gait normal
- DTR 2+ and symmetrical throughout

Question 3.
What are the pertinent positives and negatives on examination?

Question 4.
What is your differential diagnosis at this time?

Question 5.
What laboratory studies should be obtained at this time?

LABORATORY RESULTS:
- WBC = normal with a normal differential; platelets normal
- HCT = 29%; MCV = normal; MCHC = slightly decreased; RDW = markedly increased; reticulocyte count <2%
- Smear with mixed microcytic/hypochronic and macrocytic/normochromic red blood cells; WBC and platelets appear normal
- PT/PTT, liver function tests, electrolytes, and amylase normal
- Upper endoscopy with 2 cm duodenal ulcer with evidence of recent but no acute hemorrhage

Question 6.
What might the hematologic findings indicate and what should be done to further evaluate them?

ADDITIONAL LABORATORY RESULTS:
- Serum iron, total iron binding capacity, saturation, and ferritin all reduced
- Bone marrow biopsy with megaloblastic changes and low iron stores
- Serum folate and red cell folate low; B_{12} normal

Question 7.

Based on these findings, what are the diagnoses for this patient?

Question 8.

How should this patient be managed?

CHAPTER 13

BLEEDING DISORDERS

DEFINITION

- Bleeding disorders can be divided into platelet disorders or coagulation disorders.

- They include many possible etiologies; a few common selected ones include the following:

<u>Platelet disorders</u>
    Thrombocytopenia
    Platelet dysfunction

<u>Coagulation disorders</u>
    Hemophilia
    von Willebrand syndrome
    Liver dysfunction
    Disseminated intravascular coagulation (DIC)

PATHOPHYSIOLOGY

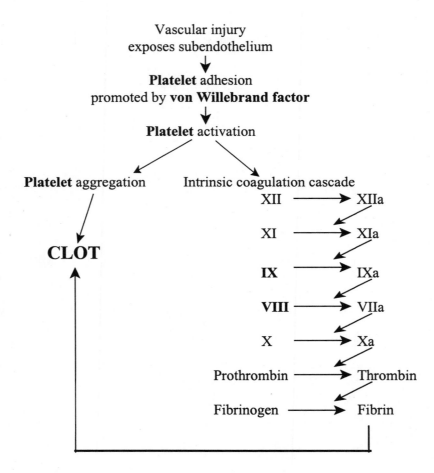

Vascular injury
exposes subendothelium

↓

Platelet adhesion
promoted by **von Willebrand factor**

↓

Platelet activation

Platelet aggregation   Intrinsic coagulation cascade

XII ⟶ XIIa

XI ⟶ XIa

IX ⟶ IXa

VIII ⟶ VIIa

X ⟶ Xa

Prothrombin ⟶ Thrombin

Fibrinogen ⟶ Fibrin

CLOT

- The preceding figure is an overview of the clotting cascade with the components that are frequently involved in bleeding disorders indicated by bold type (see Tables 13-1 and 13-2).

- Bleeding disorders result from a defect in one or more of the steps in clot formation.

- Defects can be due to inadequate quantities of platelets and/or clotting factors, or to the abnormal function of these elements.

- Defects in clotting can be inherited or acquired.

PATIENT PRESENTATION

- In general, platelet disorders present with petechiae. Bleeding usually stops easily with local pressure and does not recur once the pressure is removed, unless the platelet count is very low.

- In general, coagulation factor disorders present with ecchymoses and deep tissue hemorrhages (hematomas, menarthroses). Bleeding is slow to stop with local pressure and tends to recur when pressure is removed.

- History:

  History of easy bruising; history of bleeding after surgery or dental work; family history of bleeding disorder; history of alcohol abuse; history of medication use; history of one of the many diseases listed in Tables 13-1 and 13-2.

- Symptoms:

  "Rashes" (petechaie); bruises (purpura and ecchymoses); mucosal membrane bleeding; gum bleeding with tooth brushing; epistaxis; deep soft tissue hematomas; bleeding into joints; sustained bleeding after injury or surgery; menorrhagia; hematuria; symptoms of liver disease or other underlying systemic illness as in Tables 13-1 and 13-2.

- Examination:

  Petechiae; purpura and ecchymoses; hematomas; heme positive stools; hemathroses; evidence of liver disease or other underlying systemic illness as in Tables 13-1 and 13-2.

DIFFERENTIAL DIAGNOSIS

- See Tables 13-1 and 13-2

Table 13-1. Selected Platelet Problems

THROMBOCYTOPENIA

A. It first must be differentiated from pseudothrombocytopenia (spuriously low platelet count obtained from an automated complete blood count [CBC] counter) and dilutional thrombocytopenia caused by a transfusion greater than 10 to 12 units of red blood cells (RBC)
B. "True" thrombocytopenia can be divided into three major causes:
    1. Diminished production
        a. Congenital
        b. Acute viral infections (cytomegalovirus [CMV], rubella, Epstein-Barr virus [EBV])
        c. Vitamin B_{12}, folate, or iron deficiency
        d. Aplastic anemia
        e. Malignant marrow replacement (e.g., leukemia, metastases)
        f. Drugs (chemotherapeutic agents, estrogens, thiazide diuretics)
        g. Toxins (ethanol, cocaine)
    2. Altered distribution
        a. Hypersplenism (cirrhosis, heart failure, portal vein obstruction).
    3. Increased destruction
        a. Primary autoimmune (immune thrombocytopenic purpura [ITP], HIV-related)
        b. Secondary autimmune (systemic lupus erythematosus, malignancy, drug-induced [heparin, gold, quinidine, furosemide, anticonvulsants, penicillin, sulfonylurea, cimetidine], and infection-induced)
        c. Disseminated intravascular coagulation
        d. Thrombotic thrombocytopenic purpura
        e. Extracorporeal circulation

PLATELET DYSFUNCTION

A. It can be divided into three main categories
    1. Hereditary
        a. Defects in platelet adhesion (Bernard-Soulier syndrome)
        b. Defects in platelet aggregation (Glanzmann's thrombasthenia)
    2. Acquired
        a. Uremia
        b. Myeloproliferative syndromes (leukemia, multiple myeloma)
        c. Autoimmune diseases (collagen vascular disease, platelet antibodies)
        d. Disseminated intravascular coagulation
        e. Liver disease
    3. Drug-induced
        a. Nonsteroidal antiinflammatory drugs
        b. Aspirin
        c. Antibiotics
        d. Psychiatric drugs
        e. Cardiovascular drugs
        f. Anesthetics
        g. Antihistamines

Table 13-2. Selected Coagulation Disorders

HEMOPHILIA

A. Inherited coagulation factor deficiency; sex-linked recessive, primarily affecting males
B. 30% of cases are due to new mutations with no family history
   1. Hemophilia A—factor VIII deficiency
   2. Hemophilia B—factor IX deficiency
   3. Several more rare hereditary factor deficiencies

von WILLEBRAND SYNDROME

A. von Willebrand factor is necessary for proper adhesion between platelets and vascular subendothelial structures and between adjacent platelets
B. Is a carrier for factor VIII; without von Willebrand factor, factor VIII has a very short half life
   1. Inherited
      a. It is the most common inherited bleeding disorder in humans
      b. It is autosomal dominant with variable penetrance
      c. There are three types
         - Type I (moderate decrease in von Willebrand factor and factor VIII)
         - Type II (functional abnormality in von Willebrand factor)
         - Type III (severe decrease in von Willebrand factor and factor VIII)
   2. Acquired
      a. Antibodies to von Willebrand factor
      b. It is associated with many disease states and some drugs: lymphoproliferative disease (leukemia, lymphoma); autoimmune disease (collagen vascular); solid tumors (Wilms tumor); hyperthyroidism; valvular heart disease; dextrans; and valproate

LIVER DYSFUNCTION

A. The liver synthesizes most of the factors of the clotting system except for von Willebrand factor
B. It is also responsible for the clearance of activated clotting or fibrinolytic factors
C. Vitamin K is important in hepatic synthesis of functioning clotting factors
D. Liver disease causes coagulopathy
   1. Impaired factor synthesis
   2. Abnormally functioning clotting factors
   3. Increased consumption of coagulation factors
   4. Disturbed clearance of circulating components of the coagulation system

DISSEMINATED INTRAVASCULAR COAGULATION

A. Disseminated intravascular coagulation is associated with infection, trauma, shock, anoxia, burns, transfusion reactions, and obstetric emergencies.
B. It results in diffuse clotting with depletion of clotting factors, increased clot lysis and production of fibrin degradation products, and subsequent bleeding.
C. Fibrin degradation products are anticoagulants and exacerbate the bleeding disorder.

KEYS TO ASSESSMENT

- The approach to the patient with bleeding disorders should be systematic and include a logical selection of laboratory evaluations.

- Alcohol can cause thrombocytopenia, platelet dysfunction, and coagulation disorders and should be suspected in any bleeding patient.

- After a careful history, family history, and physical exam, obtaining basic laboratories in the majority of patients should include the following:

  - CBC with platelet count

  - Hematocrit (HCT) and hemoglobin (HGB) with RBC indices (mean corpuscular volume [MCV], mean corpuscular hemoglobin concentration [MCHC])

  - Chemistries including blood urea nitrogen (BUN) and creatinine (Cr)

  - Liver function tests (LFTs)

  - Prothrombin time (PT) and partial thromboplastin time (PTT)

- **If thrombocytopenia is found**

  - A blood smear should be obtained
    1) If the smear is normal and PT/PTT are normal, suspect autoimmune or drug-induced thrombocytopenia.
    2) If the smear is normal and the PT/PTT are abnormal, suspect liver dysfunction and evaluate for acute or chronic hepatic disease, and alcohol abuse.
    3) If the smear is abnormal and hemolysis is present, suspect disseminated intravascular coagulation or autoimmune destruction.
    4) If the smear is abnormal and the white blood cell (WBC) and RBC number or appearance is abnormal, suspect bone marrow disease and obtain bone marrow biopsy for diseases such as aplastic anemia, metastases, or leukemia.

- **If platelet disorder is suspected, but platelet count is normal, suspect platelet dysfunction**

  - Template bleeding time in adults or petechiometer test in children confirms platelet dysfunction.

  - Review medication history carefully, check BUN and Cr.

  - Other specific tests of platelet function include aggregation to adenosine, epinephrine, collagen arachidonate, and thrombin; lumiaggregation; and cyclooxygenase.

- **Platelets are normal in number and function but PT and/or PTT are abnormal**

  - If both PT and PTT are abnormal suspect liver disease.

  - If only the PT is abnormal, suspect warfarin use.

  - If only PTT is abnormal, suspect inherited disease or heparin treatment; look again for a family history and measure von Willebrand antigen and factor VIII and IX levels.

KEYS TO MANAGEMENT

- The control of hemorrhage and the stabilization of the patient are of primary importance in acute bleeding.

- All patients should discontinue alcohol intake and nonessential medications especially nonsteroidal antiinflammatory drugs.

- The choice of therapy is based on the underlying causes as follows:

  - Thrombocytopenia
    1) Treat underlying marrow disease; replace nutritional deficit; discontinue causative medication if possible; avoid toxins
    2) Hematopoietic growth factors (IL-3, IL-6, IL-11)
    3) Platelet transfusion—for platelet count ≤10,000/µL; recheck counts at 1 hour and again at 12 to 20 hours after transfusion with a goal of 50,000/µL; single-donor platelets are preferred
    4) Antifibrinolytic therapy with aminocaproic acid can be effective for patients with chronic mucosal bleeding but who do not require frequent platelet transfusions.
    5) Treat underlying disease as appropriate.

  - Platelet dysfunction
    1) Hereditary defects are treated with platelet concentrates.
    2) Acquired defects require discontinuation of associated drugs; dialysis for uremia; or treatment of the underlying systemic illness.

  - Hemophilia
    1) Replacement with concentrated factor VIII or IX for acute hemorrhage
    2) 1-deamino-(8-D-arginine)-vasopressin (DDAVP) will increase factor VIII in mild cases of Hemophilia A.
    3) Antifibrinolytic agents
    4) Liver transplant is effective but not easily available.
    5) Gene therapy is promising.

  - von Willebrand syndrome
    1) The goal is to raise the factor VIII and von Willebrand factor up to 50% of normal levels.
    2) DDAVP indirectly releases von Willebrand factor from endothelial cell storage sites; it is useful for type I and type II; side effects include facial flushing and headache.
    3) Plasma-derived products are used in patients who have type III or who do not respond to DDAVP. They contain factor VIII concentrates with von Willebrand factor multimers.
    4) Fibrinolytic inhibitors and estrogens have been used as adjunctive therapy in some patients.

  - Liver dysfunction
    1) Discontinuation of alcohol and drugs with hepatic toxicity.
    2) Fresh frozen plasma for acute bleeding.
    3) Vitamin K replacement when indicated.
    4) Antifibrinolytic therapy during hepatic surgery.

  - Disseminated intravascular coagulation (DIC)
    1) Reverse underlying pathophysiologic condition.
    2) Support circulation, oxygenation and ventilation, and fluid and electrolyte balance.
    3) Avoid transfusion of blood products unless life-threatening exsanguination occurs.
    4) Heparin or antithrombin III infusion, and plasmapheresis have been used in extreme cases with mixed success.

Pathophysiology →

What is going on in the disease process that influences how the patient presents and how he or she should be managed?

Clinical Link

What should you do now that you understand the underlying pathophysiology?

Platelets and von Willebrand factor are activated by exposure of the vascular subendothelium.	Bleeding from trauma will be excessive and prolonged in both platelet and coagulation factor disorders.
Platelet aggregation is responsible for forming the initial hemostatic barrier; this is subsequently stabilized by fibrin derived form the coagulation factor cascade.	In platelet disorders, bleeding will respond easily to local pressure and will not recur. In coagulation factor disorders, bleeding is slow to respond to local pressure and will recur when the pressure is removed.
Thrombocytopenia can result from the inability to produce platelets or from rapid destruction of platelets.	The differential diagnosis of a decreased platelet count includes toxins, marrow disease, nutritional deficiencies, as well as autoimmune diseases and disseminated intravascular coagulation.
Platelet function can be abnormal even when there are adequate quantities of platelets; this is usually the result of uremia or drug-induced.	Patients with bleeding and petechiae should be evaluated for renal disease and for drug use, especially nonsteroidal antiinflammatories.
Coagulation factor disorders are often inherited (hemophilia and von Willebrand syndrome), resulting in specific factor deficiencies.	Patients with bleeding and an abnormal partial thromboplastin time (PTT) as their only laboratory abnormality should have a careful family history and a measurement of serum factor levels.
Ethanol can affect platelet number and function, as well as the production and function of coagulation factors.	In a patient with bleeding and multiple laboratory abnormalities (decreased platelets, increased bleeding time, abnormal PT and PTT), alcohol abuse and/or liver disease should be suspected.

BIBLIOGRAPHY

Aledort, L. M. (1996). Hemophilia: Yesterday, today, and tomorrow [review, 21 refs]. *Mount Sinai Journal of Medicine, 63*(3-4), 225-235.

Aledort, L. M. (1997). von Willebrand disease: From the bedside to therapy [review, 36 refs]. *Thrombosis and Haemostasis, 78*(1), 562-565.

Berntorp, E. (1996). The treatment of haemophilia, including prophylaxis, constant infusion and DDAVP [review, 54 refs]. *Baillieres Clinical Haematology, 9*(2), 259-271.

Bick, R. L. (1994). Platelet function defects associated with hemorrhage or thrombosis [review, 240 refs]. *Medical Clinics of North America, 78*(3), 577-607.

Bick, R. L. (1996). Disseminated intravascular coagulation: Objective clinical and laboratory diagnosis, treatment, and assessment of therapeutic response [review, 181 refs]. *Seminars in Thrombosis and Hemostasis, 22*(1), 69-88.

Boyd, G. L., Diethelm, A. G., Gelman, S., Langner, R., Laskow, D., Deierhoi, M., & Barber, W. H. (1996). Correcting prolonged bleeding during renal transplantation with estrogen or plasma. *Archives of Surgery, 131*(2), 160-165.

Cahill, M. R., & Colvin, B. T. (1997). Haemophilia [review, 43 refs]. *Postgraduate Medical Journal, 73*(858), 201-206.

Castillo, R., Escolar, G., Monteagudo, J., Aznar-Salatti, J., Reverter, J. C., & Ordinas, A. (1997). Hemostasis in patients with severe von Willebrand disease improves after normal platelet transfusion and normalizes with further correction of the plasma defect. *Transfusion, 37*(8), 785-790.

Chakraverty, R., Davidson, S., Peggs, K., Stross, P., Garrard, C., & Littlewood, T. J. (1996). The incidence and cause of coagulopathies in an intensive care population. *British Journal of Haematology, 93*(2), 460-463.

Chuansumrit, A., Hathirat, P., Pintadit, P., & Isarangkura, P. (1993). Response of patients with bleeding disorder to DDAVP administration. *Southeast Asian Journal of Tropical Medicine and Public Health, 24*(Suppl 1), 174-179.

Connelly, S., & Kaleko, M. (1997). Gene therapy for hemophilia A [review, 70 refs]. *Thrombosis and Haemostasis, 78*(1), 31-36.

DeLoughery, T. G., Liebler, J. M., Simonds, V., & Goodnight, S. H. (1996). Invasive line placement in critically ill patients: Do hemostatic defects matter? *Transfusion, 36*(9), 827-831.

DiMichele, D. (1996). Hemophilia 1996. New approach to an old disease [review, 158 refs]. *Pediatric Clinics of North America, 43*(3), 709-736.

Ewenstein, B. M. (1996). The pathophysiology of bleeding disorders presenting as abnormal uterine bleeding [review, 50 refs]. *American Journal of Obstetrics and Gynecology, 175*(3 Pt 2), 770-777.

Ewenstein, B. M. (1997). von Willebrand's disease [review, 118 refs]. *Annual Review of Medicine, 48*, 525-542.

Gando, S., Kameue, T., Nanzaki, S., & Nakanishi, Y. (1996). Disseminated intravascular coagulation is a frequent complication of systemic inflammatory response syndrome. *Thrombosis and Haemostasis, 75*(2), 224-228.

Gelb, A. B., Roth, R. I., Levin, J., London, M. J., Noall, R. A., Hauck, W. W., Cloutier, M., Verrier, E., & Mangano, D. T. (1996). Changes in blood coagulation during and following cardiopulmonary bypass: Lack of correlation with clinical bleeding. *American Journal of Clinical Pathology, 106*(1), 87-99.

Giannelli, F., & Green, P. M. (1996). The molecular basis of haemophilia A and B [review, 64 refs]. *Baillieres Clinical Haematology, 9*(2), 211-228.

Goad, K. E., & Gralnick, H. R. (1996). Coagulation disorders in cancer [review, 308 refs]. *Hematology Oncology Clinics of North America, 10*(2), 457-484.

Jamieson, G. A. (1997). Pathophysiology of platelet thrombin receptors [review, 49 refs]. *Thrombosis and Haemostasis, 78*(1), 242-246.

Kleinert, D., Orto, C., Gioia, K., & Hannan, M. (1997). Von Willebrand disease: A nursing perspective [review, 14 refs]. *Journal of Obstetric, Gynecologic, and Neonatal Nursing, 26*(3), 271-276.

Ljung, R. C. (1996). Prenatal diagnosis of haemophilia [review, 23 refs]. *Baillieres Clinical Haematology, 9*(2), 243-257.

Lusher, J. M. (1996). Recombinant clotting factor concentrates [review, 51 refs]. *Baillieres Clinical Haematology, 9*(2), 291-303.

Lusher, J. M. (1996). Screening and diagnosis of coagulation disorders [review, 25 refs]. *American Journal of Obstetrics and Gynecology, 175*(3 Pt 2), 778-783.

Mannucci, P. M. (1996). The choice of plasma-derived clotting factor concentrates [review, 75 refs]. *Baillieres Clinical Haematology, 9*(2), 273-290.

Mazurier, C., & Meyer, D. (1996). Molecular basis of von Willebrand disease [review, 58 refs]. *Baillieres Clinical Haematology, 9*(2), 229-241.

Menache, D., & Aronson, D. L. (1997). New treatments of von Willebrand disease: Plasma derived von Willebrand factor concentrates [review, 37 refs]. *Thrombosis and Haemostasis, 78*(1), 566-570.

Miller, J. L. (1996). Platelet-type von Willebrand disease [review, 42 refs]. *Thrombosis and Haemostasis, 75*(6), 865-869.

Nichols, W. C., & Ginsburg, D. (1997). von Willebrand disease [review, 265 refs]. *Medicine, 76*(1), 1-20.

Nishino, M., & Yoshioka, A. (1997). The revised classification of von Willebrand disease including the previously masqueraded female hemophilia A (type 2N) [review, 64 refs]. *International Journal of Hematology, 66*(1), 21-30.

Noris, M., Benigni, A., Boccardo, P., Aiello, S., Gaspari, F., Todeschini, M., Figliuzzi, M., & Remuzzi, G. (1993). Enhanced nitric oxide synthesis in uremia: Implications for platelet dysfunction and dialysis hypotension. *Kidney International, 44*(2), 445-450.

Ono, S., Mochizuki, H., & Tamakuma, S. (1996). A clinical study on the significance of platelet-activating factor in the pathophysiology of septic disseminated intravascular coagulation in surgery. *American Journal of Surgery, 171*(4), 409-415.

Or, R., Elad, S., Shpilberg, O., & Eldor, A. (1996). Low molecular weight heparin stimulates megakaryocytopoiesis in bone-marrow transplantation patients. *American Journal of Hematology, 53*(1), 46-48.

Pasi, K. J. (1996). Gene therapy for haemophilia [review, 31 refs]. *Baillieres Clinical Haematology, 9*(2), 305-317.

Pereira, S. P., Langley, P. G., & Williams, R. (1996). The management of abnormalities of hemostasis in acute liver failure [review, 193 refs]. *Seminars in Liver Disease, 16*(4), 403-414.

Rodeghiero, F., Castaman, G., & Mannucci, P. M. (1996). Prospective multicenter study on subcutaneous concentrated desmopressin for home treatment of patients with von Willebrand disease and mild or moderate hemophilia A. *Thrombosis and Haemostasis, 76*(5), 692-696.

Rohaly-Davis, J., & Johnston, K. (1996). Hematologic emergencies in the intensive care unit [review, 23 refs]. *Critical Care Nursing Quarterly, 18*(4), 35-43.

Schwarz, H. P., Turecek, P. L., Pichler, L., Mitterer, A., Mundt, W., Dorner, F., Roussi, J., & Drouet, L. (1997). Recombinant von Willebrand factor [review, 29 refs]. *Thrombosis and Haemostasis, 78*(1), 571-576.

Scott-Timperley, L. J., & Haire, W. D. (1997). Autoimmune coagulation disorders [review, 53 refs]. *Rheumatic Diseases Clinics of North America, 23*(2), 411-423.

Sham, R. L., & Francis, C. W. (1994). Evaluation of mild bleeding disorders and easy bruising [review, 73 refs]. *Blood Reviews, 8*(2), 98-104.

Smith, M. P., Rice, K. M., Bromidge, E. S., Lawn, M., Beresford-Webb, R., Spence, K., Khair, K., Hann, I., & Savidge, G. F. (1997). Continuous infusion therapy with very high purity von Willebrand factor concentrate in patients with severe von Willebrand disease. *Blood Coagulation and Fibrinolysis, 8*(1), 6-12.

Staudinger, T., Locker, G. J., & Frass, M. (1996). Management of acquired coagulation disorders in emergency and intensive-care medicine [review, 192 refs]. *Seminars in Thrombosis and Hemostasis, 22*(1), 93-104.

Tallman, M. S. (1996). Deciphering the pathogenesis of coagulation dysfunction in leukemia [see comments]. *Leukemia Research, 20*(1), 13-16.

Vajo, Z., & Sreter, L. (1996). Management of hemophilias—Gene therapy to come? [review, 27 refs]. *Acta Physiologica Hungarica, 84*(2), 191-198.

Wahba, A., Black, G., Koksch, M., Rothe, G., Preuner, J., Schmitz, G., & Birnbaum, D. E. (1996). Cardiopulmonary bypass leads to a preferential loss of activated platelets. A flow cytometric assay of platelet surface antigens. *European Journal of Cardio-Thoracic Surgery, 10*(9), 768-773.

Zauli, G., & Catani, L. (1995). Human megakaryocyte biology and pathophysiology [review, 304 refs]. *Critical Reviews in Oncology Hematology, 21*(1-3), 135-157.

CASE STUDY*

BLEEDING DISORDERS

INITIAL HISTORY:
- Mr. H. is a 58-year-old male who has just been transferred in stable condition at 2:15 p.m. from the operating room to the intensive care unit (ICU) after undergoing an uncomplicated but lengthy (5 hour) right lung decortication procedure.
- His estimated blood loss during the procedures was 550 cc, and he received approximately 2500 cc of IV fluid during the operation.
- The initial drainage amount from his right pleural chest tube on arrival to the ICU is 120 cc.

Question 1.

What essential information do you want to be sure to receive in report from the anesthesiologist and surgeon?

ADDITIONAL HISTORY:
- Mr. H. has a previous medical history significant for a right lower lobectomy for a benign tumor resection, complicated by right empyema.
- He has a 40 pack/year smoking history (quit 3 years ago).
- He is otherwise in good health.
- Mr. H.'s home medications include only PRN albuterol inhaler use.
- He has no medication allergies.
- His surgery progressed with moderate difficulty as the visceral pleura was badly scarred.

HIS INITIAL PHYSICAL EXAMINATION ON ARRIVAL TO THE ICU FROM THE OPERATING ROOM:
- Rectal T is 35.8°C; P = 90 and regular
- No spontaneous respirations on ventilator at intermittent mandatory ventilation (IMV) 10 breaths/minute
- BP via right radial arterial line 112/60, correlates with cuff

Skin
- Grossly intact, pale, cool, dry
- 3 second capillary refill throughout
- Good turgor
- Right thoracotomy surgical dressing intact with scant bloody drainage present

---

* **Kathryn Ballenger, RN, MSN, CCRN, FNP, contributed this case study.**

Pulmonary
- #8.0 oral endotracheal tube, 23 cm @ lips
- Fully ventilated with FIO_2 = 1.00, IMV = 10, positive end-expiratory pressure (PEEP) = 5; O_2 sat = 100%
- No spontaneous respirations present
- Bilateral breath sounds present, slightly diminished in the bases
- Right lateral pleural chest tube at 20 cm H_2O suction via pleurovac system with 120 cc bloody drainage present, no air leak

Cardiovscular
- S_1 S_2 clear; no murmurs or gallops present
- Pulses full throughout

Gastrointestinal
- Left nasogastric tube to low constant suction, minimal drainage
- Hypoactive bowel sounds

Genitourinary
- Foley draining clear yellow urine
- Specific gravity 1.010

Neurological
- Remains anesthetized and sedated, unable to communicate
- Glasgow coma scale = 2T; PERRL = 2 mm

ADDITIONAL ASSESSMENTS:
- Endotracheal suction reveals scant, thin white secretions
- Initial arterial blood gas: pH = 7.45; $PaCO_2$ = 36; PaO_2 = 433
- Electrocardiogram monitor lead II shows normal sinus rhythm, no ectopy, rate = 92

VASCULAR ACCESS:
- Right subclavian triple lumen catheter—proximal port with D_5W @ KVO, middle heparin locked, distal with central venous pressure (CVP) monitor and flush per protocol, CVP = 6 mmHg
- Bilateral upper extremity IV is with normal saline infusing at KVO from operating room

POSTOPERATIVE COURSE:
- Mr. H. is stable and receives the routine postoperative care and monitoring. He is placed on an FIO_2 of 50% to begin normalizing his arterial blood gases after transport.
- At 2:45 p.m. (after 30 minutes), you note that his chest tube output is an additional 175 cc.

Question 2.
What will you evaluate related to his blood loss at this time?

RAPID ASSESSMENT AND LABORATORY RESULTS:
- No evidence of hypovolemia.
- Postoperative chest radiograph reveals proper endotracheal tube and chest tube placement, bilateral lung expansion, and no evidence of hemothorax.
- Initial postoperative laboratory results:
    - Hemoglobin = 6.8 mg/dl; hematocrit = 20%
    - Platelets = 85,000/mm^3
    - PT/PTT are normal
    - His electrolytes are within normal limits, except for potassium of 3.4 mEq/l and an ionized calcium of 3.8 mg/dl

Question 3.
What do these values represent?

Question 4.
What is your primary concern related to this patient's chest tube drainage?

Question 5.
What actions should be taken at this time to attempt to reduce his postoperative hemorrhage?

CONTINUED POSTOPERATIVE COURSE:
- At 3:00 p.m., he has an additional 200 cc of chest tube drainage (postoperative total = 495 cc).
- In addition to the normal postoperative volume resuscitation, the patient receives a rapid transfusion of 2 units packed red blood cells, 2 units fresh frozen plasma, 1 unit single donor platelets, and 1 ampule of calcium chloride intravenously.

ADDITIONAL POSTOPERATIVE DEVELOPMENTS:
- At 4:00 p.m., his chest drainage equals 275 cc (770 cc total). His hematological studies at this time are:
  - Hemoglobin = 7.0 mg/dl; HCT = 21%
  - PLTs = 65,000/mm^3
  - PT = 15 sec; PTT = 42 sec
- Mr. H. additionally receives 1 unit packed red blood cells and 2 units fresh frozen plasma.

Question 6.
What is your assessment of the situation at this time?

Question 7.
What other laboratory information will guide your decision-making at this time?

CONTINUED POSTOPERATIVE COURSE:
- At 4:30 p.m., Mr. H.'s chest tube drainage is 220 ccs (postoperative total = 990 ccs). Due to his continued excessive bleeding, he is emergently returned to the operating room for re-exploration.
- While Mr. H. is in the operating room undergoing re-exploration, his blood work returns as follows:
  - Hemoglobin = 6.2 mg/dl; HCT = 19%
  - PLTs = 48,000/mm^3
  - PTT = 47 sec; PT = 19 sec
  - Fibrinogen = 120 mg/dl
  - Fibrinogen degradation products = 150 mcg/ml
  - D-dimer = 220 ng/ml
  - Ca^{++} = 3.9 mg/dl

Question 8.

What does this lab work indicate?

Question 9.

What are the possible causes for Mr. H.'s bleeding problem?

Question 10.

Based on this information, what other information do you want to acquire?

Question 11.

What are the recommended therapeutic approaches in the management of Mr. H.'s DIC-like coagulopathy?

AFTER RETURNING FROM THE OPERATING ROOM:

- Mr. H. returns from the operating room at 5:15 p.m., after his re-exploration procedure.
- The surgeon reports that no single source of bleeding could be identified, and that there was heavy generalized diffuse oozing of blood from the chest wall. The surgeon's diagnosis of the bleeding problem is DIC, and orders that all blood products be placed on hold.
- Care of Mr. H.'s bleeding problem is supportive in nature, with administration of crystalloid fluids as needed to maintain adequate volume status.

CONTINUED POSTOPERATIVE CARE:

- Over the next 6 hours, Mr. H.'s chest tube drainage improves from 210 cc per hour to 45 cc per hour.
- He does not demonstrate other evidence of a transfusion reaction.
- His hematocrit reaches a low of 17, and on the first postoperative day he is gently transfused 2 units of packed red blood cells without complication to bring his hematocrit over 30.
- He is placed on an iron supplement, and he is instructed in dietary measures which will help improve his postoperative anemia.

CHAPTER 14

URINARY TRACT INFECTION*

DEFINITION

- Urinary tract infection (UTI) is an inflammation of the urinary tract epithelium in response to a pathogen.

- Cystitis is an infection of the bladder producing characteristic symptoms including dysuria, lower abdominal or suprapubic discomfort, and frequency of urination.

- Bacteriuria is the presence of bacteria in the urine; this condition may or may not be associated with UTI symptoms.

- Pyelonephritis is an infection of the upper urinary tracts, including the renal pelvis and renal parenchyma, also called afebrile UTI or upper tract UTI.

- Urosepsis is a systemic extension of febrile UTI; urine and blood cultures are positive for a common pathogen.

- Isolated urinary tract infection is an initial infection or an infection that is remote in time from previous episodes.

- Recurrent urinary tract infection is a new infection following successful resolution of previous episode(s).

- Persistant urinary infection is continued bacteriuria caused by inappropriate or incomplete therapy, or arising from bacterial persistence within some focus within the urine, such as a calculus or a foreign object.

- Nosocomial urinary infection is a hospital-acquired UTI.

- Complicated urinary tract infection is associated with hematuria, fever, or an infection in the patient with an indwelling catheter, obstruction, urinary calculus, or anatomic abnormality of the urinary system.

EPIDEMIOLOGY

- 6% of young adult women have bacteriuria at any given time; the majority are asymptomatic.

- Incidence of symptomatic urinary tract infections among young adult women are approximately 0.2 per month.

---

* Mikel Gray, PhD, CUNP, CCCN, FAAN, contributed this chapter.

- Prevalence increases to approximately 20% to community-dwelling elderly women (>65 years of age).

- Prevalence of young adult men is <1%; it increases to approximately 10% of community-dwelling elderly men.

- Prevalence of bacteriuria among functionally-impaired elderly women and men is 24%, as compared to 12% of nonfunctionally-impaired residents.

PATHOPHYSIOLOGY

- Routes of infection—ascending urethral course is most common

- The pathogen typically arises from the intestinal bacterial reservoir—it may arise from vaginal flora or cutaneous source.

- Pyelonephritis occurs when bacteria ascends from lower to upper urinary tract via the ureter.

- UTI via a hematogenous route is uncommon; it occasionally occurs with septicemia from *Staphlacoccus aureus* from oral infections or from *Candida fungemia*; lymphogenous infection rarely occurs from severe bowel infection or retroperitoneal abscess, particularly when obstruction is present.

Source	Common Pathogen
Community-acquired	Intestinal flora *Escherichia coli* (accounts for 85% of all infections) *Proteus* *Klebsiella* *Enterococcus fecalis* *Staphylococcus saprophytics* Cutaneous/vaginal flora *Staphylococcus epidermidis* *Candida albicans*
Nosocomial infections	*Eschericia coli* (accounts for 50% of all infections) *Klebsiella* *Enterobacter* *Citrobacter* *Pseudomonas aeruginosa* *Providencia* *Enterococcus fecalis* *Staphylococcus epidermidis*

- Virulence of pathogen is directly related to its ability to adhere to epithelial cells.

- Adherence is related to host epithelial cell recpetivity; this genotypic predisposition primary affects women.

- Urine osmolality, urea concentration, and pH influence bacterial reproduction; a dilute urine or a concentrated urine with a low pH are bacteriostatic

- Glucosuria associated with diabetes may increase bacterial reproduction and urinary tract infection risk.

- The average urinary pH of a pregnant woman tends to favor bacterial reproduction more than the average urinary pH of a nonpregnant woman.

- Pyelonephritis leads to immunoglobulin synthesis and antibodies in the urine; cystitis produces little or no detectable serologic response.

- Obstruction and vesicoureteral reflux increase the risk of febrile urinary infection.

- Voiding dysfunction (particularly detrusor sphincter dyssynergia) increases risk of cystitis and febrile urinary tract infection.

PATIENT PRESENTATION

- History:

  Previous urinary tract infection; history of "gastroenteritis" as child; congenital defect of urinary system; urinary retention; recent onset of sexual activity (women).

- Symptoms:

  Lower abdominal discomfort or nausea in child; dysuria, urinary frequency, lower abdominal, or suprapubic discomfort in young adult; lower abdominal discomfort or urinary incontinence in elderly adult; symptoms of cystitis and flank pain with chills and sweating, nausea, and vomiting with pyelonephritis; urine may or may not be odorous or cloudy.

- Examination:

  Suprapubic discomfort or no physical findings with cystitis, costovertebral angle tenderness, fever, dehydration with pyelonephritis.

DIFFERENTIAL DIAGNOSIS

- Vaginitis

- Urethritis

- Interstitial cystitis

- Pelvic pain

- Prostatitis

- Gastroenteritis (particularly in children with pylonephritis)

- Urinary calculus

- Urinary system tumor (may be confused with hemorrhagic cystitis)

KEYS TO ASSESSMENT

- Urine specimen collection—clean catch urine adequate for community-dwelling patients; catheterized specimen for patients with complicated infection, persistent bacteriuria, immobile patient, individual with urinary or fecal incontinence requiring incontinent brief

- Centrifuge urine for 5 minutes at 2000 rpm prior to dipstick urinalysis and microscopic examination.

- Urine culture and sensitivity if:

    - Patient with first febrile infection, recurrent afebrile infection (more than 1 per year), complicated urinary tract infection, history of urinary system conditions including congenital defect, urinary calculi

    - The dipstick urinalysis shows nitrates and leukocytes

    - Bacteriuria and pyuria are seen on microscopic examination

- An ultrasound and voiding cystourethrogram for an infant or child with first febrile urinary tract infection or recurrent cystitis

- Imaging study in otherwise healthy adult with first febrile UTI, persistent bacteriuria, or suspicion of foreign body or obstruction

KEYS TO MANAGEMENT

- **Prevention**

    - Avoid dehydration; the recommended daily allowance (RDA) for fluids is 30 ml/kg/day

    - Avoid constipation (encourage fluids, dietary fiber, and recreational exercise)

    - Manage urinary retention or bladder outlet obstruction

    - Teach women about proper hygiene after toileting and urination after intercourse

    - Treat infections early, particularly in patients with compromised immune function or those with urinary retention, or voiding dysfunction

- **Acute urinary tract infection**

    - Empiric treatment is for first time infection in otherwise healthy, young women; begin empiric treatment before the culture and sensitivity results for complicated or febrile urinary tract infection.

    - Antipyretics and hospitalization with intravenous fluids is necessary if pyelonephritis is associated with significant nausea and vomiting or urosepsis.

    - Select an antibiotic according to the culture and sensitivity report (when indicated), frequency of administration, risk of associated vaginitis, cost to the patient, and risk of promoting bacterial resistance (Table 14-1).

    - Emphasize compliance with antibiotic course; treat uncomplicated infection for 3 days, complicated infection for 7 days, and febrile infections for 14 days

    - Supplement antibiotic treatment with urinary analgesic (Pyridium is available as over-the-counter medication) or a combination agent such as Urised.

    - Begin prophylactic treatment using an antifungal cream for woman with a history of vaginitis when receiving antibiotic therapy, unless nitrofurantion is administered.

    - Encourage adequate fluid intake

    - Avoid bladder irritants

Table 14-1.

Antibiotic	Typical Dosage and Administration Schedule	Implications
Trimethoprim-Sulfamethoxazole (TMP-SMX)	1 double strength tablet PO BID	- BID dosage promotes compliance - Relatively inexpensive - Risk of secondary vaginitis
Nitrofurantoin (Macrodantin or Macrobid)	Macrodantin given as 50 to 100 mg PO QID; Macrobid given as 1 capsule PO BID	- BID dosage promotes compliance - More expensive than TMP-SMX - Risk of vaginitis negligible
Ampicillin	500 mg QID	- QID dosage may reduce compliance - Relatively inexpensive - Risk of secondary vaginitis
Amoxicillin	500 mg PO TID	- TID dosage may slightly reduce compliance - Relatively inexpensive compared to TMP-SMX, other penicillins
Cephalexin	500 mg PO QID	- QID dosage may reduce compliance - Relatively expensive when compared to penicillins, TMX-SMZ - Risk of secondary vaginitis
Ciprofloxacin	500 mg PO BID	- BID dosage promotes compliance - Relatively expensive - Risk of secondary vaginitis - Reserved for complicated infections
Norfloxacin	400 mg PO BID	- BID dosage promotes compliance - Relatively expensive - Risk of secondary vaginitis - Reserved for complicated infections

- **Prevention of recurrent infection**
  - Obtain a culture and sensitivity with persistent symptoms.
  - Obtain an imaging study (ultrasound, kidneys/ureter/bladder [KUB], intravenous pyelogram) of hematuria if it persists, or refer the patient to a urologist.
  - Refer to urologist if infection with *Proteus, Klebsiella* or *Pseudomonas* species or obtain imaging study to rule out urinary calculi.
  - Rule out prostatitis in men.
  - Refer to a urologist when an explanation of persistent bacteriuria is not identified.
  - Obtain an upper urinary tract imaging (ultrasonography, intravenous pyelography) study with febrile urinary tract infection.
  - Consider low-dose, suppressive therapy for recurrent, febrile infections
  - Consider self-start, intermittent therapy (where the patient is taught to obtain a culture with a dip-slide device followed by empiric treatment)
  - Consider postintercourse suppressive antibiotic therapy when the relation between intercourse and UTI is established

Pathophysiology

What is going on in the disease process that influences how the patient presents and how he or she should be managed?

→

Clinical Link

What should you do now that you understand the underlying pathophysiology?

Bacterial adherence is influenced by genotypic epithelial cell receptivity.	There is a risk for recurrent urinary tract infections, particularly among otherwise healthy adult women.
Ascending urethral course is the most common route of bacterial invasion.	Risk of recurrent infection is increased with sexual intercourse; teach the patient to urinate immediately following intercourse and to have proper hygiene following urination. Teach postcoital suppression antibiotic therapy if indicated.
Dilute urine is bacteriostatic.	Adequate fluid intake.
Gastrointestinal flora account for the majority of pathogens in the community-dwelling population.	Maintain proper hygiene following urination and avoid constipation, which increases intestinal bacterial reservoir.
Risk of pyelonephritis is greater in patients with voiding dysfunction, foreign object in urinary system (including indwelling catheter), viscoureteral reflux, and diabetics.	Identify and manage risk factors. Treat UTI promptly in the patient at-risk; treat complicated infection for 7 days and febrile UTI for 14 days.

BIBLIOGRAPHY

Barry, H. C., Ebell, M. H., & Hickner, J. (1997). Evaluation of suspected urinary tract infection in ambulatory women: A cost utility analysis of office-based strategies. *Journal of Family Practice, 44*, 49-60.

Bjornson, D. C., Rovers, J. P., Burian, J. A. & Hall, N. L. (1997). Pharmacoepidemiology of urinary tract infection in Iowa medicaid patients in long-term care facilities. *Annals of Pharmacotherapy, 31*, 837-841.

Childs, S. J., & Egan, R. J. (1996). Bacteriuria and urinary infections in the elderly. *Urologic Clinics of North American, 23*, 45-54.

Cockerill, F. R., & Edson, R. S. (1991). Trimethoprim-sulfamethoxazole. *Mayo Clinic Proceedings, 66*, 1249-1251.

Gray, M. L. (1992). *Genitourinary disorders* (pp. 52-63). St. Louis: Mosby.

Gray, M. L. (1997). Genitourinary system. In S. M. Thompson, G. K. MacFarland, J. E. Hirsh, & S. Tucker (Eds.), *Clinical Nursing* (pp. 1007-1014). St. Louis: Mosby.

Hassay, K. A. (1995). Effective management or urinary discomfort. *Nurse Practitioner, 20*, 36, 39-40, 41-44.

Leiner, S. (1995). Recurrent urinary tract infection in otherwise healthy adult women. Rational strategies for work-up and management. *Nurse Practitioner, 20*, 48, 51-52, 54-56.

Loening-Bacucke, V. (1997). Urinary incontinence and urinary tract infection and their resolution with treatment of chronic constipation of childhood. *Pediatrics, 100*, 228-232.

Mikhail, M. S., & Anyaegbunam, A. (1995). Lower urinary tract dysfunction in pregnancy: A review. *Obstetrical and Gynecological Survey, 50*, 675-683.

Millar, L. K., & Cox, S. M. (1997). Urinary tract infections complicating pregnancy. *Infectious Disease Clinics of North America, 11*, 13-26.

Nicolle, L. E. (1997). A practical guide to the management of complicated urinary tract infection. *Drugs, 53*, 583-592.

Sale, P. G. (1995). Genitourinary infection in older women. *Journal of Obstetric, Gynecologic, and Neonatal Nursing, 24*, 769-775.

Schaeffer, A. J. (1996). Urinary tract infections. In J. Y. Gillenwater, J. T. Grayuhack, S. S. Howards, & J. D. Duckett (Eds.), *Adult and pediatric urology* (pp. 219-288). St. Louis: Mosby.

Schaeffer, A. J. (1998). Infections of the urinary tract. In P. C. Walsh, A. B. Retik, E. D. Vaughan, & A. J. Wein (Eds.), *Campbell's Urology* (pp. 533-613). Philadeliphia: Saunders.

Webb, J. A. (1997). The role of imaging in adult acute urinary tract infection. *European Radiology, 7*, 837-843.

CASE STUDY

URINARY TRACT INFECTION*

INITIAL HISTORY:
- 27-year-old woman
- Symptoms of urgency to urinate, frequent urination, and urethral burning during urination has persisted for 48 hours
- She awoke from sleep with urgency and suprapubic discomfort 2 nights ago.
- Urine now has strong odor and cloudy appearance

Question 1.
What is your differential diagnosis based on the information you have now?

Question 2.
What other questions would you like to ask now?

ADDITIONAL HISTORY:
- Recurring urinary tract infections since she married at age 22 years.
- Prior UTI associated with similar symptoms.
- Denies history of febrile or hemorrhagic UTI.
- Three previous episodes over past 2 years.
- May be associated with strenuous physical exertion and sexual intercourse.
- No other medical history.
- She reports an allergy to penicillin which causes a "rash" and "trouble breathing."

---

* **Mikel Gray, PhD, CUNP, CCCN, FAAN, contributed this case study.**

Question 3.
Now what do you think of her history?

PHYSICAL EXAMINATION:
- Well-nourished female experiencing mild discomfort
- Tenderness on palpation of abdominal pelvic area; physical examination otherwise unremarkable
- T = 98.6 orally; BP = 114/64; P = 68; RR = 12 BPM

Question 4.
What laboratory studies are indicated in this patient?

LABORATORY RESULTS:
- Dipstick urinalysis:
  - Color: dark yellow
  - Specific gravity = 1.030
  - pH = 6.5
  - Protein: negative
  - Glucose: negative
  - Ketones: negative
  - Bilirubin: negative
  - Trace occult blood
  - Leukocytes: Large amount
  - Nitrates: positive
  - Urobilinogen: negative

- Microscopic examination:
  - WBC: too numerous to count (TNTC)/HPF (high power field)
  - Bacteria: TNTC
  - RBC: 3 to 4/HPF
  - Casts: negative
- Urine culture:
  - *Escherichia coli*: >104 cfu/ml
  - Organism sensitive to ampicillin, nitrofurantoin, TMX-SMZ, ciprofloxacin, cephalexin

Question 5.

What additional studies are indicated in this patient?

Question 6.

Based on these findings, what therapy would you initiate?

Question 7.

What measures would you recommend to reduce the risk of a recurrence?

CHAPTER 15

PEPTIC ULCER DISEASE

DEFINITION

- Peptic ulcer disease (PUD) is defined as defects in the gastrointestinal mucosa extending through the muscularis mucosae occurring in the esophagus, stomach, or duodenum.

- Peptic ulcers are associated with a number of conditions, however, there are two common forms:
    - Those associated with *Helicobacter pylori* (*H. pylori*) infection
    - Those associated with nonsteroidal antiinflammatory drug (NSAID) intake

- NSAIDS and alcohol may exacerbate ulcers of *H. pylori* origin.

- Other less common forms occur with acid hypersecretory syndromes (gastrinoma, mastocytosis), herpes simplex virus [HSV] type I, cytomegalovirus [CMV], duodenal obstruction, vascular insufficiency, and radiation and chemotherapy associated ulcers.

EPIDEMIOLOGY

- Lifetime prevalence of PUD is 5% to 10%; there is increasing risk with age.

- Duodenal ulcer (DU) is more common than gastric ulcer (GU) and occurs in younger patients; it affects males more often than females.

- Gastric ulcers have a peak incidence at age 55 to 65 and are rare before age 40; they occur in men at the same rate as women.

- Hospitalization rates for PUD are declining, but complication rates (perforation, hemorrhage, and death) are relatively stable.

- Genetics appear to play a role with definite familial aggregation , but no specific genetic markers have been identified.

- Psychological stress has been associated with PUD and increased gastric acid secretion with acute gastric erosions.

- *H. pylori* can be identified in 95% of DU and 85% of GU.

- *H. pylori* prevalence varies with age and socioeconomic group:
    - In developed countries, seroprevalence increases with age (85% by age 60)
    - Seroprevalence is inversely correlated with socioeconomic status (lowest income class = 100% prevalence; highest = <1%)

- The prevalence is higher in African Americans and Hispanics.
- The spread of infection through unsanitary conditions is recognized, but the specific mode of transmission is unknown.

- NSAID use is estimated to cause 100,000 hospitalizations and 10,000 to 20,000 deaths per year due to NSAID-related gastrointestinal (GI) complications in the United States.
- Risk of gastric and duodenal ulceration is 11% to 13% for patients on daily NSAIDS; it is much higher if patients are also on corticosteroids.
- Other risk factors include type O blood group, smoking, alcohol, chronic pulmonary disease, reflux esophagitis, cirrhosis, and renal failure and transplantation.
- There are no clear links between diet (including coffee) and PUD risk.

PATHOPHYSIOLOGY

- Ulcers form when there is a breakdown in the mucosal defense and repair mechanisms that normally protect the stomach and duodenum from the acid and peptic environment of the upper GI tract.
- Defense mechanisms:
  - A layer of mucus and bicarbonate over the surface of the mucosa provides a buffer and prevents pepsin diffusion into the mucosal layer.
  - A mucosal barrier of tight cellular junctions, growth factors, and membrane transport systems removes excess ions, preventing back-diffusion of hydrogen ions into the mucosa.
  - A vigorous supply of blood to the mucosa removes excess hydrogen ion and maintains nutrient flow for normal cellular function and repair.
- *H. pylori* and NSAIDs cause tissue injury resulting in defects in one or more of these defense mechanisms with subsequent exposure of the mucosa to acid and pepsin.
- *H. pylori* causes tissue injury via:
  - Production of lipopolysaccharide (LPS, endotoxin), other toxic proteins (VacA)
  - Stimulation of the release of inflammatory mediators (IL-1, IL-8, TNF)
  - Induction of chronic active gastritis and atrophic gastritis
  - Increasing gastrin, pepsin, and acid secretion
- NSAIDs cause tissue injury via local irritative effects and systemic effects mediated by cyclooxygenase inhibition resulting in decreased prostaglandin synthesis.
  - NSAIDs are concentrated inside cells and can cause direct toxicity to surface mucosal cells
  - Inhibit bicarbonate secretion from the gastric and duodenal mucosa
  - Decreased mucus cell secretion
  - Inhibit mucosal proliferation and healing
  - Cause microvascular ischemia
  - Inhibit physiologic regulation of acid secretion
  - Stimulate neutrophil adhesion to the splanchnic endothelium

- Gastric ulcers can occur in the absence of hyperacidity, whereas duodenal ulcers occur only in association with hyperacidity and are associated with both increased basal and postprandial acid secretion.
- Gastric hypermotility and duodenal hypomotility have been implicated in DU, whereas gastric hypomotility and pyloric reflux have been associated with GU.
- PUD can be complicated by bleeding, perforation and peritonitis, penetration into surrounding tissues such as pancreas and colon, and pyloric obstruction.

PATIENT PRESENTATION

- History:

    Family history of PUD; smoking; alcohol; stress; older age; low socioeconomic status; NSAID use; chronic pulmonary hepatic, or renal disease.

- Uncomplicated symptoms:

    Epigastric burning or "hunger" sensation occurring 2 to 3 hours after meals and at night, temporarily relieved with antacids, food, and milk; occasionally the epigastric discomfort is exacerbated rather than relieved by eating; "irritable stomach" to certain foods; belching; bloating; nausea; vomiting; regurgitation; fatty food intolerance; early satiety; weight loss or weight gain.

- Complicated symptoms:

    Severe unremitting pain; pain radiating to the back; projectile vomiting; hematemesis; melena; fever; hypotension.

- Examination:

    The exam is often nonspecific and unrevealing in uncomplicated PUD with only epigastric tenderness; guarding, decreased bowel sounds, fever, heme + stools indicate complications.

DIFFERENTIAL DIAGNOSIS

- Gastroesophageal reflux
- Cholelithiasis/cholecystitis
- Pancreatitis
- Diverticulitis
- Appendicitis
- Gastric carcinoma
- Drug-induced dyspepsia
- Crohns disease
- Intestinal ischemia
- Infectious gastritis (HSV, CMV, tuberculous, strongyloidiasis, giardiasis)

KEYS TO ASSESSMENT

- Complete blood cell (CBC) count, liver function tests (LFTs), amylase, bilirubin, and chemistries including calcium stool guaiac

- Assessment can follow three basic pathways:

  - New onset mild dyspeptic symptoms in patients under the age of 50 with good follow-up: a 2-week trial of empiric therapy (histamine-2 receptor antagonists [H2 blockers]) can be considered

  - Patient with no history of NSAID use and history of recurrent symptoms: noninvasive *H. pylori* testing and therapy if indicated (serology [serum] or urea breath test [15% false-positive and false-negative rate])

  - Patient with "alarm" markers (anemia, gastrointestinal bleeding, anorexia, early satiety, weight loss): upper gastrointestinal endoscopy

- Upper gastrointestinal endoscopy allows for diagnosis and differentiation of benign from malignant gastric ulceration; can simultaneously culture and stain for *H. pylori*.

- Upper gastrointestinal radiography is less sensitive and specific than endoscopy.

- If endoscopy is not definitive, ultrasonography, computed tomography (CT) scanning, and lower gastrointestinal endoscopy may be indicated.

KEYS TO MANAGEMENT

- Prevention

  - Smoking cessation; decrease alcohol consumption

  - Avoid milk and foods that give dyspeptic symptoms (does not induce or prevent ulcers but decreases symptoms and is recommended by virtually every reference as part of a nonpharmocologic ulcer prevention regimen)

  - Avoid NSAIDs if possible; if not, consider misoprostol, which reduces NSAID-induced ulcer occurrence by 40%; if patient cannot tolerate misoprostol (diarrhea, cramping), then a proton pump inhibitor (PPI) (omeprazole) is indicated, but has not been proven effective; salsalate is the NSAID with the least GI toxicity; etodolac and nabumetone are also associated with less risk of PUD than other NSAIDs

- Pharmacologic management of PUD

  - *H. pylori* negative ulcers:
    1) H2 blockers (cimetidine, ranitidine, famotidine, nizatidine) are effective for healing acute ulcers but may result in tolerance and rebound hyperacidity in some patients.
    2) PPI (omeprazole, lansoprazole, pantoprazole) provide better 24-hour acid inhibition, and have a higher rate of ulcer healing at 2 to 4 weeks than H2 blockers.
    3) Antacids are effective in ulcer healing, but have much lower rates of patient compliance and have more side effects than either H2 blockers or PPIs.
    4) Sucralfate has similar healing rates to cimetidine and is well tolerated, it but requires qid dosing.
    5) Prostaglandin (misoprostol) does result in ulcer healing, but it is not superior to any of the other choices and is associated with significant side effects.

6) Recurrences are common (up to 100% in smokers) at 3 months and therapy must be continued for 4 to 6 weeks, with a maintenance regimen of half-therapeutic doses at bedtime (e.g., 150 mg ranitidine at bedtime) for up to 5 years.

- *H. pylori* positive ulcers:
    1) The most effective therapy is a combination of clarithromycin and tetracycline (or amoxicillin or metronidazole) plus a PPI for 7 to 14 days.
    2) Other possible regimens include two antibiotics plus bismuth.
    3) Recurrence and reinfection rates are low after these regimens, and no further treatment is indicated unless symptoms recur.

- Treatment of ulcer complications:

    - Acute upper gastrointestinal bleeding from PUD requires rapid patient stabilization and possible transfusion while preparing for emergent endoscopy and medical or surgical intervention.

    - PUD perforation or penetration is a surgical emergency. Surgery for complicated or refractory ulcers includes vagotomy (truncal or selective), and a variety of gastric and duodenal resection procedures; complications include gastric hypomotility, reflux esophagitis, dumping syndrome, and diarrhea.

Pathophysiology

What is going on in the disease process that influences how the patient presents and how he or she should be managed?

$\rightarrow$

Clinical Link

What should you do now that you understand the underlying pathophysiology?

The majority of PUD is associated with *H. pylori* infection with mucosal injury.	Patients must be evaluated of *H. pylori*, and adequate management must include antibiotics.
NSAIDs cause mucosal tissue injury and are associated with a significant risk of PUD.	Patients who do not need to take NSAIDs should be encouraged to stop, and those that must continue their use should be considered for misoprostol therapy.
H. pylori and NSAID use cause defects in the mucosal defense mechanisms and must be treated directly; however, healing can be facilitated by reducing gastric and duodenal acidity.	In addition to antibiotics for *H. pylori* and discontinuing NSAID use, management should include H2 blockers or PPIs.
Once the initial therapeutic regimen has been completed, ulcer recurrence is common with NSAID-associated ulcer, but not with *H. pylori* infection.	For NSAID-associated ulcer, initial management must be continued for 4 to 6 weeks, with maintenance therapy for up to 5 years; *H. pylori*-associated ulcers do not require maintenance therapy.
PUD can be complicated by hemorrhage, perforation, pyloric obstruction, or penetration.	Increasing symptoms such as melena, hematemesis, back pain, fever, or hypotension require immediate and aggressive evaluation and possible emergent surgical intervention.

BIBLIOGRAPHY

Anonymous. (1997). Drugs for treatment of peptic ulcers. *Medical Letter on Drugs and Therapeutics, 39*(991), 1-4.

Berg, A. O. (1996). Helicobacter pylori in peptic ulcer disease: Report of an NIH consensus conference [see comments][review, 4 refs]. *Journal of the American Board of Family Practice, 9*(3), 205-207.

Bianchi, P. G., Parente, F., Imbesi, V., Montrone, F., & Caruso, I. (1996). Role of Helicobacter pylori in ulcer healing and recurrence of gastric and duodenal ulcers in longterm NSAID users. Response to omeprazole dual therapy. *Gut, 39*(1), 22-26.

Blum, A. L. (1996). Helicobacter pylori and peptic ulcer disease [review, 24 refs]. *Scandinavian Journal of Gastroenterology*, (Suppl 214), 24-27, discussion 42-43.

Blum, R. A. (1996). Lansoprazole and omeprazole in the treatment of acid peptic disorders [see comments] [review, 174 refs]. *American Journal of Health-System Pharmacy, 53*(12), 1401-1415.

Brozenec, S. A. (1996). Ulcer therapy update [review, 14 refs]. *RN, 59*(9), 48-50, 52-53, quiz 54.

Bulut, O. B., Rasmussen, C., & Fischer, A. (1996). Acute surgical treatment of complicated peptic ulcers with special reference to the elderly. *World Journal of Surgery, 20*(5), 574-577.

Casas, A. T., & Gadacz, T. R. (1996). Laparoscopic management of peptic ulcer disease [review, 23 refs]. *Surgical Clinics of North America, 76*(3), 515-522.

Cook, D. J., Reeve, B. K., Guyatt, G. H., Heyland, D. K., Griffith, L. E., Buckingham, L., & Tryba, M. (1996). Stress ulcer prophylaxis in critically ill patients. Resolving discordant meta-analyses. *Journal of the American Medical Association, 275*(4), 308-314.

Crabtree, J. E. (1996). Immune and inflammatory responses to Helicobacter pylori infection [review, 78 refs]. *Scandinavian Journal of Gastroenterology*, (Suppl 215), 3-10.

Ekstrom, P., Carling, L., Wetterhus, S., Wingren, P. E., Anker-Hansen, O., Lundegardh, G., Thorhallsson, E., & Unge, P. (1996). Prevention of peptic ulcer and dyspeptic symptoms with omeprazole in patients receiving continuous non-steroidal anti-inflammatory drug therapy. A Nordic multicentre study [see comments]. *Scandinavian Journal of Gastroenterology, 31*(8), 753-758.

Engler-Pinto, J. P., Gama-Rodrigues, J., Lopasso, F. P., Cordeiro, A. C., Saez-Alquezar, A., Laudanna, A. A., & Pinotti, H. W. (1996). Site of peptic ulcer. comparison of hydrochloric acid output, pepsinogen and gastrin serum levels. *Hepato-Gastroenterology, 43*(12), 1671-1677.

Fass, R., Hixson, L. J., Ciccolo, M. L., Gordon, P., Hunter, G., & Rappaport, W. (1997). Contemporary medical therapy for gastroesophageal reflux disease [review, 46 refs]. *American Family Physician, 55*(1), 205-212.

Fendrick, A. M., Chernew, M. E., Hirth, R. A., & Bloom, B. S. (1996). Immediate endoscopy or initial Helicobacter pylori serological testing for suspected peptic ulcer disease: Estimating cost-effectiveness using decision analysis. *Yale Journal of Biology and Medicine, 69*(2), 187-195.

Fletcher, D. R. (1997). Peptic disease: Can we afford current management? [review, 39 refs]. *Australian and New Zealand Journal of Surgery, 67*(2-3), 75-80.

Garnett, W. R. (1996). Lansoprazole: A proton pump inhibitor [review, 108 refs]. *Annals of Pharmacotherapy, 30*(12), 1425-1436.

Gomollon, F., Gimeno, L., Valdeperez, J., Yus, C., Marzo, J., & Perez-Caballero, M. C. (1996). Eradication of helicobacter pylori among patients from a primary care practice. *Journal of Family Practice, 43*(6), 551-555.

Graham, D. Y. (1996). Nonsteroidal anti-inflammatory drugs, Helicobacter pylori, and ulcers: Where we stand [review, 92 refs]. *American Journal of Gastroenterology, 91*(10), 2080-2086.

Hatton, J., Lu, W. Y., Rhoney, D. H., Tibbs, P. A., Dempsey, R. J., & Young, B. (1996). A step-wise protocol for stress ulcer prophylaxis in the neurosurgical intensive care unit. *Surgical Neurology, 46*(5), 493-499.

Hein, H. O., Suadicani, P., & Gyntelberg, F. (1997). Genetic markers for peptic ulcer. A study of 3387 men aged 54 to 74 years: The Copenhagen Male Study. *Scandinavian Journal of Gastroenterology, 32*(1), 16-21.

Hojgaard, L., Mertz, N. A., & Rune, S. J. (1996). Peptic ulcer pathophysiology: Acid, bicarbonate, and mucosal function [review, 62 refs]. *Scandinavian Journal of Gastroenterology*, (Suppl 216), 10-15.

Howden, C. W. (1997). Optimizing the pharmacology of acid control in acid-related disorders [review, 27 refs]. *American Journal of Gastroenterology, 92*(4 Suppl), 17S-19S, discussion 19S-21S.

Hunt, R. H. (1997). Peptic ulcer disease: Defining the treatment strategies in the era of *Helicobacter pylori* [review, 56 refs]. *American Journal of Gastroenterology, 92*(4 Suppl), 36S-40S, discussion 40S-43S.

Kurata, J. H., & Nogawa, A. N. (1997). Meta-analysis of risk factors for peptic ulcer. Nonsteroidal antiinflammatory drugs, Helicobacter pylori, and smoking. *Journal of Clinical Gastroenterology, 24*(1), 2-17.

Marshall, R., & Owen, W. J. (1997). Role of duodenal juice in the pathogenesis of gastroesophageal reflux disease [letter; comment]. *Annals of Surgery, 225*(1), 135-136.

Molloy, R. M., & Sonnenberg, A. (1997). Relation between gastric cancer and previous peptic ulcer disease. *Gut, 40*(2), 247-252.

O'Keefe, G., & Maier, R. V. (1996). Current management of patients with stress ulceration [review, 95 refs]. *Advances in Surgery, 30*, 155-177.

Peura, D. A. (1996). *Helicobacter pylori* and ulcerogenesis [review, 78 refs]. *American Journal of Medicine, 100*(5A), 19S-25S, discussion 25S-26S.

Reilly, T. G., Poxon, V., Sanders, D. S., Elliott, T. S., & Walt, R. P. (1997). Comparison of serum, salivary, and rapid whole blood diagnostic tests for *Helicobacter pylori* and their validation against endoscopy based tests. *Gut, 40*(4), 454-458.

Sachs, G. (1997). Proton pump inhibitors and acid-related diseases [review, 112 refs]. *Pharmacotherapy, 17*(1), 22-37.

Sanders, S. W. (1996). Pathogenesis and treatment of acid peptic disorders: Comparison of proton pump inhibitors with other antiulcer agents [review, 178 refs]. *Clinical Therapeutics, 18*(1), 2-34, discussion 1.

Sartori, S., Trevisani, L., Nielsen, I., Tassinari, D., & Abbasciano, V. (1996). Misoprostol and omeprazole in the prevention of chemotherapy-induced acute gastroduodenal mucosal injury. A randomized, placebo-controlled pilot study. *Cancer, 78*(7), 1477-1482.

Soll, A. H. (1996). Consensus conference. Medical treatment of peptic ulcer disease. Practice guidelines. Practice Parameters Committee of the American College of Gastroenterology [published erratum appears in *Journal of the American Medical Association*, 1996 May 1, 275(17):1314] [review, 99 refs]. *Journal of the American Medical Association, 275*(8), 622-629.

Sonnenberg, A., & Everhart, J. E. (1997). Health impact of peptic ulcer in the United States. *American Journal of Gastroenterology, 92*(4), 614-620.

Taniguchi, D. K., & Kowdley, K. V. (1996). Helicobacter pylori and peptic ulcer disease: Issues for primary care providers [review, 20 refs]. *Comprehensive Therapy, 22*(7), 434-439.

Telford, J. L., & Ghiara, P. (1996). Prospects for the development of a vaccine against *Helicobacter pylori* [review, 36 refs]. *Drugs, 52*(6), 799-804.

Thomason, M. H., Payseur, E. S., Hakenewerth, A. M., Norton, H. J., Mehta, B., Reeves, T. R., Moore-Swartz, M. W., & Robbins, P. I. (1996). Nosocomial pneumonia in ventilated trauma patients during stress ulcer prophylaxis with sucralfate, antacid, and ranitidine. *Journal of Trauma, 41*(3), 503-508.

Velanovich, V. (1997). Long-term quality of life outcome after treatment for *Helicobacter pylori* gastric infection. *American Surgeon, 63*(6), 551-554.

Webb, D. D. (1996). Practice guidelines for treatment of peptic ulcer disease [letter]. *Journal of the American Medical Association, 276*(14), 1136, discussion 1136-1137.

Wyncoll, D. L., Roberts, P. C., Beale, R. J., & McLuckie, A. (1997). H2 blockers in the intensive care unit: Ignoring the evidence? Telephone survey. *British Medical Journal, 314*(7086), 1013.

CASE STUDY

PEPTIC ULCER DISEASE

INITIAL HISTORY:
- 58-year-old male complaining of 3-week history of increasing epigastric pain
- Has had "heartburn" in the past for which he took "Tums," but this is much worse and only partially relieved with chewable antacids

Question 1.
What is your differential diagnosis based on this limited history?

Question 2.
What questions would you like to ask this patient about his symptoms?

ADDITIONAL HISTORY:
- Pain has a burning quality
- Relieved with eating, especially drinking milk, but recurs about 2 hours later
- Denies radiation to his back, melena, hematemesis, or fever
- Denies early satiety, anorexia, or weight loss
- Denies fatty food intolerance or change in stools
- Denies jaundice, increasing abdominal girth, or easy bruising
- Denies shortness of breath or pain with exercise

Question 3.
What questions would you like to ask about his recent and past medical history?

MORE HISTORY:
- Has been taking ibuprofen for the past 2 months for a sore knee
- Drinks approximately 3 mixed drinks each day
- Smokes ½ pack of cigarettes a day
- Has had recent job change with a great deal of stress
- Has been feeling a little tired lately but no recent illnesses or hospitalization
- Has a history of mild hypertension treated with diet
- No medications or allergies

PHYSICAL EXAMINATION:
- Thin white male in no acute distress
- T = 37 orally; P = 90 and regular; RR = 16 and unlabored; BP = 148/96 sitting right arm

HEENT, Neck
- PERRLA, fundi without vascular changes
- Pharynx clear
- No thyromegaly
- No bruits
- No adenopathy

Lungs, Cardiac
- Lungs clear to auscultation and percussion
- Cardiac with RRR without murmurs or gallops

Abdomen
- Abdomen not distended
- Bowel sounds present
- Liver percusses to 8 cm at the midclavicular line, one fingerbreadth below the right costal margin
- Epigastric tenderness without rebound or guarding
- Spleen not palpable

Rectal
- No hemorrhoids seen or felt
- Prostate not enlarged and soft
- Stool grossly normal but weakly heme+

<u>Extremeties, Neurological</u>
- No edema
- Pulses full, no bruits
- Oriented x4
- Normal strength, sensation, and DTR

Question 4.
What are the pertinent positives and negatives on the physical exam?

Question 5.
What initial diagnostic tests would you obtain now?

LABORATORY RESULTS:
- Chemistries including calcium and BUN/Cr normal
- WBC = 9000 with normal differential
- HCT = 45%
- Liver function test including bilirubin normal
- Amylase normal
- ECG = normal sinus rhythm without evidence of ischemic changes

Question 6.
What test should be chosen to best evaluate for peptic ulcer disease in this patient?

ENDOSCOPY RESULTS:

- Normal esophageal mucosa
- Gastric mucosa with superficial gastritis without ulceration
- 0.5 cm duodenal ulcer with evidence of recent bleeding, but no acute hemorrhage and no visible vessels in the ulcer crater
- *H. pylori* testing negative

Question 7.

What management would you recommend?

CHAPTER 16

HEPATITIS B AND C

DEFINITION

- Inflammation of the liver due to viral infection with the hepatitis B or hepatitis C virus
- Epidemiology, pathophysiology, and clinical manifestations are dependent on the causative virus and the host inflammatory and immunologic response to infection.

EPIDEMIOLOGY

- Hepatitis B (HBV)

  - 5% of the world's population are carriers of chronic HBV infection.

  - Over 1 million people in the United States have chronic HBV infection; overall prevalence of HBV infection is 2% to 3%, but prevalence is approximately 6.4% in Alaskan native population and 14% is in African-Americans—high risk for cirrhosis and hepatocellular carcinoma.

  - Risk of developing chronic HBV infection varies inversely with age at infection (90% of infants infected by birth become carriers; approximately 5% if older than 5 years).

  - Other high prevalence groups include intravenous (IV) drug users, first generation immigrants from endemic areas such as Southeast Asia, men having sex with men, household contacts and sexual partners of HBV carriers, heterosexuals with multiple partners, people requiring hemodialysis, patients in custodial institutions, and health care workers.

  - Alcohol appears to be a cofactor for the development of chronic disease.

  - There are no known risk factors in 30% to 40% of cases.

  - Males are affected more than females; peak age is 10 to 29.

  - Incidence has decreased by almost 50% over the past 10 years.

  - It is spread by parenteral transmission of virus via blood or blood products, sexual contact, or prenatal exposure.

- Hepatitis C (HCV)

  - Prevalence in the United States is 0.4% to 1.1%; incidence declined by 50% between 1989 and 1991.

  - It is the cause of more than 85% of post-transfusion hepatitis; risk of transfusion-related hepatitis is now approximately 0.6% per patient; risk will be even less with new modes of donor screening.

- It is also associated with IV drug use (prevalence is 48% to 90%), individuals with needle-stick injury (incidence of infection after exposure to antiHCV-positive source is 4% to 10%), persons with hemophilia, people requiring hemodialysis, health care workers, and household and sexual contacts of chronically infected persons.

- Alcohol appears to be a cofactor for the development of chronic disease.

- Chronic HCV infection occurs in up to 22% of all dialysis patients, 28% of renal transplant patients, and 25% of liver transplant patients, with some reduction in long-term survival in these groups.

- There are no known risk factors in 40% of cases.

- It is spread by direct parenteral inoculation, sexual contact, transplantation of an infected organ, or perinatal exposure.

PATHOPHYSIOLOGY

- Hepatitis B

  - Hepatocyte injury is mediated by the immune response rather than direct cytopathic effects by the virus.

  - Hepatocyte injury is mediated by CD8 lymphocyte (T cytotoxic cell) killing of infected cells and by release of inflammatory cytokines.

  - A vigorous immune response will decrease the likelihood of chronic infection, but increases the likelihood of hepatocellular necrosis.

  - The inflammatory cytokines tumor necrosis factor alpha (TNF-α) and interferon gamma (INF-γ) are vital to clearance of HBV.

  - Circulating antigen-antibody complexes may result in a serum sickness-like syndrome with angioneurotic edema, polyarteritis nodosa, systemic vasculitis with bowel ischemia, renal disease, neuropathy, and arthritis.

  - Although most acute infections resolve without sequelae, approximately 5% to 10% of patients will develop chronic infection with varying degrees of ongoing hepatocyte injury; the risk of complications can approach 90% in infants:
    1) Chronic active hepatitis with active viral replication, widespread inflammation, and sustained increases in aspartate aminotransferase (AST); 15% to 20% of these will develop cirrhosis within 5 years
    2) Chronic persistent hepatitis in which the inflammation is limited to portal areas and long-term prognosis is very good
    3) True carrier state is characterized by normal liver enzymes and normal liver histology; only about 2% of these patients will develop progressive disease

  - The mechanism of long-term asymptomatic carrier state is believed to be immunologic tolerance to the virus—the virus is not cleared but hepatocyte injury is minimal and the carrier state is life-long; this is especially common in infants in whom the immune system is immature and unable to eradicate the virus.

  - Chronic HBV infection is associated with a 10 to 100 fold risk of hepatocellular carcinoma.

- Hepatitis C

    - Direct viral cytopathicity is a primary mode of hepatocyte injury, and the viral load positively correlates with the amount of inflammation seen on liver biopsy.

    - The virus can evade immunity by its rapid mutation rate, thus it quickly develops resistant strains to antibodies; CD8 lymphocyte-mediated cellular destruction of infected cells is the primary means of effective immune response to HCV.

    - Autoimmune hepatitis is also commonly associated with HCV infection. Many patients develop anti-liver-kidney microsomal antibodies that can destroy uninfected hepatocytes. This autoimmune component of HCV results in multiple extrahepatic manifestations of the disease including membranous glomerulonephritis, cryoglobulinemia, vasculitis, dermatitis, pulmonary fibrosis, and rheumatoid arthritis.

    - Chronic hepatitis occurs in over half of the cases; disease progression is usually clinically silent and characterized by ongoing inflammation leading to cirrhosis.

    - Cirrhosis occurs in 8% to 42% of cases, and may be evident as early as 15 months after the acute infection, although the average time to cirrhosis is 20 years.

    - Hepatocellular carcinoma (HCC) occurs in 1% to 5% of patients with chronic HCV infection, but generally does not occur until 20 to 30 years after the initial infection. The pathogenesis of HCC is unknown, but is believed to be related to the high level of hepatocellular regeneration that accompanies chronic HCV hepatitis.

PATIENT PRESENTATION

- History:

    Needle-stick injury; hemodialysis; blood transfusion; organ transplant; homosexual contact with an infected individual; alcohol abuse.

- Symptoms:

    Acute infection is often asymptomatic with both HBV and HCV; incubation periods from time of exposure to development of symptoms can be as long as 6 months; if acute symptoms occur, they include fatigue, fever, myalgias and arthralgias, jaundice, anorexia, abdominal discomfort, and nausea; some cases of acute HBV infection will present with fulminant hepatic failure, including encephalitis, coagulopathy, and ascites; symptoms of chronic infection are most common in HCV and include fatigue, nausea, anorexia, coagulopathy, ascites, encephalopathy, and gastrointestinal bleeding; extra hepatic manifestations of both HBV and HCV may occur including rashes, severe abdominal pain, renal dysfunction, dyspnea , joint pain, and Raynaud phenomenon.

- Examination:

    The examination is often normal in the absence of significant hepatic failure; when liver dysfunction is severe, exam findings may include asterixis, decreased mental status, jaundice, ecchymoses, ascites, edema, pectoral alopecia, palmer erythema, spider angiomata, gynecomastia, and heme+ stools; evidence of extraarticular disease may be seen in HCV including skin lesions, arthritic changes, pulmonary crackles, and corneal ulcers.

DIFFERENTIAL DIAGNOSIS

- Hepatitis A, D, E, or G

- Hepatitis due to other viruses (Epstein-Barr [EBV], cytomegalovirus [CMV], herpes, coxsackievirus)

- Alcoholic hepatitis or cirrhosis

- Autoimmune hepatitits

- α_1-antitrypsin deficiency

- Biliary cirrhosis

- Toxins or drugs (isoniazid, rifampin, acethaminophen)

- Hemochromatosis

- Sclerosing cholangitis

KEYS TO ASSESSMENT

- History of exposures is important, but the incubation period is long and the acute infection is usually asymptomatic, so that even a careful history may not pinpoint the time or source of initial infection.

- The examination will be relatively unrevealing until late in the course of the disease; diagnosis prior to hepatic failure is dependent on serologic testing.

- Serologic testing

  - HBV
    1) Three viral antigens and three antibodies can be detected—HBsAg, HBcAg, and HBeAg; anti-HBs, anti-HBc (IgM or IgG), and anti-HBe.
    2) In acute infection, HBsAg is positive, but could represent a previous carrier state; the diagnosis of acute HBV infection is confirmed with a positive HbeAg and IgM anti-HBc antibody.
    3) Chronic infection is diagnosed by the presence of HBsAg in serum for 6 months or longer after initial detection; IgM and IgG anti-HBc are usually present; and anti-HBs and anti-HBe are present in most, but not all, cases and may take months to become detectable.
    4) HBV deoxyribonucleic acid (DNA) by polymerase chain reaction (PCR) testing is now available and can detect active viral replication in both acute and chronic infection; it is used primarily to follow response to antiviral treatment for research protocols.

  - HCV
    1) PCR testing for viral ribonucleic acid (RNA) is the only way of detecting acute infection.
    2) Anti-HCV testing has evolved rapidly and the "second and third generation" testing techniques have fewer problems with specificity and sensitivity than did the older assays; antibody titers still may not be detectable for several months after the original infection.

- Serum alanine aminotransferase (ALT) and aspartate aminotransferase (AST) levels usually rise 2 to 3 months after the initial infection.

- Diagnosis of liver failure is evidenced by increased bilirubin, prolonged coagulation times, decreased albumin, and evidence of ascites and portal hypertension with the possibility of finding esophageal varices on endoscopy.

KEYS TO MANAGEMENT

- Prevention

    - HBV
        1) Behavior changes in sexual practices, universal precautions in health care, and discontinuation of IV drug use
        2) Passive immunoprophylaxis is recommended for:
            - Perinatal exposure to an infected mother
            - Prolonged contact of a less than 12-month-old infant with an infected primary care deliverer
            - Needle-stick from an infected patient
            - Sexual exposure to an infected individual
            - Organ transplant if infected prior to transplantation
        3) Hepatitis B immunoglobulin (HBIG) is given within 12 hours of delivery or 14 days of other exposures followed by the three-dose vaccination series.
        4) Active immunoprophylaxis is recommended for all children and for other high risk groups such as health care workers and IV drug users; a three-dose regimen at 0, 1, and 6 months results in 95% of patients developing antibody with a subsequent rate of HBV infection of 3.2% compared to 26% in controls.

    - HCV
        1) Changes in sexual behavior as with HBV
        2) Trials of passive immunoprophylaxis have not been effective thus far.
        3) Vaccine development is difficult due to the high mutation rate of the virus.

- Pharmacologic treatment

    - Interferon-alpha (INF-α):
        1) Currently the only FDA-approved drug for chronic HBV or HCV.
        2) Results in approximately 35% of patients with HBV demonstrating a sustained response with loss of HBV DNA after 3 months of therapy.
        3) Results in a sustained response in approximately 20% of patients with HCV.
        4) Indications and contraindications: elevated ALT for at least 6 months with evidence of continued viral replication; no evidence of significant hepatic decompensation; no active alcohol abuse; no blood dyscrasias; no poorly controlled psychiatric disorders; no concurrent autoimmune diseases.
        5) Side effects are frequent and include an influenza-like illness with fever, chills, myalgias, and headache 4 to 8 hours after injection; fatigue; myalgias; anorexia; weight loss; bone marrow suppression; psychological side effects such anxiety, depression, and irritability; and autoimmune phenomena such as autoimmune thyroiditis, hemolytic anemia, and collagen vascular disease.
        6) Patients with HBV may experience a "flare" of their disease with interferon treatment characterized by a dramatic rise in ALT. This is a good prognostic sign indicating an increased likelihood of response; this is not seen with HCV.

    - Other drugs:
        1) Lamivudine is being tried in both HBV and HCV; early results are promising.
        2) Other antivirals such as ribavirin and famciclovir have had some success when used in combination with INF-α for HCV; results are mixed with HBV.
        3) Antiinflammatories and phlebotomy (to reduce hepatic iron stores) have improved the response to INF-α in HCV.

- Liver transplant:

  - Survival rates are now 70% to 85% at 5 years.

  - Indications include severe symptoms, decreased quality of life, and sustained jaundice and coagulopathy.

  - HBV is associated with a high risk of recurrence after transplantation (close to 100% in some studies) unless the patient is also treated with HBIG; postoperative treatment with lamivudine further improves outcomes with overall results now equivalent to all other indications for liver transplant.

  - HCV accounts for about ⅓ of all liver transplants performed in the United States; recurrence after transplant is 100%, but it is usually associated with only mild increases in ALT. Postoperative survival is excellent.

Pathophysiology →

What is going on in the disease process that influences how the patient presents and how he or she should be managed?

Clinical Link

What should you do now that you understand the underlying pathophysiology?

HBV causes liver injury primarily through immune-dependent mechanisms rather than through direct viral cytopathicity.	Patients with an effective immune response are less likely to become carriers but will present with a more fulminant clinical presentation and a high ALT.
Some patients are immunologically tolerant to HBV and will have persistent viral replication and chronic hepatitis.	HBV carrier state occurs in approximately 5% of patients and is associated with persistent infectivity, chronic liver damage, and a risk of hepatocellular carcinoma.
Treatment of HBV with INF-α may result in a transient flare in immunologic activity that indicates effective HBV killing.	Patients may experience an increase in ALT and experience a flu-like illness after therapy with INF-α.
Both active and passive immunoprophylaxis for HBV are effective in preventing infection.	Postexposure HBIG and vaccination with the three-dose regimen are effective in preventing active infection.
HCV mutates rapidly and can avoid the immune system and can develop resistance to vaccines.	Chronic HCV infective is common, and both passive and active immunoprophylaxis have been ineffective so far.
HCV has direct cytopathicity on the hepatocytes with significant hepatocellular injury and necrosis.	HCV is associated with a significant risk of cirrhosis and hepatocellular carcinoma.
HCV is associated with autoantibodies that can attack the kidney, the skin, joints, and the thyroid.	HCV infection may be associated with membranous glomerulonephritis, rashes, collagen vascular disease, and an autoimmune thyroiditis.

BIBLIOGRAPHY

Anonymous. (1997). Hepatitis C [review, 0 refs]. *Weekly Epidemiological Record, 72*(10), 65-69.

Berg, T., Dirla, U., Naumann, U., Heuft, H. G., Kuther, S., Lobeck, H., Schreier, E., & Hopf, U. (1996). Responsiveness to interferon alpha treatment in patients with chronic hepatitis C coinfected with hepatitis G virus. *Journal of Hepatology, 25*(5), 763-768.

Booth, R. (1997). Hepatitis C [review, 16 refs]. *Professional Nurse, 12*(4), 287-290.

Botte, C., & Janot, C. (1996). Epidemiology of HCV infection in the general population and in blood transfusion [review, 8 refs]. *Nephrology, Dialysis, Transplantation, 11*(Suppl 4), 19-21.

Brumage, L. K., & Wright, T. L. (1997). Treatment for recurrent viral hepatitis after liver transplantation [review, 19 refs]. *Journal of Hepatology, 26*(2), 440-445.

Caselmann, W. H., & Alt, M. (1996). Hepatitis C virus infection as a major risk factor for hepatocellular carcinoma [review, 65 refs]. *Journal of Hepatology, 24*(2 Suppl), 61-66.

Chauveau, P. (1996). Epidemiology of hepatitis C virus infection in chronic haemodialysis [review, 16 refs]. *Nephrology, Dialysis, Transplantation, 11*(Suppl 4), 39-41.

Chisari, F. V. (1997). Cytotoxic T cells and viral hepatitis [review, 50 refs]. *Journal of Clinical Investigation, 99*(7), 1472-1477.

Cirelli, R., Herne, K., McCrary, M., Lee, P., & Tyring, S. K. (1996). Famciclovir: Review of clinical efficacy and safety [review, 54 refs]. *Antiviral Research, 29*(2-3), 141-151.

Cosserat, J., Cacoub, P., & Bletry, O. (1996). Immunological disorders in C virus chronic hepatitis [review, 26 refs]. *Nephrology, Dialysis, Transplantation, 11*(Suppl 4), 31-35.

De, L. X. (1996). Serological and molecular biology screening techniques for HVC infection [review, 17 refs]. *Nephrology, Dialysis, Transplantation, 11*(Suppl 4), 9-11.

Dienstag, J. L. (1997). The natural history of chronic hepatitis C and what we should do about it [editorial; comment] [review, 37 refs]. *Gastroenterology, 112*(2), 651-655.

Diepolder, H. M., Zachoval, R., Hoffmann, R. M., Jung, M. C., Gerlach, T., & Pape, G. R. (1996). The role of hepatitis C virus specific CD4+ T lymphocytes in acute and chronic hepatitis C [review, 54 refs]. *Journal of Molecular Medicine, 74*(10), 583-588.

Dusheiko, G. M. (1996). Summary: Antiviral treatment of hepatitis C virus [review, 30 refs]. *Antiviral Research, 29*(1), 77-82.

Eddleston, A. L. (1996). Hepatitis C infection and autoimmunity [review, 36 refs]. *Journal of Hepatology, 24*(2 Suppl), 55-60.

Eickhoff, T. C. (1996). Adult immunizations: How are we doing? [review, 12 refs]. *Hospital Practice, 31*(Office Edition), 107-108.

Fattovich, G., Giustina, G., Favarato, S., & Ruol, A. (1996). A survey of adverse events in 11,241 patients with chronic viral hepatitis treated with alphfa interferon. *Journal of Hepatology, 24*(1), 38-47.

Feitelson, M. A., & Duan, L. X. (1997). Hepatitis B virus X antigen in the pathogenesis of chronic infections and the development of hepatocellular carcinoma [review, 164 refs]. *American Journal of Pathology, 150*(4), 1141-1157.

Fried, M. W. (1996). Therapy of chronic viral hepatitis [review, 75 refs]. *Medical Clinics of North America, 80*(5), 957-972.

Gretch, D. R., Polyak, S. J., Willson, R. A., & Carithers, R. L. J. (1996). Treatment of chronic hepatitis C virus infection: A clinical and virological perspective [review, 121 refs]. *Advances in Experimental Medicine and Biology, 394*, 207-224.

Hall, A. J. (1996). Viral hepatitis: Control, seroepidemiology and surveillance. *Transactions of the Royal Society of Tropical Medicine and Hygiene, 90*(1), 1-2.

Hollinger, F. B. (1996). Comprehensive control (or elimination) of hepatitis B virus transmission in the United States [review, 24 refs]. *Gut, 38*(Suppl 2), S24-S30.

Hoofnagle, J. H., & di, B. A. M. (1997). The treatment of chronic viral hepatitis [review, 106 refs]. *New England Journal of Medicine, 336*(5), 347-356.

Inchauspe, G. (1996). Protection and defense mechanisms in HCV infection [review, 21 refs]. *Nephrology, Dialysis, Transplantation, 11*(Suppl 4), 6-8.

Jonas, M. M. (1996). Interferon-alpha for viral hepatitis [review, 149 refs]. *Journal of Pediatric Gastroenterology and Nutrition, 23*(2), 93-106.

Jonas, M. M. (1996). Hepatitis C virus infection: Clinical aspects and treatment with interferon alphfa [review, 127 refs]. *Clinical Therapeutics, 18*(Suppl B), 110-125.

Kiszkis, H. (1996). Primary hepatocellular carcinoma in patients with chronic hepatitis B virus infection [review, 50 refs]. *Archivum Immunologiae et Therapiae Experimentalis, 44*(5-6), 315-323.

Korgaonkar, A., Verenkar, M. P., Savio, R., Pinto, M. J., & Singh, I. (1996). Evaluation of HBsAg carrier rate in acute viral hepatitis and high risk individuals using RPHA and ELISA. *Indian Journal of Pathology and Microbiology, 39*(4), 277-280.

Koziel, M. J. (1996). Immunology of viral hepatitis. *American Journal of Medicine, 100*(1), 98-109.

Kroes, A. C. (1996). Role of testing for antibody to hepatitis B core antigen to prevent transmission of hepatitis B virus in organ and tissue transplantation [review, 12 refs]. *Transplantation Proceedings, 28*(5), 2937-2938.

Kurstak, E., Hossain, A., & Kurstak, C. (1996). Progress in diagnosis of viral hepatitis A, B, C, D and E [review, 73 refs]. *Acta Virologica, 40*(2), 107-115.

Lemon, S. M., & Thomas, D. L. (1997). Vaccines to prevent viral hepatitis [review, 117 refs]. *New England Journal of Medicine, 336*(3), 196-204.

McMurray, R. W., & Elbourne, K. (1997). Hepatitis C virus infection and autoimmunity [review, 125 refs]. *Seminars in Arthritis and Rheumatism, 26*(4), 689-701.

Mills, P., McPeake, J., & McCruden, E. (1996). A rational approach to hepatitis C [review, 5 refs]. *Practitioner, 240*(1560), 172-176.

Mondelli, M. U. (1996). Is there a role for immune responses in the pathogenesis of hepatitis C? [review, 52 refs]. *Journal of Hepatology, 25*(2), 232-238.

Najm, W. (1997). Viral hepatitis: How to manage type C and D infections [review, 20 refs]. *Geriatrics, 52*(5), 28-30.

Neiblum, D. R., & Boynton, R. F. (1996). Evaluation and treatment of chronic hepatitis C infection [review, 65 refs]. *Primary Care; Clinics in Office Practice,* (3), 535-549.

Nolte, F. S. (1997). Laboratory diagnosis of hepatitis C [review, 43 refs]. *Immunological Investigations, 26*(1-2), 199-207.

Ohara, H., Ebisawa, I., & Naruto, H. (1997). Prophylaxis of acute viral hepatitis by immune serum globulin, hepatitis B vaccine, and health education: A sixteen year study of Japan overseas cooperation volunteers. *American Journal of Tropical Medicine & Hygiene, 56*(1), 76-79.

Olsson, R. (1996). Hepatitis and cancer: Genetic aspects [review, 53 refs]. *Scandinavian Journal of Gastroenterology, 220*(Suppl), 115-120.

Piccinino, F., Scolastico, C., Glielmo, A., Piccinino, R., & Sagnelli, E. (1997). HBV and HCV chronic hepatitis and cirrhosis [review, 29 refs]. *Research in Virology, 148*(2), 135-138.

Rensen, P. C., de, V. R. L., & van, B. T. J. (1996). Targeting hepatitis B therapy to the liver. Clinical pharmacokinetic considerations [review, 190 refs]. *Clinical Pharmacokinetics, 31*(2), 131-155.

Roggendorf, M., Lu, M., Meisel, H., Riffelmann, M., Schreier, E., & Viazov, S. (1996). Rational use of diagnostic tools in hepatitis C [review, 68 refs]. *Journal of Hepatology, 24*(2 Suppl), 26-34.

Saracco, G., & Rizzetto, M. (1997). A practical guide to the use of interferons in the management of hepatitis virus infections [review, 74 refs]. *Drugs, 53*(1), 74-85.

Sjogren, M. H. (1996). Serologic diagnosis of viral hepatitis [review, 107 refs]. *Medical Clinics of North America, 80*(5), 929-956.

Spengler, U., Lechmann, M., Irrgang, B., Dumoulin, F. L., & Sauerbruch, T. (1996). Immune responses in hepatitis C virus infection [review, 41 refs]. *Journal of Hepatology, 24*(2 Suppl), 20-25.

Terrault, N. A., & Wright, T. L. (1996). Therapy for chronic hepatitis B infection [review, 129 refs]. *Advances in Experimental Medicine & Biology, 394*, 189-205.

Trepo, C., Bailly, F., & Bizollon, T. (1996). Treatment of chronic hepatitis C: Another therapeutic option [review, 9 refs]. *Nephrology, Dialysis, Transplantation, 11*(Suppl 4), 62-64.

Van, D. P., Kane, M., & Meheus, A. (1997). Integration of hepatitis B vaccination into national immunisation programmes. Viral Hepatitis Prevention Board [see comments] [review, 18 refs]. *Briutish Medical Journal, 314*(7086), 1033-1036.

Wen, Y. (1996). Hepatitis B virus variants and their significance in pathogenesis, prevention and treatment [review, 11 refs]. *Chinese Medical Journal, 109*(1), 39-41.

Werman, H. A., & Gwinn, R. (1997). Seroprevalence of hepatitis B and hepatitis C among rural emergency medical care personnel [review, 15 refs]. *American Journal of Emergency Medicine, 15*(3), 248-251.

Williams, R. (1996). Classification, etiology, and considerations of outcome in acute liver failure [review, 39 refs]. *Seminars in Liver Disease, 16*(4), 343-348.

Woo, M. H., & Burnakis, T. G. (1997). Interferon alfa in the treatment of chronic viral hepatitis B and C [review, 59 refs]. *Annals of Pharmacotherapy, 31*(3), 330-337.

Younossi, Z. M. (1997). Chronic hepatitis C: A clinical overview [review, 48 refs]. *Cleveland Clinic Journal of Medicine, 64*(5), 259-268.

Zein, N. N., & Persing, D. H. (1996). Hepatitis C genotypes: Current trends and future implications [review, 50 refs]. *Mayo Clinic Proceedings, 71*(5), 458-462.

Zuckerman, A. J. (1996). Developing new hepatitis B immunisation strategies [review, 6 refs]. *Gut, 38*(Suppl 2), S60-S62.

Zuckerman, J. N. (1996). Nonresponse to hepatitis B vaccines and the kinetics of anti-HBs production [review, 62 refs]. *Journal of Medical Virology, 50*(4), 283-288.

CASE STUDY

HEPATITIS B AND C

INITIAL HISTORY:
- 37-year-old IV drug abuser
- Several days of increasing fatigue and anorexia
- Now with fever, abdominal discomfort, and myalgias

Question 1.
What questions would you like to ask this patient about his symptoms?

ADDITIONAL HISTORY:
- Discomfort is dull and located over the right upper quadrant.
- Patient denies jaundice, easy bruising, increasing abdominal birth, edema, or confusion.
- Stools are normal; no bloody or dark stools.
- No rashes; no hot, swollen joints
- No dyspnea; no decrease in urination

Question 2.
What questions would you like to ask this patient about his lifestyle or past medical history?

MORE HISTORY:

- Patient lived in Philadelphia and has been using IV drugs for years; he was in a needle exchange program.
- Moved to this area 6 months ago; no needle exchange program is available here.
- Lives alone; has not had a sexual encounter since moving here.
- Doesn't know of anyone who has had hepatitis.
- No dyspnea; no decrease in urination.
- Denies history of significant illnesses or any hospitalizations except for drug rehabilitation.
- Drinks alcohol "occasionally."
- On no medications; no allergies.

PHYSICAL EXAMINATION:

- Ill appearing alert male in mild distress
- T = 38 orally; P = 90 and regular; RR = 18 and unlabored; BP = 128/82 right arm sitting

HEENT, Neck, Skin
- PERRLA, fundi without lesions
- Nares clear
- No mouth lesions
- Pharynx clear without erythema or exudate
- No thyromegaly
- No adenopathy
- Nonicteric
- No rashes; no petechia or ecchymoses

Lungs, Cardiac
- Lungs clear to auscultation and percussion
- Cardiac exam with regular rate and rhythm without murmurs or gallops

Abdomen
- Nondistended
- Bowel sounds present
- Liver percusses to 12 cm at the midclavicular line
- Tenderness over the right upper quadrant without guarding or rebound
- Spleen not palpable

Rectal
- No hemorrhoids felt
- Prostate not enlarged or tender
- Stool heme negative

Extremities
- No edema
- No joint swelling or erythema

Neurological
- Alert and oriented
- No sensory or motor deficits
- DTR 2+ and symmetrical

Question 3.
What are the pertinent positives and negatives on examination?

Question 4.
What is the differential diagnosis based on the history and physical examination?

Question 5.
What laboratory assessment would you do now?

LABORATORY RESULTS:
- WBC = 15,000 with a mild increase in lymphocytes
- Chemistries normal including albumin
- PT/PTT normal
- ALT >700 and AST >300 IU/L
- Total bilirubin upper limit of normal, alkaline phosphatase mildly elevated
- Serum ferritin normal
- HBsAg positive, IgM anti-HBc positive, HBeAg positive
- IgM anti-HAV negative, HCV RNA negative by polymerase chain reaction (PCR) testing
- HIV RNA by PCR negative, anti-HIV ELSIA negative

Question 6.
What do these laboratory results mean?

Question 7.
What should you do for the patient now?

RETURN VISIT 8 MONTHS LATER:

- Patient states he recovered slowly without therapy; finally feeling back to "normal" 3 months after his initial visit.
- Did not see why he needed to return for follow-up (as instructed) until now.
- Heard he might still be infectious and wants to be checked.
- Has no complaints at this time; has been sexually active for the past 2 months.

Question 8.
What tests would you do now?

LABORATORY RESULTS:

- AST and ALT upper limit of normal
- Total bilirubin normal
- HIV ELISA negative
- HBsAg still positive
- HBV DNA (PCR) low level

Question 9.
What does this mean and what should you tell the patient?

CHAPTER 17

ALCOHOLIC HEPATIC CIRRHOSIS AND PORTAL HYPERTENSION

DEFINITION

- Alcoholic cirrhosis:

  - A chronic disease of the liver caused by alcohol intake characterized by steatosis (fatty infiltration), inflammation, and fibrosis

  - Destroys normal hepatic architecture and results in fibrous bands of connecting tissue separating lobules with nodules of regenerating liver cells unrelated to the normal vasculature

- Portal hypertension:

  - Increased pressure in the portal system due to increased portal blood flow and increased resistance to hepatic perfusion

  - Results in dilation of collateral veins and is associated with liver dysfunction, splenomegaly, and fluid and electrolyte imbalances

EPIDEMIOLOGY

- There are 15.3 million alcoholics in the United States.

- 26,000 people per year develop cirrhosis in the United States; it is estimated that 90% of the cases are due to alcohol abuse.

- In developed countries, viral hepatitis (especially hepatitis C) is the second most common cause of hepatic cirrhosis.

- Cirrhosis requires a cumulative intake of approximately 600 kg of ethanol for men and 150 to 300 kg for women; however, of those who consume this much alcohol, only 40% develop cirrhosis.

- Additional cofactors for alcoholic cirrhosis include genetic polymorphisms of the enzymes responsible for ethanol metabolism, female gender, poor nutrition, and viral hepatitis (hepatitis B or C).

- In the United States, portal hypertension is most commonly the result of alcoholic cirrhosis, followed by chronic viral hepatitis (especially hepatitis C).

PATHOPHYSIOLOGY

- Alcoholic cirrhosis:

  - Ethanol is metabolized by several enzymes. When alcohol intake is excessive, these enzymatic reactions result in the release of toxic oxygen radicals; in addition, alcohol intake reduces the activity of endogenous antioxidants (vitamins E and A, glutathione).

  - Oxygen radicals in the hepatocytes cause lipid peroxidation and deoxyribonucleic acid (DNA) damage.

  - One of the major metabolites of ethanol is acetaldehyde, which affects protein synthesis and can stimulate hepatic fibrosis.

  - Ethanol also directly affects mitochondria with intrahepatocyte accumulation of microvesicular fat described as alcoholic foamy steatosis. This process is reversible with discontinuation of alcohol intake and does not necessarily lead to cirrhosis.

  - Ethanol and hepatic injury stimulates production of inflammatory cytokines including IL-1, IL-6, IL-8, and tumor necrosing factor (TNF) released primarily from the hepatic macrophages (Kupffer cells); these result in further hepatocyte injury.

  - Ethanol increases intestinal permeability leading to alcohol-associated endotoxemia and further inflammation of the liver.

  - Fibrosis results from activation of the hepatic stellate cells, which proliferate and produce large amounts of collagen.

  - The pathologic characteristics of established alcoholic cirrhosis include steatosis, ballooning degeneration of hepatocytes, Mallory bodies (crescent shaped bunches of intracellular filaments), neutrophilic inflammation, and pericellular fibrosis.

  - Hepatocyte injury results in loss of the normal hepatic functions resulting in the risk for many complications including encephalopathy, jaundice, ascites, coagulopathy, pancytopenia, hypoalbuminemia (with resultant edema), and hyperestrinism (decreased estrogen metabolism leads to increased circulating estrogen levels).

- Portal Hypertension:

  - Increased portal pressure results from resistance to portal flow into the liver, and from increased portal blood flow.

  - Increased resistance:
    1) Alcoholic cirrhosis with inflammation causes hepatocyte swelling and collagen deposition with obstruction of the hepatic sinusoids.
    2) Myofibroblasts (found in cirrhotic livers) have some contractile function; their constriction further obstructs portal inflow to the sinusoids (and provides some response to vasodilator therapy).
    3) Intrahepatic vasoactive mediators such as endothelin and nitric oxide cause further changes in hepatic resistance to portal blood flow.

  - Increased portal blood flow:
    1) A complex interaction of neurohumoral factors (sympathetic nervous system, glucagon, serotonin, adenosine, angiotensin, atrial natriuretic factor, adenosine, nitric oxide, etc.) results in splanchnic vasodilation, increased cardiac output, decreased systemic peripheral resistance, and sodium retention.

- The result of all of these interactions is increased pressure in the portal system, with a systemic hyperdynamic state (increased cardiac output and tachycardia but decreased systemic arterial pressure).

- Once portal pressure exceeds a level of 10 to 12 mmHg above the pressure in the hepatic vein, portal collaterals begin shunting portal blood.
  1) Portal hypertension persists due to further increases in portal flow and increases in collateral resistance modulated by serotonin and nitric oxide.
  2) The major portal collaterals include those around the esophagus, stomach, rectum, and umbilicus; patients that have undergone previous abdominal surgery may also have collaterals around the small and large bowel.
  3) Dilation of these collaterals (esophageal and gastric varices, caput medusa, and hemorrhoids) results in considerable risk for serious hemorrhage.

- Increased portal pressure plus the likely associated increases in aldosterone and decreases in serum albumin result in ascites and edema.

- Ascites and relative immune compromise (decreased T cell activity) from cirrhosis and portal hypertension creates a risk for spontaneous bacterial peritonitis.

PATIENT PRESENTATION

- History:

  Alcohol abuse (40 to 80 g of ethanol a day, or about 2 to 4 drinks); female gender; poor diet; history of hepatitis.

- Symptoms:

  Confusion; jaundice; easy bruising; increasing abdominal girth; decreased exercise tolerance; hematemesis; hematochezia; melena; anorexia; weight loss; edema.

- Examination:

  Hepatomegaly; hard nodular surface to the liver; splenomegaly; jaundice; ascites; encephalopathy; asterixis; fever; edema; ecchymoses; gynecomastia; palmar erythema; testicular atrophy; spider nevi; caput medusae; hemorrhoids; heme positive stools.

DIFFERENTIAL DIAGNOSIS

- Viral or toxic hepatitis
- Nonalcoholic steatohepatitis:
  - Parenteral nutrition
  - Obesity
  - Diabetes
  - Diethylstilbestrol
  - Glucocorticoids
  - Amiodarone

- Hemochromatosis

- Primary biliary fibrosis

- Hepatic carcinoma

- Portal vein thrombosis

- Polycystic liver

KEYS TO ASSESSMENT

- Laboratory findings include macrocytic anemia, leukocytosis, modest elevations in aspartate aminotransferase (AST) and alanine aminotransferase (ALT) with an AST/ALT ratio >2, increased bilirubin, elevated prothrombin time (PT) and partial thromboplastin time (PTT), and decreased albumin.

- Other markers of alcoholic cirrhosis include laminin, hyaluronan, type III procollagen, type IV collagen, tissue inhibitor of metalloproteinase, and prolyl hydroxylase (these are not used clinically at this time).

- Patients at high risk for early mortality: 4.6X[PT(seconds) - control] + bilirubin (mg/dL) >32 indicates a 1 month mortality of 50%.

- Liver biopsy is indicated for clinical evidence of cirrhosis with a minimal alcohol intake.

- Abdominal computed tomography (CT) should be considered for evaluation of possible hepatic carcinoma.

- Ultrasound and pulsed doppler are used to evaluate biliary tree and portal vein blood flow if suspected portal hypertension.

- If portal hypertension is present, endoscopy is indicated to evaluate for varices.

- Magnetic resonance angiography can be used to further evaluate the portal vein if surgery is contemplated.

- Direct portal vein pressure measurements of the portal circulation are rarely needed, but can be done in selected cases prior to surgical intervention.

KEYS TO MANAGEMENT

- Abstinence is the most important intervention and can improve survival in most patients; it does not guarantee improvement, but improvement will not occur without it.

- Malnutrition is correlated with poor prognosis in alcoholic cirrhosis, and although nutritional supplementation has not been clearly shown to improve outcomes, it is reasonable to provide some nutritional support to malnourished and anorexic patients. Protein supplements are important to raise albumin levels, but must be given with caution in patients with a history of encephalopathy.

- Bedrest with <u>careful</u> administration of diuretics can improve edema and ascites; however, high doses of diuretics can result in intravascular hypovolemia, hypotension, and renal toxicity.

- Pharmacologic intervention includes propylthiouracil, corticosteroids, colchicine, and antioxidants, which reduce hepatic inflammation and fibrosis. All of these have shown some benefit in alcoholic cirrhosis, but results are not dramatic and side effects are common.

- Liver transplant for alcoholic cirrhosis requires evaluation for strict preoperative criteria including 6 months confirmed abstinence; survival rates after transplant are equivalent for nonalcoholic liver disease and recidivism is less than 10%.

- Propranolol has been used in portal hypertension with some improvement in portal pressures and decreased risk of variceal bleeding; nitrates can be tried in patients that are intolerant of beta blockade.

- Endoscopic prophylactic sclerosis or ligation of esophageal varices is widely used but remains controversial. Some studies have shown less bleeding and improved survival; others have shown up to a two fold increase in mortality with prophylactic sclerosis.

- Management of acute variceal hemorrhage requires emergent endoscopy and sclerotherapy and/or administration of vasopressin plus nitroglycerin or somatostatin (or its analog octreotide).

- Balloon tamponade can be used to control bleeding until the patient can undergo one of several surgical interventions, including esophageal devascularization or shunt operations such as a splenorenal shunt.

- A transjugular intrahepatic portosystemic shunt (TIPS) can be placed percutaneously, but this procedure is associated with significant risk of encephalopathy, accelerated liver failure, and restenosis and it has a 15% mortality at 1 month—it should be used only to manage acute and recurrent hemorrhage, not as a prophylactic procedure.

Pathophysiology → Clinical Link

What is going on in the disease process that influences how the patient presents and how he or she should be managed?

What should you do now that you understand the underlying pathophysiology?

Pathophysiology	Clinical Link
Ethanol is responsible for the steps in primary hepatic damage that lead to cirrhosis.	A history of alcohol intake is common in patients with cirrhosis, and abstinence is the key to management.
The process of cirrhosis includes the release of inflammatory cytokines that results in collagen synthesis and deposition.	Antiinflammatories and drugs that block collagen deposition are used in cirrhosis with some success (steroids, colchicine).
Hepatic dysfunction due to cirrhosis results in inability to excrete bilirubin, inability to make coagulation factors, inability to make albumin, inability to metabolize ADH and estrogen, and suppresses the bone marrow.	Patients with severe cirrhosis may present with jaundice, coagulopathy, edema and ascites, feminization, and anemia.
Increased portal pressure is not only due to increased hepatic resistance to perfusion by the portal vein but also to sustained increases in portal blood flow.	Therapy for portal hypertension includes shunting procedures and drugs that influence the neuro-humorally-mediated increases in portal blood flow (propranolol, somatostatin).
Increased portal pressure dilates collateral veins around the esophagus, stomach, rectum, and umbilicus.	Dilated collaterals form esophageal and gastric varices, hemorrhoids, and caput medusae; varices and hemorrhoids can bleed spontaneously with considerable morbidity and mortality.
Portal hypertension is associated with systemic hemodynamic changes such as decreased peripheral resistance, increased cardiac output, and decreased arterial pressure; the edema or cirrhosis is due to decreased intravascular oncotic pressure.	Although the patient may have considerable edema and ascites, they are often intravascularly depleted and may respond to diuretics with hypotension and oliguria.

BIBLIOGRAPHY

Boldys, H., Romanczyk, T., Hartleb, M., & Nowak, A. (1996). Short-term effects of variceal sclerotherapy on portal hypertensive gastropathy. *Endoscopy, 28*(9), 735-739.

Brecher, A. S., Hinko, A., & Twining, S. S. (1996). A proposed sequence of reactions leading to collagen biosynthesis, fibrosis, and hypertension in alcoholics [review, 107 refs]. *Journal of Investigative Medicine, 44*(2), 36-41.

Brown, R. S. J., & Lake, J. R. (1997). Transjugular intrahepatic portosystemic shunt as a form of treatment for portal hypertension: Indications and contraindications [review, 17 refs]. *Advances in Internal Medicine, 42*, 485-504.

Caregaro, L., Alberino, F., Amodio, P., Merkel, C., Bolognesi, M., Angeli, P., & Gatta, A. (1996). Malnutrition in alcoholic and virus-related cirrhosis. *American Journal of Clinical Nutrition, 63*(4), 602-609.

Combis, J. M., Vinel, J. P., Badia, P., Barange, K., Payen, J. L., Combis, F., Desmorat, H., & Pascal, J. P. (1996). Haemodynamic effects of molsidomine and propranolol in patients with cirrhosis. *British Journal of Clinical Pharmacology, 41*(5), 409-413.

Conn, H. O., Lebrec, D., & Terblanche, J. (1997). The treatment of esophageal varices: A debate and a discussion [review, 27 refs]. *Journal of Internal Medicine, 241*(2), 103-108.

Corrao, G., Ferrari, P., Zambon, A., & Torchio, P. (1997). Are the recent trends in liver cirrhosis mortality affected by the changes in alcohol consumption? Analysis of latency period in European countries. *Journal of Studies on Alcohol, 58*(5), 486-494.

Elsayed, S. S., Shiha, G., Hamid, M., Farag, F. M., Azzam, F., & Awad, M. (1996). Sclerotherapy versus sclerotherapy and propranolol in the prevention of rebleeding from esophageal varices: A randomised study. *Gut, 38*(5), 770-774.

Escorsell, A., Bandi, J. C., Moitinho, E., Feu, F., Garcia-Pagan, J. C., Bosch, J., & Rodes, J. (1997). Time profile of the haemodynamic effects of terlipressin in portal hypertension. *Journal of Hepatology, 26*(3), 621-627.

Fabrega, F., Foster, P. F., Sankary, H. N., Karademir, S., Kociss, K., McChesney, L. P., & Williams, J. W. (1997). Liver transplantation for patients with alcoholic cirrhosis. *Transplantation Proceedings, 29*(1-2), 465-466.

Fantin, A. C., Zala, G., Risti, B., Debatin, J. F., Schopke, W., & Meyenberger, C. (1996). Bleeding anorectal varices: Successful treatment with transjugular intrahepatic portosystemic shunting (TIPS). *Gut, 38*(6), 932-935.

Garcia-Pagan, J. C., Escorsell, A., Feu, F., Bandi, J. C., Moitinho, E., Casado, M., Bosch, J., & Rodes, J. (1996). Propranolol plus molsidomine vs propranolol alone in the treatment of portal hypertension in patients with cirrhosis. *Journal of Hepatology, 24*(4), 430-435.

Garcia-Pagan, J. C., Santos, C., Barbera, J. A., Luca, A., Roca, J., Rodriguez-Roisin, R., Bosch, J., & Rodes, J. (1996). Physical exercise increases portal pressure in patients with cirrhosis and portal hypertension. *Gastroenterology, 111*(5), 1300-1306.

Gerhardt, T. C., Goldstein, R. M., Urschel, H. C., Tripp, L. E., Levy, M. F., Husberg, B. S., Jennings, L. W., Gonwa, T. A., & Klintmalm, G. B. (1996). Alcohol use following liver transplantation for alcoholic cirrhosis. *Transplantation, 62*(8), 1060-1063.

Grellier, L. F., & Dusheiko, G. M. (1997). The role of hepatitis C virus in alcoholic liver disease [review, 58 refs]. *Alcohol and Alcoholism, 32*(2), 103-111.

Groszmann, R. J. (1996). Pharmacological treatment of portal hypertension [review, 30 refs]. *Digestion, 57*(Suppl 1), 103-106.

Grove, J., Daly, A. K., Bassendine, M. F., & Day, C. P. (1997). Association of a tumor necrosis factor promoter polymorphism with susceptibility to alcoholic steatohepatitis [see comments]. *Hepatology, 26*(1), 143-146.

Hamberg, K. J., Carstensen, B., Sorensen, T. I., & Eghoje, K. (1996). Accuracy of clinical diagnosis of cirrhosis among alcohol-abusing men. *Journal of Clinical Epidemiology, 49*(11), 1295-1301.

Hartigan, P. M., Gebhard, R. L., & Gregory, P. B. (1997). Sclerotherapy for actively bleeding esophageal varices in male alcoholics with cirrhosis. Veterans Affairs Cooperative Variceal Sclerotherapy Group [see comments]. *Gastrointestinal Endoscopy, 46*(1), 1-7.

Ho, H., Zuckerman, M. J., Ho, T. K., Guerra, L. G., Verghese, A., & Casner, P. R. (1996). Prevalence of associated infections in community-acquired spontaneous bacterial peritonitis. *American Journal of Gastroenterology, 91*(4), 735-742.

Homann, C., Hansen, M. B., Graudal, N., Hasselqvist, P., Svenson, M., Bendtzen, K., Thomsen, A. C., & Garred, P. (1996). Anti-interleukin-6 autoantibodies in plasma are associated with an increased frequency of infections and increased mortality of patients with alcoholic cirrhosis. *Scandinavian Journal of Immunology, 44*(6), 623-629.

Homann, C., Varming, K., Hogasen, K., Mollnes, T. E., Graudal, N., Thomsen, A. C., & Garred, P. (1997). Acquired C3 deficiency in patients with alcoholic cirrhosis predisposes to infection and increased mortality. *Gut, 40*(4), 544-549.

Jaffe, D. L., Chung, R. T., & Friedman, L. S. (1996). Management of portal hypertension and its complications [review, 82 refs]. *Medical Clinics of North America, 80*(5), 1021-1034.

Jung, K. (1997). Plasma but not serum should be used for determining tissue inhibitor of metalloproteinase in blood [letter]. *Alcoholism, Clinical and Experimental Research, 21*(6), 1155-1156.

Korner, T., Kropf, J., & Gressner, A. M. (1996). Serum laminin and hyaluronan in liver cirrhosis: Markers of progression with high prognostic value. *Journal of Hepatology, 25*(5), 684-688.

Kuo, P. C., Johnson, L. B., Plotkin, J. S., Howell, C. D., Bartlett, S. T., & Rubin, L. J. (1997). Continuous intravenous infusion of epoprostenol for the treatment of portopulmonary hypertension. *Transplantation, 63*(4), 604-606.

La, V. G., Lazzeri, C., Pascale, A., Sestini, S., Bisi, G., Sciagra, R., Vecchiarino, S., Raggi, V. C., Barletta, G., Laffi, G., & Gentilini, P. (1997). Cardiovascular and renal effects of low-dose atrial natriuretic peptide in compensated cirrhosis. *American Journal of Gastroenterology, 92*(5), 852-857.

Laso, F. J., Madruga, J. I., Lopez, A., Ciudad, J., Alvarez-Mon, M., San, M. J., & Orfao, A. (1996). Distribution of peripheral blood lymphoid subsets in alcoholic liver cirrhosis: Influence of ethanol intake. *Alcoholism, Clinical and Experimental Research, 20*(9), 1564-1568.

Li, M. K., Sung, J. J., Woo, K. S., Sanderson, J., Leung, N. W., Yu, L. M., Tsui, C. P., Chung, S. C., & Leung, F. W. (1996). Somatostatin reduces gastric mucosal blood flow in patients with portal hypertensive gastropathy: A randomized, double-blind crossover study. *Digestive Diseases and Sciences, 41*(12), 2440-2446.

Lieber, C. S. (1997). Pathogenesis and treatment of liver fibrosis in alcoholics: 1996 update [review, 175 refs]. *Digestive Diseases, 15*(1-2), 42-66.

Luca, A., Garcia-Pagan, J. C., Bosch, J., Feu, F., Caballeria, J., Groszmann, R. J., & Rodes, J. (1997). Effects of ethanol consumption on hepatic hemodynamics in patients with alcoholic cirrhosis. *Gastroenterology, 112*(4), 1284-1289.

McCullough, A. J., & Bugianesi, E. (1997). Protein-calorie malnutrition and the etiology of cirrhosis [editorial; comment] [review, 77 refs]. *American Journal of Gastroenterology, 92*(5), 734-738.

McEwen, D. R. (1996). Management of alcoholic cirrhosis of the liver [review, 64 refs]. *AORN Journal, 64*(2), 209-216.

Miyakawa, H., Liu, J., Noguchi, O., Marumo, F., & Sato, C. (1996). Effect of alcohol drinking on gene expression of hepatic O6-methylguanine DNA methyltransferase in chronic liver diseases. *Alcoholism, Clinical and Experimental Research, 20*(9 Suppl), 297A-300A.

Moller, S., Brinch, K., Henriksen, J. H., & Becker, U. (1997). Effect of octreotide on systemic, central, and splanchnic haemodynamics in cirrhosis. *Journal of Hepatology, 26*(5), 1026-1033.

Naveau, S., Giraud, V., Borotto, E., Aubert, A., Capron, F., & Chaput, J. C. (1997). Excess weight risk factor for alcoholic liver disease. *Hepatology, 25*(1), 108-111.

Nevens, F., Lijnen, P., VanBilloen, H., & Fevery, J. (1996). The effect of long-term treatment with spironolactone on variceal pressure in patients with portal hypertension without ascites. *Hepatology, 23*(5), 1047-1052.

Ohhira, M., Fujimoto, Y., Matsumoto, A., Ohtake, T., Ono, M., & Kohgo, Y. (1996). Hepatocellular carcinoma associated with alcoholic liver disease: A clinicopathological study and genetic polymorphism of aldehyde dehydrogenase 2. *Alcoholism, Clinical and Experimental Research, 20*(9 Suppl), 378A-382A.

Pares, A., Deulofeu, R., Gimenez, A., Caballeria, L., Bruguera, M., Caballeria, J., Ballesta, A. M., & Rodes, J. (1996). Serum hyaluronate reflects hepatic fibrogenesis in alcoholic liver disease and is useful as a marker of fibrosis. *Hepatology, 24*(6), 1399-1403.

Reed, T., Page, W. F., Viken, R. J., & Christian, J. C. (1996). Genetic predisposition to organ-specific endpoints of alcoholism. *Alcoholism, Clinical and Experimental Research, 20*(9), 1528-1533.

Rockey, D. (1997). The cellular pathogenesis of portal hypertension: Stellate cell contractility, endothelin, and nitric oxide [review, 43 refs]. *Hepatology, 25*(1), 2-5.

Sanyal, A. J., Freedman, A. M., Luketic, V. A., Purdum, P. P., Shiffman, M. L., DeMeo, J., Cole, P. E., & Tisnado, J. (1997). The natural history of portal hypertension after transjugular intrahepatic portosystemic shunts [comment]. *Gastroenterology, 112*(3), 889-898.

Savolainen, V. T., Pajarinen, J., Perola, M., Penttila, A., & Karhunen, P. J. (1997). Polymorphism in the cytochrome P450 2E1 gene and the risk of alcoholic liver disease. *Journal of Hepatology, 26*(1), 55-61.

Schirren, C. A., Jung, M. C., Zachoval, R., Diepolder, H., Hoffmann, R., Riethmuller, G., & Pape, G. R. (1997). Analysis of T cell activation pathways in patients with liver cirrhosis, impaired delayed hypersensitivity and other T cell-dependent functions. *Clinical and Experimental Immunology, 108*(1), 144-150.

Sekiyama, T., Komeichi, H., Nagano, T., Ohsuga, M., Terada, H., Katsuta, Y., Satomura, K., & Aramaki, T. (1997). Effects of the alpha-/beta-blocking agent carvedilol on hepatic and systemic hemodynamics in patients with cirrhosis and portal hypertension. *Arzneimittel-Forschung, 47*(4), 353-355.

Shelton, W., & Balint, J. A. (1997). Fair treatment of alcoholic patients in the context of liver transplantation [review, 33 refs]. *Alcoholism, Clinical and Experimental Research, 21*(1), 93-100.

Sirikonda, P. R., Spillert, C. R., Koneru, B., Ponnudurai, R., Wilson, D. J., & Lazaro, E. J. (1996). Deceptive prothrombin and activated partial thromboplastin times in alcoholic cirrhosis. *Journal of the National Medical Association, 88*(5), 306-309.

Sogni, P., Hadengue, A., Moreau, R., Le, M. O., Soupison, T., Oberti, F., Farinotti, R., & Lebrec, D. (1997). Acute effects of propylthiouracil on hemodynamics and oxygen content in patients with alcoholic cirrhosis. *Journal of Hepatology, 26*(3), 628-633.

Soybel, D. I. (1997). TIPS versus surgical decompression of portal hypertension. *Gastroenterology, 112*(5), 1768-1770.

Stanley, A. J., Jalan, R., Forrest, E. H., Redhead, D. N., & Hayes, P. C. (1996). Long-term follow up of transjugular intrahepatic portosystemic stent shunt (TIPSS) for the treatment of portal hypertension: Results in 130 patients [see comments]. *Gut, 39*(3), 479-485.

Trevillyan, J., & Carroll, P. J. (1997). Management of portal hypertension and esophageal varices in alcoholic cirrhosis [review, 28 refs]. *American Family Physician, 55*(5), 1851-1858.

Tsutsumi, M., Takase, S., Urashima, S., Ueshima, Y., Kawahara, H., & Takada, A. (1996). Serum markers for hepatic fibrosis in alcoholic liver disease: Which is the best marker, type III procollagen, type IV collagen, laminin, tissue inhibitor of metalloproteinase, or prolyl hydroxylase? *Alcoholism, Clinical and Experimental Research, 20*(9), 1512-1517.

Vymazal, J., Babis, M., Brooks, R. A., Filip, K., Dezortova, M., Hrncarkova, H., & Hajek, M. (1996). T1 and T2 alterations in the brains of patients with hepatic cirrhosis. *American Journal of Neuroradiology, 17*(2), 333-336.

Zervos, E. E., McCormick, J., Goode, S. E., & Rosemurgy, A. S. (1997). Peritoneovenous shunts in patients with intractable ascites: Palliation at what price? *American Surgeon, 63*(2), 157-162.

CASE STUDY*

ALCOHOLIC CIRRHOSIS AND PORTAL HYPERTENSION

INITIAL HISTORY:
- 59-year-old male
- Brought into the emergency department by wife who noticed increased confusion over last 3 days
- Dark stools all week
- Increased abdominal girth and tenderness

Question 1.
What is your differential diagnosis based on initial information?

Question 2.
What additional history would you obtain?

ADDITIONAL HISTORY (via wife):
- No recent infections, fever, illnesses, falls
- Drinks 8 to 12 beers/day and more on weekends ($\pm$ 25 years); last beers yesterday
- Smoking—20 pack/year history
- Has had a "beer belly" for about 10 years, getting bigger over the last month (tender for 3 to 4 days)
- Confusion over the last 3 to 4 days
- Occasional use of Advil or Tylenol for headache; no known use of prescription or illicit drugs
- No history to suggest prior cardiac or gallbladder disease; no previous history of hepatitis

---

* Suzanne M. Burns, RN, MSN, RRT, ACNP-CS, CCRN, contributed this case study.

Question 3.
Now what do you think?

PHYSICAL EXAMINATION:
- Confused; knows his name and his wife's name; restless in bed, lying on side
- T = 36.7 orally; P = 120 beats/minute and regular; RR = 24 breaths/minute, slightly labored; BP = 138/80 lying, 120/75 sitting

HEENT, Skin, Neck
- Slight scleral icterus
- No bruises, masses, deformities on head
- Nystagmus with lateral gaze
- Pupils 3 mm, reactive to light
- Funduscopy without lesions
- Ears—cerumen in left ear canal
- Spider angiomas over upper chest and abdomen
- Palmar erythema
- Slightly diaphoretic
- Mild jaundice
- 3 to 4 bruises on lower extremities
- Supple
- No adenopathy, thyromegaly, bruits

Lungs, Chest
- Clear to auscultation
- Poor diaphragmatic excursions (rapid, shallow breathing pattern)
- Gynecomastia

Cardiac
- Tachycardia
- Grade II systolic ejection murmur
- No gallops, rubs, or clicks

Abdomen
- Large, distended
- Hyperactive bowel sounds (has just passed large, dark maroon stool, and vomited about 100 cc blood)
- Diffusely tender to palpation
- No aortic, iliac, renal bruits
- Positive fluid wave, shifting dullness
- Splenomegaly

Extremities
- Good capillary refill
- Trace—+1 edema of feet

Neurological
- Oriented to person only; confused, muttering
- Cranial nerves: II-XII grossly intact (exception noted cranial nerve VI)
- Sensory: Extremities grossly intact to pinprick and light touch
- Reflexes: Hyperreflexic
- Asterixis

Question 4.

What are the pertinent positives and significant negatives on the exam and what do they suggest?

Question 5.

What diagnostic studies and/or therapeutic interventions do you think are indicated now?

LABORATORY:
- SaO_2 = 89%, ABGs: pH = 7.43, $PaCO_2$ = 33 mmHg, PaO_2 = 58 mmHg on room air
- CBC: HGB/HCT = 9/27, WBC = 12,000, PLTs = 75,000
- Electrolytes = Na, K, MG, and phosphate decreased
- Bilirubin (direct) slightly increased
- AST and ALT both elevated (ratio = 2/1), alkaline phosphatase = normal
- PT = 20, PTT = 32 (both elevated)
- Serum ammonia = elevated
- Albumin = low; cholesterol = low
- Chest x-ray = normal
- ECG = sinus tachycardia

Question 6.

Which labs are most important for you to act on now and what will you do?

Question 7.

Do other labs suggest the etiology of Mr. Z's internal bleeding?

STATUS UPON ICU TRANSFER:

- Mr. Z is transferred to ICU
- Continues to pass maroon colored stools
- Started on octreotide
- Mr. Z is still confused and is intubated prior to sclerotherapy for airway protection.
- GI consult service performs endoscopy, which demonstrates both esophageal and gastric varices; esophageal varices (which appear to be the site of active bleeding) are sclerosed.

Question 8.

Why is octreotide used?

Question 9.

Following schlerotherapy, Mr. Z is more stable (appears to have stopped bleeding). Despite being confused, he is able to protect his airway and is extubated. What other management do you want to consider now?

HOSPITAL COURSE:

- Mr. Z does well and is transferred from the ICU to a medical floor within 48 hours of admission.
- PT is corrected; bleeding has stopped
- Mental status has improved
- Has not experienced delrium tremens
- Spontaneous bacterial peritonitis is ruled out

Question 10.

Now what should the plan be?

DAY 4 ON MEDICAL FLOOR/HOSPITALIZATION DAY 6:

- Mr. Z is ready to be discharged in the care of his wife.
- Tired but alert and oriented
- No further bleeding

Question 11.

What instructions and medications should go home with Mr. Z and his wife?

CHAPTER 18

HEADACHE

DEFINITION

- Primary headaches refer to those that fit the diagnostic criteria for one of three major categories of headache: migraine, tension-type, or cluster headache.

- Each of these major categories have subtypes as described by the 1988 International Headache Society classification system. Some of the major subtypes of headache.

  - Migraine:
    1) Migraine without aura
    2) Migraine with aura
    3) Ophthalmoplegic migraine
    4) Retinal migraine
    5) Childhood periodic syndromes that may be precursors to or associated with migraine
    6) Complications of migraine
    7) Migrainous disorder not fulfilling above criteria

  - Tension-type headache:
    1) Episodic tension-type headache associated with disorder of pericranial muscles
    2) Episodic tension-type headache unassociated with disorder of pericranial muscles
    3) Chronic tension-type headache associated with disorder of pericranial muscles
    4) Chronic tension-type headache unassociated with disorder of pericranial muscles
    5) Headache of the tension-type not fulfilling above criteria

  - Cluster headache:
    1) Episodic cluster headache
    2) Chronic cluster headache
    3) Chronic paroxysmal hemicrania
    4) Cluster headache-like disorder not fulfilling the above criteria

- Secondary headaches refer to those that are associated with an identified underlying cause such as drug-induced, cerebrovascular disease, sinusitis, ophthalmologic or otic disease, trauma and postconcussion syndrome, trigeminal neuralgia and many others.

EPIDEMIOLOGY

- 90% to 95% of the people in the United States have unprovoked headaches annually.

- It is the number one reason for seeking health care in this country.

- 35% to 40% of patients seeking treatment have chronic daily headache (CDH), meaning headache for at least 4 hours per day for at least 25 days per month.

- Many patients with CDH have both migrainous and tension-type headaches.
- Migraine:
  - Prevalence is 18% for females, and 6% for males; prevalence is increasing.
  - Onset is often in the teens; peak prevalence is in ages 35 to 45.
  - It is more common in those from low-income households.
  - There is a clear familial tendency, especially in females, with a possible association with mitochondrial deoxyribonucleic acid (DNA) and chromosome 19.
- Tension-type:
  - It is the most common type of primary headache.
  - Most CDH patients have a preceding history of episodic tension-type headaches.
- Cluster:
  - It is much less common than migraine or tension-type; incidence is <1%.
  - The male to female ratio is 5:1.
  - The incidence is highest in the late 20s or early 30s.

PATHOPHYSIOLOGY

- Migraine:
  - There are many theories of pathogenesis; a few consistent features are being identified.
    1) Many patients experience symptoms of mood change, hunger, or drowsiness during the 24 hours prior to headache, and the onset of headache is often associated with circadian rhythms, thus suggesting a central site for initiation of migraine near the hypothalamus.
    2) Preceding the headache, there is a reduction in blood flow (oligemia) and resultant cortical depression that spreads across the hemicortex at a rate of 2 to 3 mm per minute. This may or may not be associated with the symptoms of an aura including scintillating scotoma, paraesthesias, blurred vision, or other focal neurologic signs.
    3) As the headache progresses, trigeminal ganglion stimulation appears to be an important step in migraine pathogenesis causing intracerebral and extracerebral vasodilation, thus resulting in what has been called trigeminovascular pain.
    4) Neurons that arise in the trigeminal ganglion produce a variety of neurohumoral cytokines (e.g., substance P and calcitonin gene-related peptide [CGRP]) that cause perivascular neurogenic inflammation, mast cell degranulation, and changes in serotonin that further promote migraine progression.
    5) Decreased serotonin appears to be important in migraine pathogenesis. Serotonin agonists cause vasoconstriction, reduce neurogenic inflammation, and reduce pain transmission through the trigeminal system.
    6) In premenopausal women, cyclic estrogen withdrawal contributes to changes in serotonin and other neurotransmitters and causes a rise in serum prostaglandins that promote migraine pathogenesis. Thus migraines are common among women after puberty and before menopause and may present as "menstrual migraine."

- Tension-type:

  - There has been a long-standing appreciation for the presence of pericranial muscle spasm and headache in many patients, but it is clear that there are many patients who fit the criteria for tension-type headache that do not have these muscle spasms.

  - In those patients with pericranial muscle spasms, there is increased electromyographic activity in pericranial muscles, decreased blood flow and muscle ischemia especially of the temporalis muscle, and tenderness upon palpation of the head and neck muscles.

  - It has been postulated that there are several possible central mechanisms for tension-type headaches that are not associated with pericranial muscle spasms, but these are poorly understood. Recent evidence shows that serotonin levels are reduced in patients with chronic tension-type headache.

- Cluster:

  - In susceptible individuals, alterations in seasonal photoperiod may contribute to "cluster periods" lasting 2 to 4 months and affecting hypothalamic function.

  - Hypothalamic dysfunction leads to changes in chemoreceptor responses to hypoxemia, impaired autoregulation, and neuroendocrine dysfunction.

  - With "triggering" (hypoxemia, alcohol, histamine, vasodilators), unilateral extra and intracranial vasodilation occurs with increased intracerebral blood flow resulting in compression of the sympathetic plexus and release of serotonin and histamine.

  - Patients may exhibit nasal stuffiness, lacrimation, rhinorrhea, miosis, ptosis, sweating, and eyelid edema.

PATIENT PRESENTATION

- Criteria for diagnosis of each type of primary headache are listed in Table 18-1.

- Each type of primary headache is characterized by several classic features.

  - Migraine
    1) Unilateral (can be bilateral in up to 40%), pulsating headache of severe intensity associated with nausea, photophobia, phonophobia, and aggravated by physical activity lasting 4 to 72 hours; some will be preceded (less than 1 hour prior to onset of headache) by one or more fully reversible aura symptoms indicating focal cerebral cortical or brainstem dysfunction (e.g., visual blurring or scotoma, paresthesias, focal weakness or numbness); common in women in their 30s and 40s (e.g., often in association with menses); often a positive family history of migraine can be elicited.

  - Tension-type
    1) Episodic or chronic nonpulsating mild to moderate headache with or without pericranial and neck muscle pain and tenderness, that is bilateral and is not aggravated by routine physical activity and not associated with nausea, photophobia, or phonophobia.

  - Cluster
    1) Episodic clustered attacks of excruciating unilateral periorbital headache with associated conjunctival injection, lacrimation, nasal congestion and rhinorrhea, facial sweating, miosis, and ptosis, occurring up to 8 times a day lasting 15 to 180 minutes, and often awakening the patient from sleep; more common in men and may be triggered by alcohol, histamine, or vasodilators.

DIFFERENTIAL DIAGNOSIS

- Cerebrovascular accident

- Tumor

- Temporal arteritis

- Sinusitis

- Meningitis

- Subarachnoid hemorrhage

- Posttraumatic headache

- Hypertensive headache

- Medication-induced headache

- Benign exertional or cough headache

- High altitude headache

- Idiopathic stabbing headache

- Cold stimulus headache (ice cream headache); nitrate/nitrite-induced headache (hot dog headache); monsodium glutamate (MSG) headache

- Temporomandibular joint disease

- Cervical arthritis

- Cranial neuralgias

- Ophthalmologic pain (eyestrain, ophthalmoplegia with diplopia, spasm of the near reflex, corneal or conjunctival disease, glaucoma, uveitis)

- Otalgia (otis media, mastoiditis, neoplasms)

- Oral or pharyngeal pain (toothache, apthous ulcers, carcinomas)

KEYS TO ASSESSMENT

- <u>History</u>:

    - History should identify the pattern of symptoms that may help identify the cause.
        1) Onset
        2) Frequency
        3) Duration
        4) Intensity
        5) Location
        6) Quality
        7) Precipitators and exacerbators
        8) Ameliorators
        9) Associated symptoms
        10) Neurologic accompaniments

- Past medical history about childhood and adult illnesses, injuries, immunizations, medications, and allergies:
  1) Family history
  2) Lifestyle and social history
  3) Systems review

- Examination:

  - General appearance and activity (e.g., migraine patients usually lie still, cluster patients are often restless).

  - Look for fever and hypertension.

  - Do a careful physical examination for signs of infection, neoplasm, or vascular disease.

  - Perform a head exam for scalp or facial tenderness and vascular bruits.

  - Check the eyes, ears and temporomandibular joints.

  - Check the neck for mobility and tenderness.

  - Perform a careful neurologic exam for focal neurologic findings.

- Diagnostics:

  - Further studies would be indicated based on any specific findings on the physical exam.

  - If the patient has a normal examination, no more studies may be indicated.

  - Focal neurologic findings require immediate evaluation with magnetic resonance imaging (MRI), computed tomography (CT), or other specific studies.

  - If meningitis or subarachnoid hemorrhage are suspected, lumbar puncture is indicated.

  - Other suspected causes of secondary headache should be evaluated as appropriate.

KEYS TO MANAGEMENT

- Migraine

  - Avoid precipitating factors:
    1) Modify diet (e.g., decrease caffeine, highly seasoned foods, and chocolate)
    2) Maintain a regular sleeping schedule
    3) Avoid alcohol
    4) Maximize stress coping mechanisms
    5) Avoid oral contraceptives

- Acute migraine

  - **Sumatriptan or zolmitripan**—serotonin agonists with the most effective and rapid relief (>80% respond) and well tolerated (can cause coronary vasospasm); can be given SQ or PO

  - **Ergotamine** (usually in combination with caffeine)—<50% respond; also has a significant risk for coronary spasm

  - **Dihydroergotamine** (DHE)—intravenous (IV) or intramuscular (IM) injection gives rapid and effective relief (up to 90% respond); may require repeated injections; useful if patient does not respond to sumatriptan; may cause coronary spasm but less so than ergotamine

- **Others**—intranasal lidocaine (high recurrence rate); intravenous chlorpromazine or prochlorperazine; narcotics (largely ineffective)

  - Numerous new serotonin agonists are in development including naratriptan, rizatriptan, and eletriptan.

- Migraine prophylaxis is indicated when attack frequency is between 2 and 8 per month and are severe enough to impair normal life, or when patient is intolerant to abortive therapies due to side effects.

  - **β-blockers** (propranolol, metoprolol, atenolol, nadolol, and timolol only) are the first choice with 10% to 15% of patients having side effects.

  - **Calcium antagonists** (flunarizine) have frequent side effects that limit use.

  - **Valproate** is effective, but has frequent side effects.

  - **Nonsteroidal antiinflammatory drugs (NSAIDS)** (naproxen) are useful in some patients who do not tolerate β-blockers.

  - **Methysergide** should be used only for severe refractory cases due to high risk of serious side effects such as abdominal pain, nausea, and retroperitoneal fibrosis.

  - **Amitriptyline** is useful in patients with both migraine and tension-type headaches, but also has significant side effects.

- Tension-type

  - Episodic headaches can usually be managed with over-the-counter (OTC) drugs such as aspirin or acetaminophen (with or without caffeine) or nonsteroidal antiinflammatory agents.

  - CDH should be treated with antidepressants—tricyclic antidepressants have the longest track record. Rebound headache from an overuse of OTCs can be a serious problem.

  - Physical therapy including proper attention to posture (especially at work) and daily exercises to loosen up the neck and shoulder muscles can be very helpful.

  - Stress management and relaxation therapy can also be effective, sometimes in combination with biofeedback or transcutaneous electrical nerve stimulation (TENS).

  - Obtain a referral for a psychological evaluation if indicated.

- Cluster

  - Avoidance of triggers
    1) Avoid alcohol, histamine, and vasodilators
    2) Avoid prolonged contact with solvents, gasoline and oil-based paints
    3) Prophylaxis prior to airplane or high altitude travel

  - Acute cluster headache
    1) Oxygen inhalation (aborts 90% of attacks) should be started immediately at 7 L/min via mask
    2) Sublingual, medihaler, or IM ergotamine
    3) Intranasal lidocaine

  - Cluster headache prophylaxis
    1) Ergotamine daily during attack periods
    2) Verapamil daily (70% respond)
    3) Lithium if resistant to ergotamine-verapamil (70% respond)
    4) Methysergide or prednisone in highly refractory cases

Table 18-1.
Criteria for Diagnosis of Each Type of Primary Headache

DIAGNOSTIC CRITERIA FOR MIGRAINE WITHOUT AND WITH AURA

Migraine without Aura
A. At least five attacks fulfilling B-D
B. Headache attacks lasting 4 to 72 hours (untreated or unsuccessfully treated)
C. Headache has at least two of the following characteristics:
  1. Unilateral location
  2. Pulsating quality
  3. Moderate or severe intensity (inhibits or prohibits daily activities)
  4. Aggravation by walking stairs or similar routine physical activity
D. During headache, at least one of the following are present:
  1. Nausea and/or vomiting
  2. Photophobia and phonophobia.
E. At least one of the following are present:
  1. History and physical and neurologic examinations do not suggest headaches secondary to organic or systemic metabolic disease
  2. History and/or physical and/or neurologic examinations do suggest such disorder, but it is ruled out by appropriate investigations
  3. Such disorder is present, but migraine attacks do not occur for the first time in close temporal relation to the disorder

Migraine with Aura
A. At least two attacks fulfilling B
B. At least three of the following four characteristics are present:
  1. One or more fully reversible aura symptoms indicating focal cerebral cortical and/or brain stem dysfunction
  2. At least one aura symptom develops gradually over more than 4 minutes or two or more symptoms occur in succession
  3. No aura symptom lasts more than 60 minutes; if more than one aura symptom is present, accepted duration is proportionally increased
  4. Headache follows aura with a free interval of less than 60 minutes (it may also begin before or simultaneously with the aura)
C. At least one of the following are present:
  1. History and/or physical and/or neurologic examinations do not suggest headaches secondary to organic or systemic metabolic disease
  2. History and physical and/or neurologic examinations do suggest such disorder but it is ruled out by appropriate investigations

----

CRITERIA FOR VARIOUS FORMS OF TENSION-TYPE HEADACHE

Tension-type Headache
A. At least two of the following pain characteristics are present:
  1. Pressing/tightening (nonpulsing quality)
  2. Mild or moderate intensity (may inhibit but does not prohibit activities)
  3. Bilateral location
  4. No aggravation by walking stairs or similar routine physical activity
B. Both of the following occur:
  1. No nausea or vomiting (anorexia may occur); and
  2. Photophobia and phonophobia are present, or one but not the other is present
C. At least one of the following occur:
  1. History and physical and neurological examinations do not suggest headaches secondary to organic or systemic metabolic disease.

Table 18-1 continued:

2. History and/or physical and/or neurological examinations do suggest such disorders, but it is ruled out by appropriate investigations
3. Such disorder is present, but tension-type headache does not occur for the first time in close temporal relation to the disorder

Episodic Tension-type Headache
    A. Diagnostic criteria includes:
        1. At least 10 previous headache episodes; number of days with such headache is 180 per year (<15 per month)
        2. Headache lasting from 30 minutes to 7 days

Chronic tension-type Headache
    A. Diagnostic criteria includes:
        1. Average headache frequency $\geq$15 days per month ($\geq$180 days per year) for $\geq$6 months

Tension-type Headache Associated with Disorder of Pericranial Muscles
    A. At least one of the following is present:
        1. Increased tenderness of pericranial muscles demonstrated by manual palpation or pressure algometer
        2. Increased electromyographic activity of pericranial muscles at rest or during physiologic tests

Tension-type Headache Unassociated with Disorder of Pericranial Muscles
    A. There is no increased tenderness of pericranial muscles; if studied, electromyography of pericranial muscles shows normal levels of activity

---

DIAGNOSTIC CRITERIA FOR CLUSTER HEADACHE
    A. At least five attacks fulfilling B-D
    B. Severe unilateral orbital, supraorbital, and/or temporal pain lasting 15 to 180 minutes untreated
    C. Headache is associated with at least one of the following signs, which have to be present on the pain side:
        1. Conjunctival injection
        2. Lacrimation
        3. Nasal congestion
        4. Rhinorrhea
        5. Forehead and facial swelling
        6. Meiosis
        7. Ptosis
        8. Eyelid edema
    D. Frequency of attacks: from 1 every other day to 8 per day
    E. At least one of the following occurs:
        1. History and physical and neurologic examinations do not suggest headaches secondary to organic or systemic metabolic disease
        2. History and/or physical neurologic examinations do not suggest such disorder, but it is ruled out by appropriate investigations
        3. Such disorder is present but migraine attacks do not occur for the first time in close temporation relation to the disorder
    F. Cluster headache; periodicity undetermined
    G. Episodic cluster headache: attacks occur in periods lasting 7 days to 1 year separated by pain-free periods lasting $\geq$14 days
    H. Chronic cluster headache: attacks occur for more than 1 year without remission or with remissions lasting $\geq$14 days

Adapted from the 1988 International Headache Society Classification System.

Pathophysiology

What is going on in the disease process that influences how the patient presents and how he or she should be managed?

→

Clinical Link

What should you do now that you understand the underlying pathophysiology?

Migraine is possibly associated with changes in mitochondrial DNA.	Migraine is more common in females and has a familial tendency, especially from mothers to daughters.
Migraines are associated with vasoconstriction followed by vasodilation and inflammation with activation of the trigeminal ganglion and disturbances in neurotransmitters, especially serotonin.	Many migraines are preceded by an aura of neurologic symptoms such as scotoma paresthesias, followed by severe pulsating headache; serotonin agonists and vasoconstrictor medications can be used to abort an attack, and antiinflammatories help some patients.
Estrogen withdrawal just prior to menses is associated with changes in neurotransmitters in the central nervous system (CNS), especially serotonin.	Migraines are often associated with the menstrual cycle or the use of exogenous hormones.
Tension-type headaches are often associated with pericranial muscle spasms, but some are not, and there appears to be a central mechanism that may also be related to serotonin.	Many tension-type headaches are associated with poor posture and stress-related muscle tension and will respond to physical therapy and relaxation techniques; other patients have features of both tension-type and migraine and may respond to antidepressants and/or serotonin agonists.
Cluster headaches are associated with hypothalamic dysfunction, cerebral hypoxemia, and neuroendocrine dysfunction with release of histamine; intracranial vasodilation may compress the sympathetic plexus.	Seasonal "clusters" of headaches are related to changes in photoperiod; headaches are associated with nasal stuffiness and lacrimation as well as miosis and ptosis.
There are many structures in the head that can cause cranial pain such as sinuses, eyes, ears, mouth, etc., but most are associated with positive findings on physical exam.	The differential diagnosis of headache is extensive, but a primary headache is common, and patients with a normal exam do not require extensive diagnostic testing.

BIBLIOGRAPHY

Anonymous. (1996). Clinical policy for the initial approach to adolescents and adults presenting to the emergency department with a chief complaint of headache. American College of Emergency Physicians. *Annals of Emergency Medicine, 27*(6), 821-844.

Anonymous. (1996). Headache. *Current Opinion in Neurology, 9*(3), B60-B65.

Bansevicius, D., & Sjaastad, O. (1996). Cervicogenic headache: The influence of mental load on pain level and EMG of shoulder-neck and facial muscles. *Headache, 36*(6), 372-378.

Bendtsen, L., Jensen, R., & Olesen, J. (1996). Amitriptyline, a combined serotonin and noradrenaline re-uptake inhibitor, reduces exteroceptive suppression of temporal muscle activity in patients with chronic tension-type headache. *Electroencephalography and Clinical Neurophysiology, 101*(5), 418-422.

Burton, L. J., Quinn, B., Pratt-Cheney, J. L., & Pourani, M. (1997). Headache etiology in a pediatric emergency department. *Pediatric Emergency Care, 13*(1), 1-4.

Coutin, I. B., & Glass, S. F. (1996). Recognizing uncommon headache syndromes. [Review] [25 refs]. *American Family Physician, 54*(7), 2247-2252.

Cull, R. E., Price, W. H., & Dunbar, A. (1997). The efficacy of subcutaneous sumatriptan in the treatment of recurrence of migraine headache. *Journal of Neurology, Neurosurgery and Psychiatry, 62*(5), 490-495.

Drummond, P. D. (1996). The site of sympathetic deficit in cluster headache. *Headache, 36*(1), 3-9.

Duarte, J., Sempere, A. P., Delgado, J. A., Naranjo, G., Sevillano, M. D., & Claveria, L. E. (1996). Headache of recent onset in adults: A prospective population-based study. *Acta Neurologica Scandinavica, 94*(1), 67-70.

Durham, C. F., Dalton, J. A., Carlson, J., Neelon, V., Alden, K. R., & Englebardt, S. (1997). Migraine headache. *Journal of the American Academy of Nurse Practitioners, 9*(4), 179-185.

Edmeads, J. (1997). Headaches in older people. How are they different in this age-group? [review, 18 refs]. *Postgraduate Medicine, 101*(5), 91-94.

Evans, R. W. (1996). Diagnostic testing for the evaluation of headaches [review, 159 refs]. *Neurologic Clinics, 14*(1), 1-26.

Fanciullacci, M., Alessandri, M., Sicuteri, R., & Marabini, S. (1997). Responsiveness of the trigeminovascular system to nitroglycerine in cluster headache patients. *Brain, 120*(Pt 2), 283-288.

Fernandez, E., & Sheffield, J. (1996). Relative contributions of life events versus daily hassles to the frequency and intensity of headaches. *Headache, 36*(10), 595-602.

Ferrari, A., Stefani, M., Sternieri, S., Bertolotti, M., & Sternieri, E. (1997). Analgesic drug taking: Beliefs and behavior among headache patients. *Headache, 37*(2), 88-94.

Ferrari, M. D. (1997). 311C90: Increasing the options for therapy with effective acute antimigraine 5HT1B/1D receptor agonists [review, 15 refs]. *Neurology, 48*(3 Suppl 3), S21-S24.

Fettes, I. (1997). Menstrual migraine. Methods of prevention and control [review, 32 refs]. *Postgraduate Medicine, 101*(5), 67-70.

Franceschini, R., Leandri, M., Gianelli, M. V., Cataldi, A., Bruno, E., Rolandi, E., & Barreca, T. (1996). Evaluation of beta-endorphin secretion in patients suffering from episodic cluster headache. *Headache, 36*(10), 603-607.

Gallagher, R. M., Mueller, L., & Ciervo, C. A. (1996). Analgesic use in cluster headache. *Headache, 36*(2), 105-107.

Goadsby, P. J. (1997). Bench to bedside: What have we learned recently about headache? [review, 85 refs]. *Current Opinion in Neurology, 10*(3), 215-220.

Goadsby, P. J. (1997). Current concepts of the pathophysiology of migraine [review, 42 refs]. *Neurologic Clinics, 15*(1), 27-42.

Goadsby, P. J., & Lipton, R. B. (1997). A review of paroxysmal hemicranias, SUNCT syndrome and other short-lasting headaches with autonomic feature, including new cases. *Brain, 120*(Pt 1), 193-209.

Goadsby, P. J., & Olesen, J. (1997). Increasing the options for effective migraine management [review, 16 refs]. *Neurology, 48*(3 Suppl 3), S1-S3.

Hammill, J. M., Cook, T. M., & Rosecrance, J. C. (1996). Effectiveness of a physical therapy regimen in the treatment of tension-type headache. *Headache, 36*(3), 149-153.

Harden, R. N., Gracely, R. H., Carter, T., & Warner, G. (1996). The placebo effect in acute headache management: Ketorolac, meperidine, and saline in the emergency department. *Headache, 36*(6), 352-356.

Haslam, D. (1996). A pain in the head, or in the neck? *Practitioner, 240*(1569), 711.

Havelius, U., Heuck, M., Milos, P., & Hindfelt, B. (1996). Ciliospinal reflex response in cluster headache. *Headache, 36*(9), 568-573.

Hobson, W. H., Shiraki, R., Steiner, D., & Van, H. M. (1996). Spinal manipulation vs. amitriptyline for the treatment of chronic tension headache: A randomized clinical trial [letter; comment]. *Journal of Manipulative and Physiological Therapeutics, 19*(4), 278-279.

Holm, J. E., Lamberty, K., McSherry, W. C., & Davis, P. A. (1997). The stress response in headache sufferers: Physiological and psychological reactivity. *Headache, 37*(4), 221-227.

Hopkins, A. (1996). The epidemiology of headache and migraine, and its meaning for neurological services. *Schweizerische Medizinische Wochenschrift Journal Suisse de Medecine, 126*(4), 128-135.

Jensen, R. (1996). Mechanisms of spontaneous tension-type headaches: An analysis of tenderness, pain thresholds and EMG. *Pain, 64*(2), 251-256.

Labbe, E. E., Murphy, L., & O'Brien, C. (1997). Psychosocial factors and prediction of headaches in college adults. *Headache, 37*(1), 1-5.

Larsson, B., & Carlsson, J. (1996). A school-based, nurse-administered relaxation training for children with chronic tension-type headache. *Journal of Pediatric Psychology, 21*(5), 603-614.

Lewis, T. A., & Solomon, G. D. (1996). Advances in cluster headache management [see comments] [review, 35 refs]. *Cleveland Clinic Journal of Medicine, 63*(4), 237-244.

Lipchik, G. L., Holroyd, K. A., France, C. R., Kvaal, S. A., Segal, D., Cordingley, G. E., Rokicki, L. A., & McCool, H. R. (1996). Central and peripheral mechanisms in chronic tension-type headache. *Pain, 64*(3), 467-475.

Lipchik, G. L., Holroyd, K. A., Talbot, F., & Greer, M. (1997). Pericranial muscle tenderness and exteroceptive suppression of temporalis muscle activity: A blind study of chronic tension-type headache. *Headache, 37*(6), 368-376.

Lipton, R. B. (1997). Ergotamine tartrate and dihydroergotamine mesylate: Safety profiles [review, 33 refs]. *Headache, 37*(Suppl 1), S33-S41.

Lokken, C., Holm, J. E., & Myers, T. C. (1997). The menstrual cycle and migraine: A time-series analysis of 20 women migraineurs. *Headache, 37*(4), 235-239.

MacGregor, E. A. (1997). Menstruation, sex hormones, and migraine [review, 75 refs]. *Neurologic Clinics, 15*(1), 125-141.

Martelletti, P., & Giacovazzo, M. (1996). Putative neuroimmunological mechanisms in cluster headache. An integrated hypothesis [review, 44 refs]. *Headache, 36*(5), 312-315.

Martin, P. R., & Seneviratne, H. M. (1997). Effects of food deprivation and a stressor on head pain. *Health Psychology, 16*(4), 310-318.

Mathew, N. T. (1997). Dosing and administration of ergotamine tartrate and dihydroergotamine [review, 48 refs]. *Headache, 37*(Suppl 1), S26-S32.

Mathew, N. T. (1997). Serotonin 1D (5-HT1D) agonists and other agents in acute migraine [review, 127 refs]. *Neurologic Clinics, 15*(1), 61-83.

Mathew, N. T. (1997). Transformed migraine, analgesic rebound, and other chronic daily headaches [review, 54 refs]. *Neurologic Clinics, 15*(1), 167-186.

Melanson, S. W., & Raftis, J. (1996). Clinical pearls. Headache and eye pain. *Academic Emergency Medicine, 3*(9), 879-880.

Mills, T. M., & Scoggin, J. A. (1997). Intranasal lidocaine for migraine and cluster headaches. *Annals of Pharmacotherapy, 31*(7-8), 914-915.

Mongini, F., Defilippi, N., & Negro, C. (1997). Chronic daily headache. A clinical and psychological profile before and after treatment. *Headache, 37*(2), 83-87.

Moschiano, F., D'Amico, D., Grazzi, L., Leone, M., & Bussone, G. (1997). Sumatriptan in the acute treatment of migraine without aura: Efficacy of 50-mg dose. *Headache, 37*(7), 421-423.

Mueller, L., Gallagher, R. M., & Ciervo, C. A. (1997). Methylergonovine maleate as a cluster headache prophylactic: A study and review [review, 63 refs]. *Headache, 37*(7), 437-442.

Nordin, M., Fagius, J., & Waldenlind, E. (1997). Sympathetic vasoconstrictor outflow to extremity muscles in cluster headache. Recordings during spontaneous and nitroglycerin-induced attacks. *Headache, 37*(6), 358-367.

Olesen, J. (1997). International Headache Society classification and diagnostic criteria in children: A proposal for revision [letter; comment]. *Developmental Medicine & Child Neurology, 39*(2), 138.

Packard, R. C., & Ham, L. P. (1997). Pathogenesis of posttraumatic headache and migraine: A common headache pathway? [review, 114 refs]. *Headache, 37*(3), 142-152.

Pini, L. A., Bigarelli, M., Vitale, G., & Sternieri, E. (1996). Headaches associated with chronic use of analgesics: A therapeutic approach. *Headache, 36*(7), 433-439.

Pryse-Phillips, W. E., Dodick, D. W., Edmeads, J. G., Gawel, M. J., Nelson, R. F., Purdy, R. A., Robinson, G., Stirling, D., & Worthington, I. (1997). Guidelines for the diagnosis and management of migraine in clinical practice. Canadian Headache Society [review, 160 refs]. *Canadian Medical Association Journal, 156*(9), 1273-1287.

Queiroz, L. P., Rapoport, A. M., Weeks, R. E., Sheftell, F. D., Siegel, S. E., & Baskin, S. M. (1997). Characteristics of migraine visual aura. *Headache, 37*(3), 137-141.

Queiroz, L. P., Weeks, R. E., Rapoport, A. M., Sheftell, F. D., Baskin, S. M., & Siegel, S. E. (1996). Early and transient side effects of repetitive intravenous dihydroergotamine. *Headache, 36*(5), 291-294.

Ramadan, N. M. (1997). Unusual causes of headache [review, 50 refs]. *Neurology, 48*(6), 1494-1499.

Raskin, N. H. (1997). Short-lived head pains [review, 44 refs]. *Neurologic Clinics, 15*(1), 143-152.

Rubin, P. A., Chen, V. N., & Acquadro, M. A. (1996). Cluster headache presenting with orbital inflammation. *Ophthalmic Surgery and Lasers, 27*(2), 143-146.

Rubino, F. A. (1997). Initial evaluation of headache [review, 17 refs]. *Journal of the Florida Medical Association, 84*(1), 20-23.

Russell, M. B., Andersson, P. G., & Iselius, L. (1996). Cluster headache is an inherited disorder in some families. *Headache, 36*(10), 608-612.

Saper, J. R. (1997). Diagnosis and symptomatic treatment of migraine [review, 56 refs]. *Headache, 37*(Suppl 1), S1-S14.

Schachtel, B. P., Furey, S. A., & Thoden, W. R. (1996). Nonprescription ibuprofen and acetaminophen in the treatment of tension-type headache. *Journal of Clinical Pharmacology, 36*(12), 1120-1125.

Schoenen, J. (1997). Acute migraine therapy: The newer drugs [review, 38 refs]. *Current Opinion in Neurology, 10*(3), 237-243.

Schoenen, J. (1997). Clinical neurophysiology of headache [review, 140 refs]. *Neurologic Clinics, 15*(1), 85-105.

Sheftell, F. D. (1997). Role and impact of over-the-counter medications in the management of headache [review, 38 refs]. *Neurologic Clinics, 15*(1), 187-198.

Shibata, K., Osawa, M., & Iwata, M. (1997). Pattern reversal visual evoked potentials in classic and common migraine. *Journal of the Neurological Sciences, 145*(2), 177-181.

Silberstein, S. D., & Lipton, R. B. (1996). Headache epidemiology. Emphasis on migraine [review, 75 refs]. *Neurologic Clinics, 14*(2), 421-434.

Solomon, G. D. (1997). Evolution of the measurement of quality of life in migraine [review, 33 refs]. *Neurology, 48*(3 Suppl 3), S10-S15.

Solomon, G. D., Cady, R. K., Klapper, J. A., & Ryan, R. E. J. (1997). Standards of care for treating headache in primary care practice. National Headache Foundation. *Cleveland Clinic Journal of Medicine, 64*(7), 373-383.

Solomon, S. (1997). Diagnosis of primary headache disorders. Validity of the International Headache Society criteria in clinical practice [review, 22 refs]. *Neurologic Clinics, 15*(1), 15-26.

Spence, J. (1996). Migraine and other causes of headache [review, 25 refs]. *Annals of Emergency Medicine, 27*(4), 448-450.

Srikiatkhachorn, A., & Phanthumchinda, K. (1997). Prevalence and clinical features of chronic daily headache in a headache clinic. *Headache, 37*(5), 277-280.

Stewart, W. F., Staffa, J., Lipton, R. B., & Ottman, R. (1997). Familial risk of migraine: A population-based study. *Annals of Neurology, 41*(2), 166-172.

Stone, R. G., & Wharton, R. B. (1997). Simultaneous multiple-modality therapy for tension headaches and neck pain. *Biomedical Instrumentation and Technology, 31*(3), 259-262.

Strittmatter, M., Hamann, G. F., Grauer, M., Fischer, C., Blaes, F., Hoffmann, K. H., & Schimrigk, K. (1996). Altered activity of the sympathetic nervous system and changes in the balance of hypophyseal, pituitary and adrenal hormones in patients with cluster headache. *Neuroreport, 7*(7), 1229-1234.

Tfelt-Hansen, P. (1997). Prophylactic pharmacotherapy of migraine. Some practical guidelines [review, 27 refs]. *Neurologic Clinics, 15*(1), 153-165.

Ulrich, V., Russell, M. B., Jensen, R., & Olesen, J. (1996). A comparison of tension-type headache in migraineurs and in non-migraineurs: A population-based study. *Pain, 67*(2-3), 501-506.

Winner, P. K. (1997). Headaches in children. When is a complete diagnostic workup indicated? [review, 22 refs]. *Postgraduate Medicine, 101*(5), 81-85.

Wittrock, D. A. (1997). The comparison of individuals with tension-type headache and headache-free controls on frontal EMG levels: A meta-analysis. *Headache, 37*(7), 424-432.

Young, W. B. (1997). Appropriate use of ergotamine tartrate and dihydroergotamine in the treatment of migraine: Current perspectives. *Headache, 37*(Suppl 1), S42-S45.

Zwart, J. A. (1997). Neck mobility in different headache disorders. *Headache, 37*(1), 6-11.

CASE STUDY*

HEADACHE

INITIAL HISTORY:
- 34-year-old female presents with headache
- 2-day history of dull pain over the top of her head
- Unrelieved by aspirin or acetaminophen
- Admits to previous headaches of a similar nature
- Notes that they are becoming increasingly frequent

Question 1.
What is the differential diagnosis based on this history alone?

Question 2.
What further questions would you like to ask her to complete her review of symptoms?

ADDITIONAL HISTORY:
- Headache is generalized around the entire head.
- The pain sometimes wakes her from sleep but does not interfere with her daily activities.
- She denies nausea, vomiting, fever, chills, numbness or tingling, or visual changes.
- She had some neck and shoulder pain, but no neck stiffness.
- She denies photosensitivity or decreased level of consciousness.
- She has no nasal or postnasal drainage.

---

* **Leslie Buchanan, RN, MSN, FNP, contributed this case study.**

Question 3.
What other questions would you like to ask about her past medical, family, and social history?

MORE HISTORY:
- Patient denies any head injury.
- She admits to experiencing a great deal of stress recently.
- She drinks 3 to 4 beers each evening.
- Her mother had similar headaches occasionally, but nothing serious.
- Her last menstrual period was 3 weeks ago.
- She does not take oral contraceptives (OCPs) or estrogens.

PHYSICAL EXAMINATION:
- Alert, well-developed, well nourished female in no acute distress
- BP = 140/90; P = 80 and regular; RR = 16 and unlabored; T = 37.2 orally
- Skin is warm and dry; no rashes

HEENT
- No scalp tenderness
- Face nontender; no pain with percussion of the sinus cavities
- Tympanic membranes noninjected; no bulging or retraction
- Extraoccular movements full; visual acuity sharp (20/20 OU with corrective lenses)
- PERRL; no photosensitivity; conjunctiva clear; funduscopic demonstrates sharp disks and no hemorrhages
- Nasal mucosa pink; no drainage
- Throat noninjected without postnasal drainage

Neck
- Supple with full range of motion
- No palpable lymphadenopathy in the anterior or posterior chains
- No bruits heard

Lungs, Cardiovascular
- Lungs clear to auscultation and percussion
- Cardiac with RRR without murmurs or gallops

<u>Abdomen, Extremities</u>
- Abdomen without tenderness or masses
- Extremities with good pulses, no edema

<u>Neurological</u>
- Oriented x3, memory recent and remote clear
- No focal motor or sensory deficits
- Cranial nerves in tact
- Deep tendon reflexes +2 in all groups
- Negative Kernig and Brudzinski sign
- Negative Romberg

Question 4.
What are the pertinent positive and negative findings on examination?

Question 5.
What laboratory studies are indicated at this time?

Question 6.
What is your diagnosis?

Question 7.
What should your treatment plan encompass?

MANAGEMENT:
- Patient was given appropriate pharmacologic suggestions (for OTC medication).
- Patient was referred for physical therapy.
- Patient was referred for stress management therapy.

Question 8.
What further care would you recommend?

CHAPTER 19

STROKE

DEFINITION

- A stroke (cerebrovascular accident [CVA]) is defined as a focal neurological disorder developing suddenly because of a pathophysiological process in blood vessels:

    - Acute brain infarction (ABI)

    - Intracerebral hemorrhage (ICH)

    - Subarachnoid hemorrhage (SAH)

EPIDEMIOLOGY

- Third leading cause of death in the United States; 10.6% of all deaths, 500,000 deaths/year

- ABI

    - 75% of all strokes—risk increases with age.

    - Strong association with coronary artery disease—both share many risk factors.
        1) Hypertension is the most important modifiable risk factor.
        2) Smoking increases risk by 2 to 3 fold, risk returns to normal 4 to 5 years after smoking cessation.
        3) Other factors include age >67, diabetes, hyperlipidemia, male sex or a female after menopause, family history, and recent myocardial infarction.

    - Atrial fibrillation carries an 8% per year risk of embolic stroke.

    - Arteriolar obstruction and hypercoagulability—polycythemia, sickle cell disease, oral contraceptives.

    - Migraine

- ICH

    - 15% of all strokes—mortality is very high, especially if there is severe coma upon presentation.

    - Risk factors include hypertension, alcohol abuse, coagulopathies, cocaine or amphetamine abuse, blood dyscrasia, and iatrogenic anticoagulation.

- SAH

    - 10% of all strokes (25% of all stroke deaths)—incidence is higher in young adults and in women.

    - Risk factors include congenital saccular aneurysms, migraine, hypertension, smoking, polycystic kidney, Marfan's syndrome, fibromuscular dysplasia, and sickle cell disease.

PATHOPHYSIOLOGY

- <u>Cerebral circulation</u>
    - In the normal brain, cerebral blood flow is maintained despite changes in mean arterial pressure (MAP) or intracranial pressure (ICP) due to autoregulation.
    - In the injured brain, autoregulation is lost and even small changes in MAP or ICP will affect cerebral blood flow (CBF).
    - There are many collaterals for cerebral perfusion (Circle of Willis) so that the obstruction of a vessel may not lead to infarction of distal tissue, and deficits can be unpredictable.

- <u>ABI</u>
    - There are four main classifications:
        1) Atherothrombic occlusion of extracranial or intracranial arteries
        2) Cardioembolic due to atrial fibrillation, recent myocardial infarction with ventricular aneurysm, congestive heart failure, or valvular disease
        3) Lacunar due to deep cerebral infarcts of the lenticulostriate arteries
        4) Hemodynamic due to decreased global cerebral perfusion
    - Neural cellular response to ischemia (Figure 19-1)

Figure 19-1.

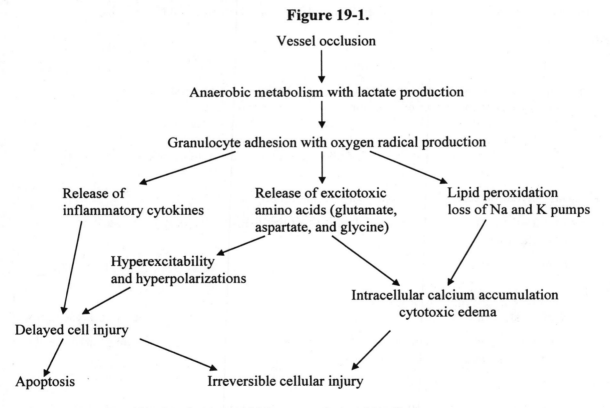

- Patterns of ischemic neuronal injury, sparing and healing
    1) Area of dense infarction and necrosis is at the center of ischemic brain tissue.
    2) Spontaneous or therapeutic reperfusion results in the limitation of infarct size, but also contributes to oxygen radical production.
    3) Selective neuronal necrosis—some neurons and glial cells survive, especially if reperfused with 12 hours; sparing may be maximized by rapid perfusion and neuroprotective therapy.

- Penumbra—tissue at the periphery of the ischemic zone
    1) Cerebral blood flow (CBF) approximately 20 ml/100 gm/min—neurons are viable but there is no synaptic function. They may be salvageable if perfusion is restored 90 minutes to several hours after initial event.
    2) Ischemic tissue contains high extracellular potassium causing multiple repetitive depolarizations, leading to ATP depletion and delayed cell death; new therapies are aimed at blocking periinfarct depolarizations.

- Delayed neuronal death
    1) Inflammation, granulocyte adhesion, oxygen radical production, and cytokine release cause not only acute neuronal damage but also delayed effects with T lymphocytes and macrophages infiltrating up to 2 weeks after the initial insult.
    2) Cytokines (TNFα, TGFβ) also induce the activation of cellular endonucleases that cleave neuronal deoxyribonucleic acid (DNA) (apoptosis); this may continue for 2 weeks after infarct.

    - Healing and functional recovery
    1) The brain surrounding the infarct is hypermetabolic; it underscores the need for maximal oxygen and nutrient delivery during the perinfarction time period.
    2) Polypeptide growth factors (neurotrophins, fibroblast growth factors) result in dendritic sprouting and new axonal growth, and they are protective against delayed neuronal injury. Trials with exogenous basic fibroblast growth factor (bFGF) are encouraging.

- Systemic responses to cerebral ischemia
    1) Arrhythmias (tachy or brady, arrhythmias, ST-T wave changes, increased creatinine phosphokinase MB [CPK-MB], wall motion abnormalities) are believed to be due to a burst of catecholamines.
    2) Neurogenic pulmonary edema (adult [acute] respiratory distress syndrome [ARDS])
    3) Peptic ulcer disease (Cushing ulcer)
    4) Endocrine abnormalities (syndrome of inappropiate antidiuretic hormone [SIADH])

- ICH

    - Rupture of artery or arteriole with hematoma formation under arterial pressure

    - It was once thought to be caused by microaneurysms (Charcot-Bouchard), but recent studies discount this; some are caused by congenital saccular aneurysms deep in the fissures (see SAH).

    - Cerebral amyloid angiopathy is a common cause in patients over age 65 and is associated with pathologic brain changes and dementia similar to Alzheimer disease.

    - Vascular malformations and angiomas cause hemorrhage in children and young adults.

    - Mechanisms of brain injury in ICH
        1) Direct trauma to neurons by ejection of blood into brain tissue
        2) Mass effect with mechanical compression of surrounding tissues
            - Hematoma is surrounded by an ischemic penumbra; ischemic changes of intracellular calcium accumulation, excitotoxic amino acid release, and hyperpolarization will lead to acute and delayed cell death.
            - Extravasation of blood causes vasospasm and worsening ischemia.
            - Mass effect increases ICP, which decreases CBF, and may result in shift of the brain and herniation across the midline or through the foramenae.
            - Evacuation of the hematoma within 2 to 4 hours may reduce brain injury; expansion of the hematoma occurs in 14%, usually within 6 hours, with a poor prognosis.

- SAH
  - Rupture of congenital saccular (berry) aneurysms—most common at the junction of the anterior cerebral and anterior communicating arteries; 12% to 31% have multiple aneurysms.
  - Acute presentation may be preceded by one or more promontory bleeds.
  - Mechanism of brain injury in SAH
    1) Extravasation of blood over the surface of the brain, the ventricles, and the spinal column.
    2) Results in inflammation, release of excitotoxic amino acids, and toxic oxygen radicals.
    3) Causes cerebrospinal fluid (CSF) outflow obstruction and hydrocephalus increases ICP.
    4) Delayed vasospasm:
       - Occurs in 70% of cases; symptomatic in 36%.
       - Occurs 3 to 21 days after the initial bleed (peak = days 4 to 12).
       - Increases overall mortality by 3-fold and can result in significant ischemic neuronal damage.
  - Hyponatremia
    1) Common (10% to 34%); associated with a higher rate of secondary cerebral infarctions
    2) May be due to the syndrome of inappropriate antidiuretic hormone (SIADH) or cerebral salt wasting syndrome that is mediated by atrial natriuretic factor (ANF).

PATIENT PRESENTATION

- History:

  Risk factors; history of drug abuse; recent cardiac event; palpitations; recent change in medications; previous transient painless loss of focal neurologic function (transient ischemic attack [TIA]); previous syncope or seizures; recurrent headaches.

- Symptoms:

  Abrupt painless loss of neurologic function (ABI) or severe headache and decreased level of consciousness (ICH and SAH); focal weakness or numbness; difficulty speaking; visual changes; difficulty controlling gait; intention tremor; seizures.

- Examination:

  Decreased level of consciousness; pupillary asymmetry and decreased reactiveness; papilledema; meningismus; aphasia or dysarthria; focal motor or sensory deficit; flaccid or spastic muscle tone; asymmetrical deep tendon reflexes; Babinski reflex; ataxia; other specialized neurologic test abnormalities; ventilatory abnormalities (e.g., Cheyne-Stokes respirations); tachycardia; premature beats or arrhythmias; carotid bruits; decreased peripheral pulses or peripheral bruits; evidence of hematologic disease or coagulopathy (petechiae, ecchymoses).

DIFFERENTIAL DIAGNOSIS

- Primary cardiac event with acute hypotension
- Primary seizure disorder
- Brain tumor
- Metabolic or toxic insult (hypoglycemia, drugs)

- Meningitis

- Trauma

KEYS TO ASSESSMENT

- Monitor vital signs and obtain arterial blood gases

- Quick assessment of neurologic deficit

- Electrocardiogram (ECG) and cardiovascular assessment

- Continuous blood pressure monitoring

- More thorough neurological examination

- Repetitive exams—monitor for stroke in evolution with worsening deficits

- Serum laboratory studies—arterial blood gases, glucose, electrolytes, coagulation studies, complete blood count (CBC), toxicology screen

- Computed tomography (CT) scan/magnetic resonance imagery (MRI)—CT scan is faster, but MRI is the best method for differentiation of cerebral hemorrhage from infarction acutely.

  - Diffusion-weighted MRI—location and extent of ischemia is seen immediately.

  - Perfusion imaging—evaluates blood flow and can detect perfusion deficits.

  - Magnetic resonance spectroscopy—metabolic abnormalities are associated with ischemia.

- Vascular studies

  - Angiography may be indicated urgently in SAH.

  - Noninvasive vascular studies to evaluate cerebral and carotid circulations include:
    1) Carotid duplex ultrasonography
    2) Quantitative oculopneumo plethysmography
    3) Transcranial doppler sonography
    4) Positron emission tomography (PET)

  - Echocardiography—standard or transesophageal to evaluate for cardiac source of emboli.

KEYS TO MANAGEMENT

- **Acute**

  - Oxygen—intubation and mechanical ventilation if hypoxic and/or hypercapnic.

  - Control blood pressure.
    1) CBF is directly proportional to MAP in brain injured patients.
    2) Fluid resuscitation increases blood flow and vascular volume in hypotension patient.
    3) Hypertension should be treated carefully, no more than a decrease of 20% in MAP over 1 hour—IV nitroprusside or labetalol.

  - Monitor and control ICP.
    1) Consider ICP bolt placement.
    2) Consider osmotherapy (mannitol).
    3) Consider hyperventilation—watch out for decreased CBF.

- Monitor and manage electrolyte disturbances.

- Rapid seizure intervention.

- Attention to nutrition should be begun early (malnutrition results in poorer outcomes).

- <u>ABI</u>
    1) Thrombolysis
        - Acute stroke <6 to 8 hours old; incomplete stroke; thrombus within the carotid arteries; absence of coagulopathy or concurrent antiplatelet or anticoagulant agent; absence of uncontrolled systolic or diastolic hypertension; and absence of ICH.
        - tPa works best if given early (less than 90 minutes), with less risk of hemorrhagic conversion.
        - World literature review suggests that neurologic salvage and decreased mortality is achieved in many patients.
        - Hemorrhagic conversion with neurologic worsening occurs in 2% to 17% (higher risk if thrombolysis has begun more than 8 hours after ischemic event) with a nearly 50% mortality.
    2) Heparin—primarily indicated for stroke in evolution, cardioembolism, and concurrent deep venous thrombosis (DVT)
    3) Calcium channel blockers—studies are mixed; nimodipine is promising, also in combination with free radical scavenger (eliprodil)
    4) N-methyl-D-aspartate (NMDA) receptor/channel antagonists—block release of glutamate and aspartate, thus decreasing intracellular calcium influx; examples include dextrophan, cerestat, selfotel, and remacemide. Preliminary studies are encouraging and may be used as adjuncts to thrombolysis.
    5) Insulin—hyperglycemia worsens stroke injury; it is used to control glucose in neuro ICU, but benefits are not proven.

- <u>ICH</u>
    1) Bedrest, sedate
    2) Control blood pressure—use labetalol rather than nitrates because it does not cause cerebral vasodilation
    3) Bolt for ICP monitoring—hyperventilate + osmolar therapy if indicated
    4) Surgical decompression in selected patients; < 4 hours after event for maximal effect

- <u>SAH</u>
    1) Monitor for arrhythmias and myocardial ischemia
    2) Darkened room; bedrest with head at 30 degrees
    3) Meperidine or codeine for pain—reassess mental status
    4) Ulcer prophylaxis; stool softeners; seizure prophylaxis controversial—10% to 20% seize
    5) Monitor for adequate cerebral perfusion using transcranial doppler (TCD)
    6) Monitor for increased ICP—hyperventilate + osmolar therapy
    7) Prevent rebleeding
        - Antifibrinolytic drugs—aminocaproic acid or tranexamic; drug is given on day of admission
        - Surgery—if in good condition, operate in 1 to 2 days to clip aneurysm (up to 90% successful); if in poor condition delay 7 to 14 days and reconsider (<50% improvement)
        - Intraarterial—balloons or platinum coils used to block aneurysm in the necks of selected patients; the results are very encouraging so far

8) Prevent vasospasm
- Monitor for headache, mental status changes, and new deficits.
- Triple H (hypervolemic/hypertensive/hemodilution) can be used in the absence of increased ICP; it improves perfusion pressure and reduces viscosity.
- Calcium channel blockers—nimodipine, nicardipine, nilvadipine—given IV. They clearly reduce severe neurologic deficits and work more by reducing ischemic intracellular calcium influx than by cerebral vasodilation.
- Percutaneous transluminal carotid angioplasty (PTCA)—helpful in some patients with refractory vasospasm.
- Monitor with daily transcranial doppler ultrasound.

- **Chronic**

  - Neurologic rehabilitation techniques are varied and of mixed clear therapeutic benefit but all are superior to neglect. Improvements can be seen many months after the acute event.

  - Nutrition is vitally important.

  - Monitor for depression, recurrent cerebrovascular disease, and cardiac disease, especially coronary artery disease.

  - Manage blood pressure carefully.

- **Prevention**

  - Hypertension is the single most important modifiable risk factor—up to 70% of strokes could be prevented with treatment.

  - Stopping smoking can decrease risk to normal after 2 to 5 years.

  - Cholesterol management reduces risk, especially using reductase inhibitors (e.g., pravastatin).

  - Use warfarin therapy for nonvalvular atrial fibrillation.

  - Aspirin dose is controversial; 75 mg per day is suggested.

  - Management of transient ischemic attacks (TIA)
    1) Medical therapy with antiplatelet drugs is first choice for "noncritical" stenosis.
    2) Use warfarin for a clear, cardiac source and in atrial fibrillation.
    3) Surgical intervention (carotid endarterectomy) or PTCA is the best choice for critical stenoses. It is indicated for asymptomatic carotid obstruction, as well as in TIA.

Pathophysiology

What is going on in the disease process that influences how the patient presents and how he or she should be managed?

→

Clinical Link

What should you do now that you understand the underlying pathophysiology?

Pathophysiology	Clinical Link
Ischemic stroke and coronary artery disease share many risk factors and are most often due to atherosclerosis.	Patients with stroke should be monitored for coronary artery disease and vis versa.
Subarachnoid hemorrhage occurs in young, healthy people with few risk factors; many are preceded by promontory bleeds.	Severe headache, stiff neck, and/or decreased level of consciousness must be thoroughly evaluated, even in a young, healthy person.
Acute brain infarction is characterized by both acute ischemic neural cell death and delayed cell death; both are mediated through excitotoxins, oxygen radicals, and inflammation.	New therapies aimed at reducing excitotoxins, oxygen radicals, and inflammation may reduce infarct size and improve delayed outcomes.
Intracranial hemorrhage is associated with rapid brain injury, increased intracranial pressure, and poor prognosis.	Rapid and accurate diagnosis and management of ICH is vital to patient survival.
Subarachnoid hemorrhage is characterized by a high likelihood of severe vasospasm that can result in significant ischemic injury.	Patients with SAH must be monitored closely for up to 3 weeks after bleeding and should be treated aggressively to prevent rebleeding and vasospasm.
ABI, ICH, and SAH are very different in their pathophysiology, complications, and management.	Rapid evaluation, including CT or MRI, is vital to delivering appropriate care.
Risk of stroke is related to several potentially reversible factors, and a correction of these is associated with a significant decrease in risk.	Management of hypertension, dyslipidemia, smoking, and atherosclerosis is vital to stroke prevention.

BIBLIOGRAPHY

Alexandrov, A. V., Black, S. E., Ehrlich, L. E., Caldwell, C. B., & Norris, J. W. (1997). Predictors of hemorrhagic transformation occurring spontaneously and on anticoagulants in patients with acute ischemic stroke. *Stroke, 28*(6), 1198-1202.

Anonymous. (1996). Atherosclerotic disease of the aortic arch as a risk factor for recurrent ischemic stroke. The French Study of Aortic Plaques in Stroke Group [see comments]. *New England Journal of Medicine, 334*(19), 1216-1221.

Aronow, W. S., Ahn, C., & Gutstein, H. (1996). Risk factors for new atherothrombotic brain infarction in 664 older men and 1,488 older women. *American Journal of Cardiology, 77*(15), 1381-1383.

Aronow, W. S., Ahn, C., Kronzon, I., & Gutstein, H. (1997). Association of plasma renin activity and echocardiographic left ventricular hypertrophy with frequency of new coronary events and new atherothrombotic brain infarction in older persons with systemic hypertension. *American Journal of Cardiology, 79*(11), 1543-1545.

Aronow, W. S., Ahn, C., Kronzon, I., Gutstein, H., & Schoenfeld, M. R. (1997). Association of extracranial carotid arterial disease, prior atherothrombotic brain infarction, systemic hypertension, and left ventricular hypertrophy with the incidence of new atherothrombotic brain infarction at 45-month follow-up in 1,482 older patients. *American Journal of Cardiology, 79*(7), 991-993.

Baird, A. E., Austin, M. C., McKay, W. J., & Donnan, G. A. (1997). Sensitivity and specificity of 99mTc-HMPAO SPECT cerebral perfusion measurements during the first 48 hours for the localization of cerebral infarction. *Stroke, 28*(5), 976-980.

Baron, J. C., & Marchal, G. (1996). SPECT using 99mTc-HMPAO versus neurological scales to predict outcome of acute cerebral infarction [letter; comment]. *Stroke, 27*(7), 1253-1254.

Bogousslavsky, J., Castillo, V., Kumral, E., Henriques, I., & Melle, G. V. (1996). Stroke subtypes and hypertension. Primary hemorrhage vs infarction, large- vs small-artery disease. *Archives of Neurology, 53*(3), 265-269.

Bornstein, N. M., Gur, A. Y., Treves, T. A., Reider-Groswasser, I., Aronovich, B. D., Klimovitzky, S. S., Varssano, D., & Korczyn, A. D. (1996). Do silent brain infarctions predict the development of dementia after first ischemic stroke? *Stroke, 27*(5), 904-905.

Bryan, R. N., Wells, S. W., Miller, T. J., Elster, A. D., Jungreis, C. A., Poirier, V. C., Lind, B. K., & Manolio, T. A. (1997). Infarctlike lesions in the brain: Prevalence and anatomic characteristics at MR imaging of the elderly—Data from the Cardiovascular Health Study [see comments]. *Radiology, 202*(1), 47-54.

Castillo, J., Davalos, A., Naveiro, J., & Noya, M. (1996). Neuroexcitatory amino acids and their relation to infarct size and neurological deficit in ischemic stroke. *Stroke, 27*(6), 1060-1065.

Chamorro, A., Saiz, A., Vila, N., Ascaso, C., Blanc, R., Alday, M., & Pujol, J. (1996). Contribution of arterial blood pressure to the clinical expression of lacunar infarction. *Stroke, 27*(3), 388-392.

Chamorro, A. (1997). Hemorrhagic infarct [letter; comment]. *Neurology, 48*(1), 295-296.

Chaves, C. J., Pessin, M. S., Caplan, L. R., Chung, C. S., Amarenco, P., Breen, J., Fine, J., Kase, C., Tapia, J., Babikian, V., Rosengart, A., & DeWitt, L. D. (1996). Cerebellar hemorrhagic infarction. *Neurology, 46*(2), 346-349.

Davis, P. H., Clarke, W. R., Bendixen, B. H., Adams, H. P. J., Woolson, R. F., & Culebras, A. (1996). Silent cerebral infarction in patients enrolled in the TOAST Study. *Neurology, 46*(4), 942-948.

Di Tullio,. M. R., Sacco, R. L., & Homma, S. (1996). Atherosclerotic disease of the aortic arch as a risk factor for recurrent ischemic stroke [letter; comment]. *New England Journal of Medicine, 335*(19), 1464, discussion 1464-1465.

Fazekas, F., Fazekas, G., Schmidt, R., Kapeller, P., & Offenbacher, H. (1996). Magnetic resonance imaging correlates of transient cerebral ischemic attacks. *Stroke, 27*(4), 607-611.

Franke, C. L., Palm, R., Dalby, M., Schoonderwaldt, H. C., Hantson, L., Eriksson, B., Lang-Jenssen, L., & Smakman, J. (1996). Flunarizine in stroke treatment (FIST): A double-blind, placebo-controlled trial in Scandinavia and the Netherlands. *Acta Neurologica Scandinavica, 93*(1), 56-60.

Fujikawa, T., Yokota, N., Muraoka, M., & Yamawaki, S. (1996). Response of patients with major depression and silent cerebral infarction to antidepressant drug therapy, with emphasis on central nervous system adverse reactions. *Stroke, 27*(11), 2040-2042.

Fujishima, S., Abe, I., Okada, Y., Saku, Y., Sadoshima, S., & Fujishima, M. (1996). Serial changes in blood pressure and neurohormone levels after the onset of lacunar stroke. *Angiology, 47*(6), 579-587.

Fushimi, H., Inoue, T., Yamada, Y., Udaka, F., & Kameyama, M. (1996). Asymptomatic cerebral small infarcts (lacunae), their risk factors and intellectual disturbances. *Diabetes, 45*(Suppl 3), S98-S100.

Garcia, J. H., Lassen, N. A., Weiller, C., Sperling, B., & Nakagawara, J. (1996). Ischemic stroke and incomplete infarction [review, 48 refs]. *Stroke, 27*(4), 761-765.

Giroux, C., & Scatton, B. (1996). Ischemic stroke: Treatment on the horizon [review, 12 refs]. *European Neurology, 36*(2), 61-64.

Goldstein, L. B. (1997). Influence of common drugs and related factors on stroke outcome [review, 79 refs]. *Current Opinion in Neurology, 10*(1), 52-57.

Gruber, A., Dietrich, W., Czech, T., & Richling, B. (1997). Recurrent aneurysmal subarachnoid haemorrhage: Bleeding pattern and incidence of posthaemorrhagic ischaemic infarction. *British Journal of Neurosurgery, 11*(2), 121-126.

Haapaniemi, H., Hillbom, M., & Juvela, S. (1997). Lifestyle-associated risk factors for acute brain infarction among persons of working age. *Stroke, 28*(1), 26-30.

Hoekstra-van Dalen, R. A., Cillessen, J. P., Kappelle, L. J., & van Gijn, J. (1996). Cerebral infarcts associated with migraine: Clinical features, risk factors and follow-up. *Journal of Neurology, 243*(7), 511-515.

Hornig, C. R., Haberbosch, W., Lammers, C., Waldecker, B., & Dorndorf, W. (1996). Specific cardiological evaluation after focal cerebral ischemia. *Acta Neurologica Scandinavica, 93*(4), 297-302.

Hupperts, R. M., Warlow, C. P., Slattery, J., & Rothwell, P. M. (1997). Severe stenosis of the internal carotid artery is not associated with borderzone infarcts in patients randomised in the European Carotid Surgery Trial. *Journal of Neurology, 244*(1), 45-50.

Jack, C. R. J. (1997). MR imaging of the brain in epidemiologic research: The Cardiovascular Health Study [editorial; comment]. *Radiology, 202*(1), 17-19.

Karanjia, P. N., Nelson, J. J., Lefkowitz, D. S., Dick, A. R., Toole, J. F., Chambless, L. E., Hayes, R., & Howard, V. J. (1997). Validation of the ACAS TIA/stroke algorithm. *Neurology, 48*(2), 346-351.

Kawamata, T., Speliotes, E. K., & Finklestein, S. P. (1997). The role of polypeptide growth factors in recovery from stroke [review, 30 refs]. *Advances in Neurology, 73*, 377-382.

Kazumata, K., Tanaka, N., Ishikawa, T., Kuroda, S., Houkin, K., & Mitsumori, K. (1996). Dissociation of vasoreactivity to acetazolamide and hypercapnia. Comparative study in patients with chronic occlusive major cerebral artery disease. *Stroke, 27*(11), 2052-2058.

Kittner, S. J., Stern, B. J., Feeser, B. R., Hebel, R., Nagey, D. A., Buchholz, D. W., Earley, C. J., Johnson, C. J., Macko, R. F., Sloan, M. A., Wityk, R. J., & Wozniak, M. A. (1996). Pregnancy and the risk of stroke [see comments]. *New England Journal of Medicine, 335*(11), 768-774.

Korogi, Y., Takahashi, M., Nakagawa, T., Mabuchi, N., Watabe, T., Shiokawa, Y., Shiga, H., O'Uchi, T., Miki, H., Horikawa, Y., Fujiwara, S., & Furuse, M. (1997). Intracranial vascular stenosis and occlusion: MR angiographic findings. *American Journal of Neuroradiology, 18*(1), 135-143.

Korpelainen, J. T., Sotaniemi, K. A., Huikuri, H. V., & Myllya, V. V. (1996). Abnormal heart rate variability as a manifestation of autonomic dysfunction in hemispheric brain infarction. *Stroke, 27*(11), 2059-2063.

Kothari, R., Pancioli, A., Brott, T., & Broderick, J. (1996). Thrombolytic therapy for cerebral infarction [see comments] [review, 116 refs]. *Academic Emergency Medicine, 3*(9), 881-892.

Loeb, C., Gandolfo, C., Del, S. M., Conti, M., Finocchi, C., & Calautti, C. (1996). Asymptomatic cerebral infarctions in patients with ischemic stroke. *European Neurology, 36*(6), 343-347.

Lyrer, P. A., Engelter, S., Radu, E. W., & Steck, A. J. (1997). Cerebral infarcts related to isolated middle cerebral artery stenosis. *Stroke, 28*(5), 1022-1027.

Macko, R. F., Ameriso, S. F., Barndt, R., Clough, W., Weiner, J. M., & Fisher, M. (1996). Precipitants of brain infarction. Roles of preceding infection/inflammation and recent psychological stress. *Stroke, 27*(11), 1999-2004.

Marks, M. P., de Crespigny, A., Lentz, D., Enzmann, D. R., Albers, G. W., & Moseley, M. E. (1996). Acute and chronic stroke: Navigated spin-echo diffusion-weighted MR imaging [published erratum appears in *Radiology* 1996 Jul; 200(1), 289]. *Radiology, 199*(2), 403-408.

Mochizuki, Y., Oishi, M., & Takasu, T. (1997). Cerebral blood flow in single and multiple lacunar infarctions. *Stroke, 28*(7), 1458-1460.

Morfis, L., Schwartz, R. S., Poulos, R., & Howes, L. G. (1997). Blood pressure changes in acute cerebral infarction and hemorrhage. *Stroke, 28*(7), 1401-1405.

Morris, P. L., Robinson, R. G., de Carvalho, M. L., Albert, P., Wells, J. C., Samuels, J. F., Eden-Fetzer, D., & Price, T. R. (1996). Lesion characteristics and depressed mood in the stroke data bank study. *Journal of Neuropsychiatry and Clinical Neurosciences, 8*(2), 153-159.

Nedergaard, M. (1996). Spreading depression as a contributor to ischemic brain damage. *Advances in Neurology, 71*, 75-83, discussion 83-84.

Nomura, H., Morita, C., Kuwano, S., Eto, H., Goto, H., & Kuwahara, H. (1996). Efficacy of combination antiplatelet therapy and nicardipine for chronic cerebral infarction. *Clinical Therapeutics, 18*(3), 483-490.

Rausch, M., & Eysel, U. T. (1996). Visualization of CBF changes during cortical infarction using IR thermo-encephaloscopy. *Neuroreport, 7*(15-17), 2603-2606.

Riggs, J. E. (1997). Tissue-type plasminogen activator should not be used in acute ischemic stroke. *Archives of Family Medicine, 6*(2), 102-104.

Samuelsson, M., Soderfeldt, B., & Olsson, G. B. (1996). Functional outcome in patients with lacunar infarction. *Stroke, 27*(5), 842-846.

Sander, D., & Klingelhofer, J. (1996). Extent of autonomic activation following cerebral ischemia is different in hypertensive and normotensive humans. *Archives of Neurology, 53*(9), 890-894.

Sasaki, O., Takeuchi, S., Koizumi, T., Koike, T., & Tanaka, R. (1996). Complete recanalization via fibrinolytic therapy can reduce the number of ischemic territories that progress to infarction. *American Journal of Neuroradiology, 17*(9), 1661-1668.

Schwalen, S., Altermann, A., Jorg, J., Berg, K., & Cramer, B. M. (1996). Bilateral suppression of the sympathetic nervous system in hemispheric brain infarction. *Journal of Neurology, 243*(2), 157-160.

Seil, F. J. (1997). Recovery and repair issues after stroke from the scientific perspective [review, 23 refs]. *Current Opinion in Neurology, 10*(1), 49-51.

Shephard, T. J., & Fox, S. W. (1996). Assessment and management of hypertension in the acute ischemic stroke patient. *Journal of Neuroscience Nursing, 28*(1), 5-12.

Siqueira, N. J. I., Santos, A. C., Fabio, S. R., & Sakamoto, A. C. (1996). Cerebral infarction in patients aged 15 to 40 years. *Stroke, 27*(11), 2016-2019.

Snowdon, D. A., Greiner, L. H., Mortimer, J. A., Riley, K. P., Greiner, P. A., & Markesbery, W. R. (1997). Brain infarction and the clinical expression of Alzheimer disease. The Nun Study. *Journal of the American Medical Association, 277*(10), 813-817.

So, E. L., Annegers, J. F., Hauser, W. A., O'Brien, P. C., & Whisnant, J. P. (1996). Population-based study of seizure disorders after cerebral infarction. *Neurology, 46*(2), 350-355.

Steinke, W., Schwartz, A., & Hennerici, M. (1996). Topography of cerebral infarction associated with carotid artery dissection. *Journal of Neurology, 243*(4), 323-328.

Tanahashi, N., Tomita, M., Kobari, M., Takeda, H., Yokoyama, M., & Fukuuchi, Y. (1996). Aspirin improves the enhanced erythrocyte aggregability in patients with cerebral infarction. *Journal of the Neurological Sciences, 139*(1), 137-140.

Toni, D., Fiorelli, M., Bastianello, S., Sacchetti, M. L., Sette, G., Argentino, C., Montinaro, E., & Bozzao, L. (1996). Hemorrhagic transformation of brain infarct: Predictability in the first 5 hours from stroke onset and influence on clinical outcome [see comments]. *Neurology, 46*(2), 341-345.

Wang, T. D., Wu, C. C., & Lee, Y. T. (1997). Myocardial stunning after cerebral infarction. *International Journal of Cardiology, 58*(3), 308-311.

Witte, O. W., & Stoll, G. (1997). Delayed and remote effects of focal cortical infarctions: Secondary damage and reactive plasticity [review, 139 refs]. *Advances in Neurology, 73*, 207-227.

Yamashita, K., Kobayashi, S., Yamaguchi, S., & Koide, H. (1996). Cigarette smoking and silent brain infarction in normal adults. *Internal Medicine, 35*(9), 704-706.

CASE STUDY*

STROKE

INITIAL HISTORY:
- 76-year-old man
- Describes symptoms starting 30 minutes ago
- Sudden onset of difficulty getting his mouth to form words
- Face and mouth numb; tongue felt "thick"
- Unable to hold his coffee cup in his right hand
- Right leg weak, needed to hold onto the table to stand

Question 1.
What is your differential diagnosis based on the information you have now?

Question 2.
What other questions would you like to ask?

ADDITIONAL HISTORY:
- History of essential hypertension
- Has not been taking his hydroclorothiazide because it makes him feel "bad."
- Was told he has high cholesterol.
- Has experienced several brief spells of right-sided weakness which resolved in a few minutes—thought this was his arm falling asleep.
- No head trauma or recent infections.
- Family history: mother died of stroke, father died of acute myocardial infarction (AMI).
- Smokes 1 pack/day for past 30 years

---

* Gail L. Kongable-Beckman, RN, MSN, contributed this case study.

Question 3.
Now what do you think?

PHYSICAL EXAMINATION:
- Alert and anxious white male
- Slurred speech, uses appropriate words
- T = 37 C, orally; RR = 16 and regular; HR = 86 and irregular; BP = 190/120 mmHg standing

HEENT
- Conjunctiva is clear without exudate or lesions
- Fundi is without lesions, nicking, or cotton tufts
- Nasal mucosa is pink without drainage
- Oral mucous membranes are moist
- Pharynx is pink without lesions or exudate

Skin, Neck
- Pale with senile lentigines, no lesions or bruises
- No lesions or bruises, no tenting; dry and flaky
- Supple, no lymphadenopathy or thyromegaly
- Bruit auscultated over left carotid artery

Lungs
- Chest expansion is symmetric and full
- Diaphragmatic excursion is equal at 4 cm
- Lung sounds are clear to auscultation

Cardiac
- Heart sounds: irregular; irregular rate and rhythm
- No murmurs, gallops, or clicks

Abdomen
- Nondistended; bowel sounds are present and not hyperactive
- Liver percusses 2 cm below right costal margin but overall 12 cm in size
- No tenderness or masses

Extremities
- Cool but good capillary refill at 3 seconds
- 1+ pitting edema of bilateral ankles
- Radial artery pulses full and equal; anterior pedal pulses diminished but equal
- No clubbing

Neurological

- Alert and oriented
- Facial droop on right, with loss of nasolabial fold
- Diminished gag reflex
- Strength 3/5 in the right upper extremity and 4/5 in the right lower extremity; 5/5 in the left upper and lower extremities
- Deep tendon reflexes (DTRs) 1+ on right, 2+ on left
- Sensory intact to touch

Question 4.

What studies would you initiate now while preparing your interventions?

Question 5.

What therapies would you initiate immediately while awaiting results of the lab studies?

LABORATORY:

- ECG; atrial fibrillation
- Serum glucose 130 mg%
- PT = 12.5 seconds; PTT = 28 seconds
- Platelet count 220,000/cubic mm
- Head CT without contrast was normal

EMERGENCY ROOM COURSE:

- Risks and benefits of thrombolytic therapy are explained to patient and family.
- Patient does not improve neurologically.
- BP responds to labetalol.

PHYSICAL EXAM NOW:
- Vital signs:
  - BP = 170/86; HR = 100, irregular
- Neurological exam:
  - Alert and oriented
  - Follows commands
  - Right hemiparesis worsening; strength is now 2/5 in both the upper and lower extremities on the right, still 5/5 on the left
  - Moderate dysarthria
  - Decreased sensation on right

Question 6.
What do you think is happening? Why is the hemiparesis worsening? What does his CT scan mean? Should you continue to treat his hypertension to bring it down to normal?

Question 7.
What interventions should be initiated now?

RESPONSE TO THERAPY:
- Gradual improvement of hemiparesis and dysarthria to baseline within 5 hours of treatment
- BP = 160/72 without continuous antihypertensive drugs
- No symptoms of cerebral or systemic hemorrhage

Question 8.
Now what should be done and what can the patient expect?

HOSPITAL COURSE:

- Patient does well with digoxin 0.125 mg PO daily for atrial fibrillation. He converts to normal sinus rhythm; P = 82, regular.
- Total cholesterol = 270; HDL = 25, ratio 6.6
- Antihypertensive therapy with an ACE inhibitor is initiated.
- Antiplatelet therapy; aspirin 325 mg PO QID
- He has not smoked while hospitalized.
- Cardiac echo was normal (no mural thrombus); carotid doppler showed <40% stenosis on right and <50% stenosis on the left with no hemodynamic changes (not a candidate for carotid endarterectomy at this point).

Question 9.
What instructions and medication should this patient go home with?

Question 10.
What steps can he take to prevent future attacks?

CHAPTER 20

ALZHEIMER DISEASE

DEFINITION

- Alzheimer disease (AD) is defined as a gradual onset and continuing decline of cognitive function from a previously higher level, resulting in impairment of social and occupational function.

- Impairment of recent memory occurs and at least one of the following:

  - Language disturbances

  - Word-finding difficulties

  - Disturbances of praxis

  - Visual agnosia

  - Constructional disturbances

  - Disturbances of executive function, including abstract reasoning and concentration

- Cognitive deficits are not due to other psychiatric, neurologic, or systemic diseases.

- Cognitive deficits do not exclusively occur in the setting of delirium.

EPIDEMIOLOGY

- Most common dementia of the elderly; 15% lifetime risk in the United States.

- Over the age or 65, 4% of the population is affected; over the age of 80, 20% of the population is affected.

- Over 4 million people in the United States have AD.

- There are 100,000 deaths per year.

- Risk factors:

  - Increasing age

  - Female gender

  - Genetics
      1) There is an increased risk in siblings; there is an even greater risk in identical twins.
      2) Most people with trisomy 21 (Downs syndrome) will develop AD after age 40.
      3) Several genes have been identified so far:
          - β-amyloid precursor protein gene (APP) on chromosome 21 (APP found in structural lesions commonly seen in AD brain tissue) (see below)

- Presenilin 1 gene (PS1) on chromosome 14; associated with early onset dementia in particular families
- Presenilin 2 gene (PS2) on chromosome 1; associated with early onset dementia in particular families
- ϵ 4 allele on the apolipoprotein E (ApoE) gene of chromosome 19—doubles the risk of AD and occurs in 34% to 65% of people with AD, but also occurs in 24% to 31% of people without AD; abnormal binding of ApoE protein to tau protein of neurofibrillary tangles and to amyloid-beta proteins of senile plaques (see Figure 20-1)

4) There is also evidence for a probable gene locus on chromosome 12 that has yet to be identified.

5) The primary genetic defect for sporadic AD may be located in the mitrochondrial deoxyribonucleic acid (DNA) with defects in intracellular calcium regulation and premature cell death.

- Head trauma
   1) Trauma with a loss of consciousness results in a 3-fold increase in risk, the latest studies suggest this is only true if ApoE allele is also present.

- Estrogen deficiency in postmenopausal women may be a contributing factor to the development of AD. Estrogen replacement improves cognitive function and protects against AD in older women.

- Other associated risk factors include alcohol abuse, depression, and sleep disturbance.

PATHOPHYSIOLOGY

- There are several structural abnormalities common to AD brain tissue:

   - Neurofibrillary tangles are bundles of filamentous tau proteins in the cytoplasm of neurons.

   - Neuritic plaques are clusters of degenerating nerve-terminals with a β-amyloid protein core that occur in greatest numbers in the parietal-temporal region and hippocampus (memory).

   - There is a degeneration of cholinergic neurons.

- Inflammation with the production of toxic oxygen radicals clearly plays a role, and there is some evidence for an autoimmune contribution to the disease process.

- Excitotoxins (glutamate and aspartate) are found in high levels in the structural lesions of AD, and are known to damage cells.

- Several neurotransmitters are altered; the most important change is a 40% to 90% decrease in choline acetyltransferase with decreased levels of acetylcholine (Ach) occurring even in the first year of dementia symptoms.

- Metabolic changes include decreased parietal glucose metabolism

- Pharmacologic interventions are being tested for every step of this proposed pathophysiolgic process.

- Depression

- Vascular dementia

Figure 20-1.

Theories of Alzheimer's Pathogenesis

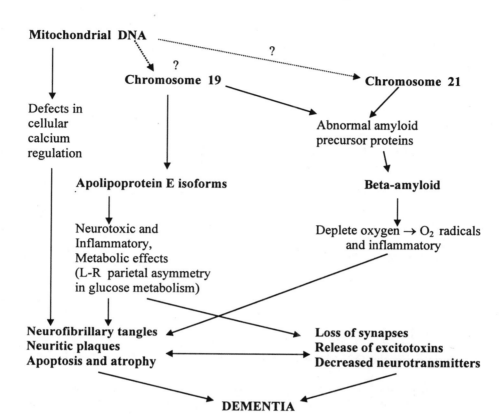

Patient Presentation

- History:

    Often obtained from family; patient may be unaware of changes; family history; history of head trauma; absence of other causes such as heavy alcohol abuse, nutritional deficits, and drug use (illicit or prescribed); seizures; other neurologic complaints (focal weakness or numbness; cerebral or meningeal infections; syphilis; thyroid disease

- Symptoms:

    Insidious and gradually progressive loss of memory with apraxias, aphasias, and visual and cognitive disturbances; clear consciousness with absence of hallucinations and delusions until late in the disease course; absence of asterixis or tremor

- Examination:

    Cognitive memory deficits without focal neurologic findings or evidence of delirium or systemic disease as the cause of mental status changes

Differential Diagnosis

- Other forms of idiopathic dementia such as Dementia Associated with Lewy Bodies (DLB)

- Alcohol and/or drug use

- Pernicious anemia

- Mass lesions

- Thyroid disorders

- Huntington chorea

- Chronic infection (syphilis, viral, fungal)

- Toxins (lead)

- Vasculitis

- Chronic subdural hematoma

- Normal pressure hydrocephalus

- Parkinson disease

KEYS TO ASSESSMENT

- Establish dementia using the DSM IV criteria:

  - Use established mental-status tests such as: Information-Orientation-Concentration Test, Mini-Mental State Examination (MMSE), Dementia Rating Scale, Mattis, Blessed Scale, etc.

- Rule out treatable causes of dementia:

  - Magnetic resonance imaging (MRI)

  - Electroencephalogram (EEG)

  - B_{12}, thyroid

  - Toxins

  - Serology

  - Lumbar puncture

  - Review drugs

  - Rule out depression (pseudodementia)

- Differentiate from delirium, which has a sudden onset, fluctuating course, reduced consciousness, globally oriented attention, visual hallucinations, fleeting delusions, complete disorientation, reduced or greatly exaggerated activity, incoherent speech, and asterixis or tremor.

- The family is an important source of information about the underlying disease process and for identifying the key issues in patient management.

- Establish the stage of AD progression:

  - Stage I: Forget where things are placed, get lost, forget appointments—both recent and remote memory; depression and anxiety.

- Stage II: Language trouble, spatial disorientation, poor problem solving, confusion, denial.
- Stage III: Aimlessness, hallucinations, agitation, aphasia.

KEYS TO MANAGEMENT

- Nonpharmacologic

    - Involve the family early on and assess the "caregiver burden" to decide on the need for alternative living options and for monitoring changes in the patient with therapy.

    - Maintain the socialization of the patient. Walking daily with a care provider has been shown to improve AD patient's cognitive abilities.

    - Prevent injury, especially in later stages when disorientation worsens.

    - Maintain good nutrition and exercise.

    - Refer families to support organizations.

- Pharmacologic

    - Treating primary cognitive deficits:
        1) Tacrine and donepezil are cholinesterase inhibitors that increase acetylcholine; they provide some improvements in memory, orientation, and ability to care for self, but it is not clear how well these improvements are maintained. The drugs are associated with fatigue, insomnia, and significant gastrointestinal (GI) distress including nausea, diarrhea, and anorexia.
        2) Estrogens improve cerebral blood flow, stimulate neural growth and activity, suppress ApoE activity, and may be protective and therapeutic in postmenopausal women.

    - Slowing disease progression:
        1) N-methyl-D-aspartate (NMDA) antagonists (block the excitotoxins aspartate and glutamate), calcium channel blockers, and nerve growth factors are all being tested without conclusive results so far.
        2) Selegiline (an anti-Parkinson drug) and hydergine (a vasodilator and metabolic enhancer) may slow the rate of functional decline in some patients with AD, but are of unproved benefit; they have few side effects and are well-tolerated.
        3) There is increasing evidence that antiinflammatory agents (nonsteroidal) help prevent AD and slow disease progression.
        4) Vitamin E (α-tocopherol) has shown some promise in slowing functional decline in AD.

    - Controlling behavior:
        1) Neuroleptics may be needed to control behavior, but most are anticholinergic and may worsen cognitive function with many side effects; newer drugs such as clozapine and risperidone decrease agitation and psychosis with fewer side effects.
        2) Anxiolytics may help with anxiety and insomnia but often result in confusion and ataxia.
        3) Antidepressants may be indicated for associated depression but also often have anticholinergic effects. The new serotonin uptake inhibitors (fluoxetime, citalopram) are undergoing testing.

Pathophysiology

What is going on in the disease process that influences how the patient presents and how he or she should be managed?

Clinical Link

What should you do now that you understand the underlying pathophysiology?

Pathophysiology	Clinical Link
Genetics of AD are very complicated and polygenic, except in the case of early-onset familial inheritance; the genetic links are still being defined.	Population screening for AD is not possible nor desirable at this time; a family history of early-onset AD (50s or younger) should be investigated.
Decreased acetylcholine is a primary feature of AD pathophysiology.	Tacrine and donepezil probably improve cognition by increasing Ach, but more effective drugs with fewer side effects are needed.
Two protein gene products, β-amyloid precursor protein and ApoE, have been identified as being key components of the structural abnormalities characteristic of AD; there are inflammatory, metabolic, and excitotoxic components to the pathophysiology of AD.	Further understanding of these processes, and identification of others, may lead to more specific AD therapies; numerous trials are underway.
The clinical manifestations of AD, especially in the late stages, can be easily confused with delirium, which is an acute state that requires rapid intervention.	Evaluation for the rapidity of onset of symptoms, amount of agitation, and severity or disorientation and reduced consciousness must be done quickly and carefully to rule out a treatable and potentially life-threatening cause of delirium.
Numerous other causes for dementia exist including vascular disease, depression, chronic infection, endocrine or metabolic disease, and drugs.	The diagnosis of AD is one of exclusion; careful exam and lab analysis is necessary to rule out treatable causes of dementia.
AD occurs in the elderly and is associated with low levels of Ach.	Although caregiver burden is very significant in AD, treatment with neuroleptics, anxiolytics, and antidepressants is associated with considerable toxicity.

BIBLIOGRAPHY

Aisen, P. S. (1997). Inflammation and Alzheimer's disease: Mechanisms and therapeutic strategies [review, 63 refs]. *Gerontology, 43*(1-2), 143-149.

Aisen, P. S., & Davis, K. L. (1997). The search for disease-modifying treatment for Alzheimer's disease [review, 89 refs]. *Neurology, 48*(5 Suppl 6), S35-S41.

Albert, M. S. (1996). Cognitive and neurobiologic markers of early Alzheimer disease [review, 62 refs]. *Proceedings of the National Academy of Sciences of the United States of America, 93*(24), 13547-13551.

Arai, H. (1996). Biological markers for the clinical diagnosis of Alzheimer's disease [review, 81 refs]. *Tohoku Journal of Experimental Medicine, 179*(2), 65-79.

Arai, H., Higuchi, S., & Sasaki, H. (1997). Apolipoprotein E genotyping and cerebrospinal fluid tau protein: Implications for the clinical diagnosis of Alzheimer's disease [review, 35 refs]. *Gerontology, 43*(Suppl 1), 2-10.

Birge, S. J. (1997). The role of estrogen in the treatment of Alzheimer's disease [review, 55 refs]. *Neurology, 48*(5 Suppl 7), S36-S41.

Bissette, G. (1997). Neuropeptides and Alzheimer's disease pathology [review, 72 refs]. *Annals of the New York Academy of Sciences, 814*, 17-29.

Borson, S., & Raskind, M. A. (1997). Clinical features and pharmacologic treatment of behavioral symptoms of Alzheimer's disease [71 refs]. *Neurology, 48*(5 Suppl 6), S17-S24.

Bourgeois, M. S., Schulz, R., & Burgio, L. (1996). Interventions for caregivers of patients with Alzheimer's disease: A review and analysis of content, process, and outcomes [review, 117 refs]. *International Journal of Aging and Human Development, 43*(1), 35-92.

Breitner, J. C. (1996). The role of anti-inflammatory drugs in the prevention and treatment of Alzheimer's disease [review, 81 refs]. *Annual Review of Medicine, 47*, 401-411.

Cacabelos, R. (1996). Diagnosis of Alzheimer's disease: Defining genetic profiles (genotype vs phenotype) [review, 104 refs]. *Acta Neurologica Scandinavica Supplementum, 165*, 72-84.

Cook, I. A., & Leuchter, A. F. (1996). Synaptic dysfunction in Alzheimer's disease: Clinical assessment using quantitative EEG [review, 42 refs]. *Behavioural Brain Research, 78*(1), 15-23.

Crawford, J. G. (1996). Alzheimer's disease risk factors as related to cerebral blood flow [review, 163 refs]. *Medical Hypotheses, 46*(4), 367-377.

Farlow, M. R. (1997). Alzheimer's disease: Clinical implications of the apolipoprotein E genotype [review, 46 refs]. *Neurology, 48*(5 Suppl 6), S30-S34.

Forloni, G. (1996). Neurotoxicity of beta-amyloid and prion peptides [review, 111 refs]. *Current Opinion in Neurology, 9*(6), 492-500.

Fratiglioni, L. (1996). Epidemiology of Alzheimer's disease and current possibilities for prevention [review, 68 refs]. *Acta Neurologica Scandinavica Supplementum, 165*, 33-40.

Geldmacher, D. S., & Whitehouse, P. J. J. (1997). Differential diagnosis of Alzheimer's disease [review, 65 refs]. *Neurology, 48*(5 Suppl 6), S2-S9.

Giacobini, E. (1996). New trends in cholinergic therapy for Alzheimer disease: Nicotinic agonists or cholinesterase inhibitors? [72 refs]. *Progress in Brain Research, 109*, 311-323.

Goedert, M. (1996). Tau protein and the neurofibrillary pathology of Alzheimer's disease [review, 26 refs]. *Annals of the New York Academy of Sciences, 777*, 121-131.

Gooch, M. D., & Stennett, D. J. (1996). Molecular basis of Alzheimer's disease [review, 122 refs]. *American Journal of Health-System Pharmacy, 53*(13), 1545-1457, quiz 1603-1604.

Gozes, I., Bardea, A., Bechar, M., Pearl, O., Reshef, A., Zamostiano, R., Davidson, A., Rubinraut, S., Giladi, E., Fridkin, M., & Brenneman, D. E. (1997). Neuropeptides and neural survival: Neuroprotective strategy for Alzheimer's disease [review, 33 refs]. *Annals of the New York Academy of Sciences, 814*, 161-166.

Haley, W. E. (1997). The family caregiver's role in Alzheimer's disease [review, 63 refs]. *Neurology, 48*(5 Suppl 6), S25-S29.

Hardy, J. (1996). New insights into the genetics of Alzheimer's disease [review, 38 refs]. *Annals of Medicine, 28*(3), 255-258.

Hardy, J. (1997). Amyloid, the presenilins and Alzheimer's disease [review, 53 refs]. *Trends in Neurosciences, 20*(4), 154-159.

Hardy, J. (1997). The Alzheimer family of diseases: Many etiologies, one pathogenesis? [comment] [review, 21 refs]. *Proceedings of the National Academy of Sciences of the United States of America, 94*(6), 2095-2097.

Hefti, F., Armanini, M. P., Beck, K. D., Caras, I. W., Chen, K. S., Godowski, P. J., Goodman, L. J., Hammonds, R. G., Mark, M. R., Moran, P., Nishimura, M. C., Phillips, H. S., Shih, A., Valverde, J., & Winslow, J. W. (1996). Development of neurotrophic factor therapy for Alzheimer's disease [review, 36 refs]. *Ciba Foundation Symposium, 196*, 54-63, discussion 63-69.

Henderson, V. W. (1997). The epidemiology of estrogen replacement therapy and Alzheimer's disease [review, 142 refs]. *Neurology, 48*(5 Suppl 7), S27-S35.

Hier, D. B. (1997). Alzheimer's disease [review, 10 refs]. *Surgical Neurology, 47*(1), 84-85.

Keefover, R. W. (1996). The clinical epidemiology of Alzheimer's disease [review, 194 refs]. *Neurologic Clinics, 14*(2), 337-351.

Kolanowski, A. (1996). Everyday functioning in Alzheimer's disease: Contribution of neuropsychological testing [see comments] [review, 68 refs]. *Clinical Nurse Specialist, 10*(1), 11-17.

Kumar, V., Goldstein, M. Z., & Doraiswamy, P. M. (1996). Advances in pharmacotherapy for decline of memory and cognition in patients with Alzheimer's disease [review, 28 refs]. *Psychiatric Services, 47*(3), 249-253.

Lannfelt, L. (1996). Genetics of Alzheimer's disease [review, 33 refs]. *Acta Neurologica Scandinavica Supplementum, 168*, 25-27.

Lendon, C. L., Ashall, F., & Goate, A. M. (1997). Exploring the etiology of Alzheimer disease using molecular genetics [review, 130 refs]. *Journal of the American Medical Association, 277*(10), 825-831.

LeBars, P. L., Katz, M. M., Berman, N., Itil, T. M., Freedman, A. M., & Schatzberg, A. F. (for the North American Egb Study Group). (1997). A placebo-controlled, double-blind, randomized trial of an extract of Ginkgo Balboa for dementia. *Journal of the American Medical Association, 278* (16) 1327-1332.

Mahley, R. W., Nathan, B. P., & Pitas, R. E. (1996). Apolipoprotein E. Structure, function, and possible roles in Alzheimer's disease [review, 24 refs]. *Annals of the New York Academy of Sciences, 777*, 139-145.

McGeer, P. L., & McGeer, E. G. (1996). Anti-inflammatory drugs in the fight against Alzheimer's disease [review, 16 refs]. *Annals of the New York Academy of Sciences, 777*, 213-220.

Morris, J. C. (1996). Classification of dementia and Alzheimer's disease [review, 77 refs]. *Acta Neurologica Scandinavica Supplementum, 165*, 41-50.

Muir, J. L. (1997). Acetylcholine, aging, and Alzheimer's disease [review, 124 refs]. *Pharmacology, Biochemistry and Behavior, 56*(4), 687-696.

Nordberg, A. (1996). Functional studies of new drugs for the treatment of Alzheimer's disease [review, 43 refs]. *Acta Neurologica Scandinavica Supplementum, 165*, 137-144.

Paganini-Hill, A. (1996). Estrogen replacement therapy and Alzheimer's disease [review, 49 refs]. *British Journal of Obstetrics and Gynaecology, 103*(Suppl 13), 80-86.

Parnetti, L., Senin, U., & Mecocci, P. (1997). Cognitive enhancement therapy for Alzheimer's disease. The way forward [review, 107 refs]. *Drugs, 53*(5), 752-768.

Pericak-Vance, M. A., Bass, M. P., Yamaoka, L. H., Gaskell, P. C., Scott, W. K., Terwedow, H. A., Menold, M. M., Conneally, P. M., Small, G. W., Vance, J. M., Saunders, A. M., Roses, A. D. , & Haines, J. L. (1997). Complete genomic screen in late-onset familial Alzheimer Disease: Evidence for a new locus on chromosome #12. *Journal of the American Medical Association, 278*(15) 1237-1241.

Peskind, E. R. (1996). Neurobiology of Alzheimer's disease [review, 53 refs]. *Journal of Clinical Psychiatry, 57*(Suppl 14), 5-8.

Plassman, B. L., & Breitner, J. C. (1997). The genetics of dementia in late life [review, 150 refs]. *Psychiatric Clinics of North America, 20*(1), 59-76.

Post, S. G., Whitehouse, P. J., Binstock, R. H., Bird, T. D., Eckert, S. K., Farrer, L. A., Fleck, L. M., Gaines, A. D., Juengst, E. T., Karlinsky, H., Miles, S., Murray, T. H., Quaid, K. A., Relkin, N. R., Roses, A. D., St., G. P. H., Sachs, G. A., Steinbock, B., Truschke, E. F., & Zinn, A. B. (1997). The clinical introduction of genetic testing for Alzheimer disease. An ethical perspective [review, 75 refs]. *Journal of the American Medical Association, 277*(10), 832-836.

Raiha, I., Kaprio, J., Koskenvuo, M., Rajala, T., & Sourander, L. (1997). Alzheimer's disease in twins [review, 32 refs]. *Biomedicine and Pharmacotherapy, 51*(3), 101-104.

Robbins, T. W., McAlonan, G., Muir, J. L., & Everitt, B. J. (1997). Cognitive enhancers in theory and practice: Studies of the cholinergic hypothesis of cognitive deficits in Alzheimer's disease [review, 34 refs]. *Behavioural Brain Research, 83*(1-2), 15-23.

Roses, A. D. (1996). Apolipoprotein E alleles as risk factors in Alzheimer's disease [review, 66 refs]. *Annual Review of Medicine, 47*, 387-400.

Roses, A. D. (1996). The Alzheimer diseases [review, 48 refs]. *Current Opinion in Neurobiology, 6*(5), 644-650.

Rossor, M. N., Fox, N. C., Freeborough, P. A., & Harvey, R. J. (1996). Clinical features of sporadic and familial Alzheimer's disease [review, 40 refs]. *Neurodegeneration, 5*(4), 393-397.

Samuels, S. C., & Davis, K. L. (1997). A risk-benefit assessment of tacrine in the treatment of Alzheimer's disease [review, 55 refs]. *Drug Safety, 16*(1), 66-77.

Schneider, L. S. (1996). New therapeutic approaches to Alzheimer's disease [review, 51 refs]. *Journal of Clinical Psychiatry, 57*(Suppl 14), 30-36.

Selkoe, D. J. (1996). Amyloid beta-protein and the genetics of Alzheimer's disease [review, 93 refs]. *Journal of Biological Chemistry, 271*(31), 18295-18298.

Selkoe, D. J. (1997). Alzheimer's disease: Genotypes, phenotypes, and treatments [review, 17 refs]. *Science, 275*(5300), 630-631.

Singh, V. K. (1997). Neuroautoimmunity: Pathogenic implications for Alzheimer's disease [review, 82 refs]. *Gerontology, 43*(1-2), 79-94.

Small, G. W., Rabins, P. V., Barry, P. P., Buckholtz, N. S., DeKosky, S. T., Ferris, S. H., Finkel, S. I., et al. (1997). Diagnosis and treatment of Alzheimer Disease and related disorders: Consensus Statement of the American Association for Geriatric Psychiatry, the Alzheimer"s Association, and the American Geriatrics Society. *Journal of the American Medical Association, 278*(16), 1363-1371.

Small, G. W. (1996). Neuroimaging and genetic assessment for early diagnosis of Alzheimer's disease [review, 41 refs]. *Journal of Clinical Psychiatry, 57*(Suppl 14), 9-13.

Terry, R. D. (1996). The pathogenesis of Alzheimer disease: An alternative to the amyloid hypothesis [review, 25 refs]. *Journal of Neuropathology & Experimental Neurology, 55*(10), 1023-1025.

Van, D. K. (1997). The possible role of peroxynitrite in Alzheimer's disease: A simple hypothesis that could be tested more thoroughly [review, 49 refs]. *Medical Hypotheses, 48*(5), 375-380.

Wallin, A., & Blennow, K. (1996). Clinical subgroups of the Alzheimer syndrome [review, 39 refs]. *Acta Neurologica Scandinavica Supplementum, 165*, 51-57.

Whitehouse, P. J. (1997). Genesis of Alzheimer's disease [review, 58 refs]. *Neurology, 48*(5 Suppl 7), S2-S7.

Yamada, K., Nitta, A., Hasegawa, T., Fuji, K., Hiramatsu, M., Kameyama, T., Furukawa, Y., Hayashi, K., & Nabeshima, T. (1997). Orally active NGF synthesis stimulators: Potential therapeutic agents in Alzheimer's disease [review, 32 refs]. *Behavioural Brain Research, 83*(1-2), 117-122.

CASE STUDY*

ALZHEIMER DISEASE

INITIAL HISTORY:
- 76-year-old woman
- Told daughter she had not been feeling well
- Shopping for groceries with daughter
- Became separated in the aisles
- Became confused and angry when store employees and others tried to assist her
- Now 30 minutes later

Question 1.
What is your differential diagnosis based on the information you now have?

Question 2.
What other questions would you like to ask now? (These questions should be asked of the patient first, and then of a reliable historian separately.)

---

* Gail L. Kongable-Beckman, RN, MSN, contributed this case study.

ADDITIONAL HISTORY:
- The daughter has noticed increased anxiety and confusion in her mother on several occasions.
- No personal or family history of psychological illness
- Daughter describes language problems such as trouble finding words
- Problems with abstract thinking
- Poor or decreased judgment
- Disorientation in place and time
- Changes in mood and behavior
- Changes in personality

FURTHER HISTORY:
- No history of trauma or recent infection
- Family history: father and brother have died from stroke and heart disease; mother had Alzheimer disease
- Current medications: aspirin, 325 mg daily; hydrochlorothiazide, 25 mg BID
- No other medical history
- No known allergies

Question 3.
Now what do you think about her history?

PHYSICAL EXAMINATION:
- Alert elderly woman in no acute distress
- T = 37 orally; P = 85 and regular; RR = 15 and unlabored; BP 158/88 right arm sitting

HEENT, Skin, Neck
- Pupils are small and react to light sluggishly.
- Ocular fundus is pale; vessels are narrow and attenuated.
- Dentures present, buccal and pharyngeal membranes are moist without lesions or exudate.
- Pale, dry with senile lentigines
- Transparent with decreased turgor
- Minor multiple ecchymosis noted on forearms.
- No other lesions or abrasions
- No lymphadenopathy, no thyromegaly
- Trachea is midline
- Carotid pulses full and equal bilaterally without bruit
- No jugular venous distension

Lungs
- Increased anterior/posterior diameter, with mild kyphosis
- No shortness of breath
- Lungs clear to ausculation throughout, bilaterally

Cardiac
- Apical pulse at 5th ICS, L MCL
- Regular rate and rhythm
- Normal S_1, S_2; no murmurs, clicks, or rubs

Abdomen, Extremities, Neurological
- Round, symmetric with no apparent masses or hernias
- No scars or lesions
- Bowel sounds present; no bruits
- Tympany to percussion in all quadrants; no masses or organomegaly
- No redness, cyanosis, skin lesions
- Symmetric with no swelling or atrophy
- Warm bilaterally
- All pulses present and equal bilaterally
- No lymphadenopathy
- Orientation to person, time, and place inconsistent
- Pinprick, light touch, vibration intact; able to identify a key
- Motor: no atrophy, weakness or tremor; rapid alternating movements smooth
- DTRs all 2+
- No Babinski

Musculoskeletal
- Gait slightly wide based; unable to tandem walk
- No Romberg
- Joints and muscles symmetric; no swelling, masses, deformities, tenderness
- Mild kyphosis of the spine
- Joints: full, smooth range of motion; no crepitance, tenderness
- Extremities: able to maintain flexion and extension against resistance without tenderness

Question 4.
What studies would you initiate now while preparing your interventions?

Question 5.
What therapies would you initiate immediately while awaiting result of the lab studies?

LABORATORY RESULTS:
- Head CT scan showed one small capsular infarction, no mass lesion or edema, no hydrocephalus.
- No significant abnormal results of chemistry, hematology, and metabolic screens.
- MMSE findings of impairment of memory and three other cognitive areas.
- Geriatric Depression Scale (GDS) is positive for memory difficulty, disrupted sleep-wake cycle, apathy, increased dependence (classic for Alzheimer disease).

Question 6.
What does Alzheimer dementia look like on CT scan?

EMERGENCY ROOM COURSE:
- Patient is cooperative, in no apparent distress.
- Becomes less confused with repeated explanation of circumstances.
- Physical exam now: unchanged
- Repeat lab studies: None

Question 7.
What do you think is happening?

Question 8.
Now what should be done and what can the patient expect?

HOSPITAL COURSE:

- Response to therapy: stable condition
- Discharged to home in the care of daughter after 24 hours

Question 9.
What instructions and medications should this patient go home with?

Question 10.
What steps can she take to prevent future problems?

CHAPTER 21

EPILEPSY*

DEFINITION

- Epilepsy, as defined by the Commission on Epidemiology and Prognosis of Epilepsy, is the occurrence of at least two unprovoked seizures with at least a 24-hour separation between those seizures.

- Neither seizures nor epilepsy is a diagnosis or disease entity itself; it is a symptom of other processes that affect the brain in a variety of ways, but has the final common clinical expression of a seizure.

- Seizures are the cardinal manifestation of epilepsy, though not all patients with seizures have epilepsy.

- A seizure is an excessive or abnormal sudden, high frequency discharge of the brain's neurons.

- Seizures lasting longer than 20 minutes are labeled as status epilepticus and constitute a medical emergency requiring immediate intervention.

CLASSIFICATION

- The diagnosis, treatment, and prognosis of seizure disorders depend on the correct identification of types of seizures and epilepsy. There are two currently accepted classification schemes: the International Classification of Epileptic Seizures [ICES] and the International Classification of Epilepsies and Epileptic Syndromes [ICEES].

- **Overview of ICES**

  - Partial seizures—begin in a focal or restricted part of the cortex
    1) Simple partial seizures—consciousness is not impaired
       - They are further subdivided into various categories based on signs and symptoms produced by the seizure.
    2) Complex partial seizures—consciousness is impaired
       - Complex partial seizures can arise from any cortical area, yet they are frequently considered equivalent to temporal lobe seizures; they are frequently preceded by an aura.
    3) Partial seizures—evolve into secondarily generalized seizures
       - The secondarily generalized seizures are usually tonic-clonic.

  - Generalized seizures—begin with epileptiform activity over the entire cortex
    1) Absence seizures are brief generalized seizures without prominent motor manifestations and are typically associated with a generalized 3-Hz spike-and-wave pattern on the electroencephalogram (EEG).

---

* Lucy R. Deivert, RN, BA, BSN, coauthored this chapter.

    2) Myoclonic seizures appear as singular or successive shock-like body jerks; the EEG would show generalized discharges.

    3) Clonic seizures result in a relatively symmetric, bilateral, synchronous, and semirythmic jerking of the upper and lower extremities, increasing in amplitude and decreasing in frequency as the seizure progresses.

    4) Tonic seizures cause sudden, sustained tone, and are frequently manifested as flexor or extensor posturing. They may be accompanied by a guttural cry as air is forced out of closed vocal cords.

    5) Tonic-clonic seizures often evolve from tonic to clonic movements and may be preceded by brief myoclonic or clonic activity.

    6) Atonic seizures, also know as "drop attacks," result from a sudden brief loss of tone.

- Unclassified epileptic seizures—in practice, seizures may not always fall clearly into one category, although it is important to remember that a single patient may present with several different seizure types.

- **Overview of ICEES**

  - Like ICES, ICEES divides seizure types into partial, generalized, and undetermined. While ICES categorizes seizure type, ICEES expands this classification scheme to include more information about the cause and clinical manifestations of the seizure. Subcategories of the epilepsies and epileptic syndromes include the following:
    1) Idiopathic—most common; no obvious underlying cause or pathological alteration other than a presumed genetic predisposition
    2) Symptomatic—occur as a result of a defined cerebral disorder
    3) Cryptogenic—suspected to be symptomatic despite absence of definitive proof of the underlying cause

- Both the ICES and ICEES are useful but they also they have their limitations. Both are so detailed as to be impractical for most nonneurologists; new classification schemes are being proposed.

EPIDEMIOLOGY

- Epilepsy is one of the most common chronic neurological disorders in the United States, with a prevalence of approximately 0.5%.

- The cumulative lifetime risk of having a seizure is 8%.

- Half the lifetime risk of developing epilepsy occurs during childhood or adolescence.

- During childhood, rates are highest during the first year of life and then drop sharply; rates drop off again during adolescence; over age 50, the rate of epilepsy begins to increase again, secondary to cerebrovascular disease and cerebral vascular accidents.

- The mortality rate of a patient with epilepsy is 2 to 4 times the nonepileptic population, with the mortality being highest in the 10 years after diagnosis.

- 10% of deaths in patients with epilepsy are directly related to a seizure or status epilepticus, while 5% of deaths are secondary to a fatal accident during a seizure.

- The suicide risk in people with epilepsy is 25 times that of the general population.

PATHOPHYSIOLOGY

- A few of the familial epilepsies have been found to have a genetic basis, with mutations in the ion channels that modulate neuronal firing; however, for the vast majority of the epilepsies a genetic link has yet to be discovered.

- One or more of the following mechanisms are postulated to be involved in the genesis and spread of epileptic discharges:

  - Changes in voltage-regulated ion channels in neuronal membranes that lead to excessive depolarization or excessive action potential firing.

  - Changes in the extracellular concentrations of potassium and calcium.

  - Increased excitation or decreased inhibition at the synapse allowing for excessive neuronal firing.
    1) Excitatory Amino Acids (EAAs) are in a physiologic balance with the inhibitory neurotransmitters.
    2) Glutamate, an EAA, is the primary excitatory neurotransmitter in the central nervous system; gamma-amniobutyric acid (GABA) is the primary inhibitory neurotransmitter.
    3) The excitotoxic hypothesis of neurologic disease describes excessive release into, or defective removal from, glutamate in the synapse.
    4) Overall, the effects of GABA are depressant; impairment of GABA produces seizures, whereas enhancement results in an anticonvulsant effect. Many new antiepileptic drugs (AEDs) are targeted at enhancing GABA activity.

PATIENT PRESENTATION

- History:

  Positive family history of seizures; febrile seizures as a child; head injury; stroke; heart disease; reported lapses of consciousness; episodes of incontinence; seizure activity witnessed by others; history of motor vehicle accidents or other unexplained injuries; alcohol or drug abuse or toxicity.

- Symptoms:

  Localized seizure-like movements on one part of the body; episodic loss of consciousness; focal neurologic deficits; visual changes; headache; confusion; incontinence, tongue-biting; fatigue; tearfulness; incontinence; symptoms from injuries.

- Examination:

  Between seizures, the exam may be completely normal; witnessed seizures allow for confirmation of the diagnosis; focal neurologic findings; evidence of injury; evidence of drug or alcohol abuse.

DIFFERENTIAL DIAGNOSIS

- Not seizures:

  - Syncope—cardiac disease, orthostatic blood pressure changes, vasovagal episodes

  - Psychogenic "seizures"

  - Migraines

- Not epilepsy:

    - Alcohol abuse/withdrawal

    - Vascular pathology

    - Tumor

    - Intoxication—theophylline, tricyclic antidepressants, carbon monoxide, alcohol

    - Metabolic disarray—hypoglycemia, hypo-/hypernatremia, hypo-/hypercalcemia

    - Fever—more common in young children

    - Infections

    - Cranial trauma

    - Eclampsia

KEYS TO ASSESSMENT

- Goals of evaluation are as follows:

    - Verify that a seizure has occurred.
        1) Obtain a detailed patient interview and, if possible an interview of those who witnessed the seizure; these subjective accounts can assist in differential diagnosis, as well as establishing seizure type.
    - Rapidly identify potential life-threatening causes (trauma, myocardial infarction, stroke, metabolic disarray, drug toxicity).
        1) When a seizure occurs within well-defined circumstances, such as a stroke or head injury, the focus should be on treating the underlying cause and preventing recurrence of the seizure.
        2) An urgent metabolic and toxic screening is necessary for every patient presenting with a first generalized seizure, with particular attention paid to natremia and glycemia.
    - When the patient is known to have epilepsy and is under treatment, a seizure should not be managed in the atmosphere of an emergency; the priority should be understanding what triggered the seizure (e.g., improper medication use, alcohol, skipped meals, sleep deprivation, stress, fever).
    - Physical examination should include a thorough neurological exam to look for focal deficits; when the neuro exam is abnormal, computed tomography (CT) scan becomes urgent.
    - Following a normal neuro exam, patients should have an EEG and CT scan or magnetic resonance imaging (MRI) on an outpatient basis, with the CT or MRI scheduled as soon as possible if the EEG shows abnormal activity.
    - EEG
        1) EEG is essential for the use of the ICES and ICEES to appropriately categorize and manage epilepsy.
        2) In an isolated first seizure, EEG findings may be of little value in predicting risk of recurrence, but may be used in deciding when to initiate treatment with AEDs.
        3) Incidence of epileptiform activity in people without seizures is 0% to 3.8%.
        4) Many patients with epilepsy have a normal EEG on one or more occasion.

5) Repetition of EEGs and the use of different activations (hyperventilation, photic stimulation, sleep) increase the chances of finding paroxysmal activity in epileptic patients.

- CT or MRI
    1) Demonstrate lesions though not necessarily epileptogenic focus
    2) Crucial in presurgical evaluation
    3) Experimental fMRI (functional MRI) and MRSI (MR spectroscopic imaging)

- Positron emission tomography (PET)
    1) Identifies the foci of epileptogenesis as an area of interictal hypometabolism

- Single photon emission computed tomography (SPECT)
    1) Measures distribution of blood flow; can be applied during seizures since tracers can be mixed at the bedside

KEYS TO MANAGEMENT

- • Pharmacologic

    - Treatment is started after the first seizure only if there are epileptiform abnormalities on EEG or an associated epileptogenic condition that cannot be reversed.

    - The risk of a second seizure, following the first unprovoked tonic-clonic seizure, is 42% at 2 years; thus, in many individuals the first seizure remains an isolated episode.

    - Upon seizure recurrence (especially if less than 1 year after the first seizure), therapy should be begun.

    - Initial therapy for epilepsy is monotherapy.

    - Approximately 70% of patients can achieve seizure control with AEDs.

    - Dosing of medications:
        1) A very low dose is used for the first few days, then a gradual increase.
        2) Generalized tonic-clonic seizures typically require a lower dose than partial seizures.
        3) With an increased dose there are increased adverse drug reactions.
        4) The final decision about which dose is appropriate will take into account the individual characteristics of the patient—a complete and detailed medical and social history is helpful in choosing the appropriate AED.
        5) The best AED is the one that controls seizures without causing unacceptable side effects.
        6) The nature of the seizure that the patient is experiencing, as well as the specific epileptic syndrome, may influence the choice of AED.

    - Use of AEDs in women
        1) Women using conventional AEDs are at risk for altered bone health, disturbances in fertility, menstrual cyclicity, ovulatory function, sexuality, possible failure of hormonal contraception, and fetal malformations.

    - The role of plasma drug concentrations
        1) There is no justification for increasing drug dosage when the patient is fully controlled, even though the plasma concentration of the drug is below the lower limit of the therapeutic range.
        2) It may be useful as a measure of compliance, to rule out poor compliance as a reason for treatment failure.
        3) Many of the new AEDs do not offer correlates to plasma levels.

- Polypharmacy in drug resistant epilepsy
    1) Polypharmacy is generally utilized after failure of successive monotherapy.
    2) Combine drugs with different mechanisms of action
    3) Avoid drugs with similar adverse effects

- Brief overview of AEDs
    1) <u>Phenytoin</u>
        - It will control focal and secondary generalized seizures in 60% of patients.
        - It is a poor choice in young females, secondary to hirsutism and gum hyperplasia.
    2) <u>Carbamazepine</u>
        - It is the first choice for partial epilepsy and secondarily generalized tonic-clonic seizures; it will control focal seizures in 60% of patients.
        - It may cause mild neutropenia and/or liver toxicity.
    3) <u>Phenobarbital</u>
        - It is effective in about 60% of patients.
        - Usefulness is limited by dose-dependent sedation; it can produce depression.
    4) <u>Valproic acid</u>
        - It is effective for focal seizures with or without secondary generalization.
        - It may be a drug of choice for new onset epilepsy due to its usefulness with focal and primary generalized seizures.
        - Weight gain is a frequent reason for noncompliance.
    5) <u>Benzodiazepines</u>
        - They are the first choice in status epilepticus.
        - Otherwise, they are very sedating and patients build tolerance quickly.
    6) <u>Some new AEDS</u>
        - Gabapentin—add-on drug in patients with partial seizures with or without secondary generalization
        - Lamotrigine—partial seizures and generalized epilepsies
        - Vigabatrin—partial seizures refractory to carbamazepine and valproic acid
        - Oxcarbazepine—newly diagnosed partial seizures

- Deciding when to stop drug therapy in the seizure-free patient
    1) A patient on monotherapy who has been seizure free more than 2 years may be a candidate for drug withdrawal.
    2) An abnormal EEG offers a poor prognosis of successful medication withdrawal.
    3) Implications of drug withdrawal should be discussed with the patient, especially the probability of relapse.
    4) If withdrawal is indicated and agreed upon, it should take place gradually over no less than 6 months.

- <u>Surgical</u>

    - Surgery is typically reserved for those patients who fail medical management, but it is probably underused in the management of refractory epilepsy.

    - There must be a well-localized epileptogenic focus, and the focus must be located such that the surgery would not result in severe speech or memory deficits.

    - The prototype of surgically remediable epilepsy syndromes is temporal lobe epilepsy, one of the most common forms of epilepsy and also one of the most refractory.

    - Pediatric epilepsy surgery is increasing secondary to the delineation of certain catastrophic epileptic disorders of infants and young children, and the greater understanding of the plasticity of the developing brain, along with the damage caused by repeated seizures.

Pathophysiology

What is going on in the disease process that influences how the patient presents and how he or she should be managed?

→

Clinical Link

What should you do now that you understand the underlying pathophysiology?

Pathophysiology	Clinical Link
Seizures are categorized by their clinical appearance and EEG pattern; these categories are correlated with prognosis and response to medication.	A careful history of a seizure from observers, as well as an EEG, is essential to the appropriate identification of the seizure type and selection of the proper drug.
Seizures result from abnormal ionic exchange at the neuronal membrane, or from an imbalance of excitatory (glutamate) and inhibitory (GABA) neurotransmitters.	AEDs work primarily by stabilizing neuronal membrane ionic activity; the newer drugs are aimed at modulating glutamate and/or GABA activity.
Seizures can result from many causes, including anoxia, space-occupying lesions, infarctions, toxins, metabolic disarray, trauma, and infections.	A thorough evaluation with special emphasis on the neurologic exam and laboratories is essential in the new-onset seizure patient, and a CT or MRI should be done quickly if there is any evidence of localized neurologic disease.
An EEG can be abnormal in people without epilepsy and can be normal in patients with epilepsy.	The EEG is most useful in the evaluation of new-onset seizures if it can be correlated by observed epileptic activity; thus, activators, such as sleep deprivation, hyperventilation, and photic stimulation with observation of the patient, may be indicated to confirm the diagnosis.
The efficacy and side effects of the AEDs varies significantly between individual patients.	The selection of appropriate pharmacologic management must also be based on psychosocial information obtained from the patient and family.

BIBLIOGRAPHY

Aldenkamp, A. P. (1997). Effect of seizures and epileptiform discharges on cognitive function [review, 40 refs]. *Epilepsia, 38*(Suppl 1), S52-S55.

Andermann, F. (1997). Brain structure and epilepsy: The impact of modern imaging [comment]. *American Journal of Neuroradiology, 18,* 302-306.

Andersson, T., Braathen, G., Persson, A., & Theorell, K. (1997). A comparison between one and three years of treatment in uncomplicated childhood epilepsy: A prospective study. II. The EEG as predictor of outcome after withdrawal of treatment. *Epilepsia, 38,* 225-232.

Anonymous. (1997). ILAE Commission Report. The epidemiology of the epilepsies: Future directions. International League Against Epilepsy [review, 32 refs]. *Epilepsia, 38,* 614-618.

Anonymous. (1997). ACOG educational bulletin. Seizure disorders in pregnancy. Number 231, December 1996. Committee on Educational Bulletins of the American College of Obstetricians and Gynecologists. *International Journal of Gynaecology and Obstetrics, 56,* 279-286.

Anonymous. (1997). A global survey on epilepsy surgery, 1980-1990: A report by the Commission on Neurosurgery of Epilepsy, the International League Against Epilepsy. *Epilepsia, 38,* 249-255.

Baker, G. A., Jacoby, A., Buck, D., Stalgis, C., & Monnet, D. (1997). Quality of life of people with epilepsy: A European study. *Epilepsia, 38,* 353-362.

Baker, G. A., Nashef, L., & van Hout, B. A. (1997). Current qissues in the management of epilepsy: The impact of frequent seizures on cost of illness, quality of life, and mortality [review, 47 refs]. *Epilepsia, 38* (Suppl 1), S1-S8.

Bartolomei, F., Suchet, L., Barrie, M., & Gastaut, J. L. (1997). Alcoholic epilepsy: A unified and dynamic classification. *European Neurology, 37,* 13-17.

Bauer, G. (1994). Seizure types and epileptic syndromes in adults. *European Neurology 34*(Suppl 1), 13-17.

Baumhackl, U., Billeth, R., & Graf, M. (1994). Type-specific diagnostic analysis of first epileptic seizure in adults. *European Neurology 34*(Suppl 1), 71-73.

Beckung, E., & Uvebrant, P. (1997). Impairments, disabilities and handicaps in children and adolescents with epilepsy. *Acta Paediatrica, 86,* 254-260.

Beghi, E. & Perucca, E. (1995). The management of epilepsy in the 1990s. *Drugs 49(5),* 680-694.

Berg, A. T., Testa, F. M., Levy, S. R., & Shinnar, S. (1996). The epidemiology of epilepsy. *Neurology Clinics 14(2),* 383-398.

Braathen, G., & Melander, H. (1997). Early discontinuation of treatment in children with uncomplicated epilepsy: A prospective study with a model for prediction of outcome. *Epilepsia, 38,* 561-569.

Britton, J. W., & So, E. L. (1996). Selection of antiepileptic drugs: A practical approach. *Mayo Clinic Proceedings 71*(8), 778-786.

Buck, D., Baker, G. A., Jacoby, A., Smith, D. F., & Chadwick, D. W. (1997). Patients' experiences of injury as a result of epilepsy. *Epilepsia, 38,* 439-444.

Chadwick, D. W. (1997). An overview of the efficacy and tolerability of new antiepileptic drugs. *Epilepsia, 38* (Suppl 1), S59-S62.

Chapman, D. P., & Giles, W. H. (1997). Pharmacologic and dietary therapies in epilepsy: Conventional treatments and recent advances [review, 97 refs]. *Southern Medical Journal, 90,* 471-480.

Cockerell, O. C., Johnson, A. L., Sander, J. W., & Shorvon, S. D. (1997). Prognosis of epilepsy: A review and further analysis of the first nine years of the British National General Practice Study of Epilepsy, a prospective population-based study. *Epilepsia, 38,* 31-46.

Commission on Classification and Terminology of the International League Against Epilepsy. (1989). Proposal for Revised Classification of Epilepsies and Epileptic Syndromes. *Epilepsia 30*(4), 389-399.

Deckers, C. L., Hekster, Y. A., Keyser, A., Meinardi, H., & Renier, W. O. (1997). Reappraisal of polytherapy in epilepsy: A critical review of drug load and adverse effects [review, 41 refs]. *Epilepsia, 38,* 570-575.

Dichter, M. A. (1995). Integrated use of old and new antiepileptic drugs. *Current Opinion in Neurology 8,* 95-102.

Duncan, J. S. (1997). Imaging and epilepsy [review, 274 refs]. *Brain, 120,* 339-377.

Elmslie, F., & Gardiner, M. (1995). Genetics of the epilepsies. *Current Opinion in Neurology* 8, 126-129.

Engel, J. Jr. (1996). Surgery for seizures. *The New England Journal of Medicine 334*(10), 647-652.

Fish, D. R., & Spencer, S. S. (1995). Clinical correlations: MRI and EEG. *Magnetic Resonance Imaging 13*(8), 1113-1117.

Fried, I. (1995). Magnetic resonance imaging and epilepsy: Neurosurgical decision making. *Magnetic Resonance Imaging 13*(8), 1163-1170.

Gall, C. M., Lauterborn, J. C., Guthrie, K. M., & Stinis, C. T. (1997). Seizures and the regulation of neurotrophic factor expression: Associations with structural plasticity in epilepsy [review, 97 refs]. *Advances in Neurology, 72,* 9-24.

Garcia, P. A., Laxer, K. D., & Ng, T. (1995). Application of spectroscopic imaging in epilepsy [review]. *Magnetic Resonance Imagining 13*(8), 1181-1185.

Greenamyre, J. T., & Porter, R. (1994). Anatomy and physiology of glutamate in the CNS. *Neurology 44*(Suppl 8), S7-S12.

Henry ,T. R. (1996). Functional neuroimaging with positron emission tomography. *Epilepsia 37*(12), 1141-1154.

Henry, T. R., & Drury, I. (1997). Non-epileptic seizures in temporal lobectomy candidates with medically refractory seizures. *Neurology, 48,* 1374-1382.

Hernandez, T. D., & Naritoku, D. K. (1997). Seizures, epilepsy, and functional recovery after traumatic brain injury: A reappraisal [review, 47 refs]. *Neurology, 48,* 803-806.

Hicks, T. P., & Conti, F. (1996). Amino acids as the source of considerable excitation in the cerebral cortex [review]. *Canadian Journal of Physiology and Pharmacology 74*(4), 341-361.

Holmes, G. L. (1995). Pathogenesis of epilepsy: The role of excitatory amino acids. *Cleveland Clinic Journal of Medicine 62*(4), 240-247.

Hufnagel, A., Zentner, J., Fernandez, G., Wolf, H. K., Schramm, J., & Elger, C. E. (1997). Multiple subpial transection for control of epileptic seizures: Effectiveness and safety. *Epilepsia, 38,* 678-688.

Jalava, M.., & Sillanpaa, M. (1997). Physical activity, health-related fitness, and health experience in adults with childhood-onset epilepsy: A controlled study. *Epilepsia, 38,* 424-429.

Larkin, M. (1997). Epilepsy genes signal new targets for therapy [news]. *Lancet, 349,* 626.

Lee, J. H., Lee, B. I., Park, S. C., Kim, W. J., Kim, J. Y., Park, S. A., & Huh, K. (1997). Experiences of epilepsy surgery in intractable seizures with past history of CNS infection. *Yonsei Medical Journal, 38,* 73-78.

Leestma, J. E., Annegers, J. F., Brodie, M. J., Brown, S., Schraeder, P., Siscovick, D., Wannamaker, B. B., Tennis, P. S., Cierpial, M. A., & Earl, N. L. (1997). Sudden unexplained death in epilepsy: Observations from a large clinical development program. *Epilepsia, 38,* 47-55.

Malow, B. A., Fromes, G. A., & Aldrich, M. S. (1997). Usefulness of polysomnography in epilepsy patients. *Neurology, 48,* 1389-1394.

Morrell, M. J. (1996). The new antiepileptic drugs and women: Efficacy, reproductive health, pregnancy, and fetal outcome. *Epilepsia 37*(Suppl 6), S34-S44.

Morris, H. H. (1997). New treatment options for epilepsy. *Cleveland Clinic Journal of Medicine, 64,* 125-127.

Mosewich, R. K., & So, E. L. (1996). A clinical approach to the classification of seizures and epileptic syndromes [review]. *Mayo Clinic Proceedings 71*(4), 405-414.

Olsen, R. W., & Avoli, M. (1997). GABA and epileptogenesis [review, 85 refs]. *Epilepsia, 38,* 399-407.

Osservatorio Regionale per L'Epilepsia. (1996). ILAE classification of epilepsies: Its applicability and practical value of different diagnostic categories. *Epilepsia 37*(11), 1051-1059.

Pranzatelli, M. R., & Nadi, N. S. (1995). Mechanism of action of antiepileptic and antimyoclonic drugs [review]. *Advances in Neurology 67,* 329-360.

Radue, E. W., & Scollo-Lavizzari, G. (1994). Computed tomography and magnetic resonance imaging in epileptic seizures. *European Neurology 34*(Suppl 1), 55-57.

Ridsdale, L., Robins, D., Cryer, C., & Williams, H. (1997). Feasibility and effects of nurse run clinics for patients with epilepsy in general practice: Randomised controlled trial. Epilepsy Care Evaluation Group. *British Medical Journal, 314,* 120-122.

Schachter, S. C., & Yerby, M. S. (1997). Management of epilepsy: Pharmacologic therapy and quality-of-life issues [review, 21 refs]. *Postgraduate Medicine, 101,* 133-138.

Shorvon, S., & Stefan, H. (1997). Overview of the safety of newer antiepileptic drugs [review, 79 refs]. *Epilepsia, 38* (Suppl 1), S45-S51.

Snead, O. C. 3rd. (1995). Basic mechanisms of generalized absence seizures [review]. *Annals of Neurology 37*(2), 146-157.

Spencer, S. S. (1996). Long-term outcome after epilepsy surgery. *Epilepsia 37*(9), 807-813.

Spencer, S. S., Theodore, W. H., & Berkovic, S. F. (1995). Clinical applications: MRI, SPECT, and PET. *Magnetic Resonance Imaging 13*(8), 1119-1124.

Sperling, M. R., O'Connor, M. J., Saykin, A. J., & Plummer, C. (1996). Temporal lobectomy for refractory epilepsy. *Journal of the American Medical Association 276*(6), 470-475.

Tardy, B., Lafond, P., Convers, P., Page, Y., Zeni, F., Viallon, A., Laurent, B., Barral, F. G., & Bertrand,. J.C. (1995). Adult first generalized seizure: Etiology, biological tests, EEG, CT scan, in an ED. *American Journal of Emergency Medicine 13*(1), 1-5.

Vassella, F. (1994). Seizure types and epileptic syndromes [review]. *European Neurology 34*(Suppl 1), 3-12.

Welch, K. M., & Lewis, D. (1997). Migraine and epilepsy [review, 26 refs]. *Neurologic Clinics, 15,* 107-114.

Wieser, H. G. (1994). PET and SPECT in epilepsy. *European Neurology 34*(Suppl 1), 58-62.

Wieser, H. G. (1994). Role of surgery in the therapy of epilepsy. *European Neurology 34*(Suppl 1), 66-70.

Wilder, B. J. (1995). The treatment of epilepsy: An overview of clinical practices. *Neurology 45*(Suppl 2), S7-S11.

CASE STUDY[*]

EPILEPSY

INITIAL HISTORY:

- 15-year-old boy
- Playing touch football when symptoms developed
- Was tackled and became unreasonably angry at his friend
- Fell to the ground with sudden onset of unconsciousness
- His body stiffened with arms and legs extended
- He did not breathe for about 10 seconds
- He then began violent, rhythmic, muscular contractions accompanied by strenuous hyperventilation which lasted 2 to 3 minutes
- Incontinent of urine
- He then lay limp, breathing quietly, and woke up confused
- Now 1 hour later in the emergency room

Question 1.
What is your differential diagnosis based on the information you now have?

Question 2.
What other questions would you like to ask now?

* Gail L. Kongable-Beckman, RN, MSN, contributed this case study.

ADDITIONAL HISTORY:

- No memory of the event; first memory was of finding himself on the ground
- No history of seizures
- Denies taking any drugs or alcohol
- No recent infections
- History of minor head injury as a child with loss of consciousness
- Had complained of headache to his mother earlier in the day
- No nausea or vomiting
- Had been having a stressful time in school
- Older sister had a seizure with high fever at age 3, none since

Question 3.
What do you think about his history?

PHYSICAL EXAMINATION:

- Alert but tired teenager in no apparent distress
- BP = 115/72 mmHg, sitting; T = 37 orally; P = 72, regular; RR = 14, regular and unlabored

Skin, HEENT

- Pink, warm, dry; no lesions or abrasions
- Conjunctiva pink, moist
- Visual acuity 20/20 without glasses
- Fundi without lesions or hemorrhages
- Nasal mucosa pink, moist without lesions, no exudate
- Bite wound left lateral tongue, no exudate
- Pharynx pink without exudate

Neck

- Supple
- No adenopathy, no thyromegaly
- No bruits

Lungs

- Chest expansion full, symmetrical
- Normal diaphragmatic position and excursion
- Lung sounds clear to auscultation throughout all lobes bilaterally

Cardiac
- Apical pulse palpated at 4th intercostal space, midclavicular line
- Heart rate and rhythm regular
- No murmurs, clicks, gallops, extrasystoles

Abdomen, Extremities
- Nondistended
- Bowel sounds present and not hyperactive
- Liver percusses 2 cm below right costal margin (RCM); overall size is 8 cm
- No tenderness, masses, organomegaly
- Brisk capillary refill at 3 seconds; no edema, no clubbing

Neurological
- Alert, oriented, somewhat sleepy
- Cranial nerves II-XII intact
- Strength 5/5 throughout
- DTRs 2+ and symmetrical
- Sensory intact to touch
- No Romberg
- Able to perform rapid alternating movements (RAM) smoothly without error

Question 4.
What studies would you initiate now while preparing your interventions?

Question 5.
What therapies would you initiate immediately while awaiting results of the lab studies?

LABORATORY:
- CBC, chemistries, liver function studies, and urinalysis are all within normal ranges
- Head CT and MRI are normal

EMERGENCY ROOM COURSE:
- Patient becomes increasingly irritable and anxious.
- He experiences a second seizure with sudden loss of consciousness, generalized tonic convulsion is closely followed by alternating clonic convulsions.
- The event lasts about 3 minutes.
- The patient appears to sleep for about 5 minutes (postictal).
- The patient awakens confused.

PHYSICAL EXAMINATION NOW:
- P = 110, regular; RR = 20; BP = 130/76
- Lungs are clear to auscultation, no aspiration
- Skin diaphoretic, warm
- Patient sleepy, oriented to name only
- Neurologic exam remains normal

Question 6.
What interventions should be initiated now?

RESPONSE TO THERAPY:
- No further seizure activity over the next 4 hours
- Patient is drowsy and oriented when awakened from sleep.
- RR = 12

Question 7.
Now what should be done and what can the patient expect?

HOSPITAL COURSE:
- The patient does well with no further seizures.
- He continues to be tired, but has no other adverse effects.
- He is discharged home on the second day.

Question 8.

What instructions and medications should the patient go home with?

CHAPTER 22

ACUTE BACTERIAL MENINGITIS

DEFINITION

- Infection of the meninges by bacteria, usually with an underlying encephalitis

EPIDEMIOLOGY

- There are 3 cases per 100,00 persons per year in the United States; median age is 25 years.

- The risk factors include extremes of age, splenectomy, sickle-cell disease, alcoholism, liver disease, otitis media, sinusitis, pneumonia, diabetes, immunosuppression, ventricular shunt, cerebrospinal fluid (CSF) leak, and recent neurosurgical procedures.

- Community-acquired meningitis is preceded by nasopharyngeal colonization.

- Since the use of the *Haemophilus influenzae* (*H. influenza*) vaccine became widespread, the incidence of bacterial meningitis has declined and there has been a shift in the most likely etiologic organisms:

    - <1 month old = Group B streptococci

    - >1 month and older = *Streptococcus pneumoniae* (pneumococcus)

    - *Neisseria meningitidis* (meningococcus) is common in ages 2 to 18 years.

- Penicillin resistance of streptococcal infections is now estimated at 25% to 35% (>40% in children 6 years old), and resistance to cefotaxime is 15%.

- Staph and gram-negative organisms are more common in older patients and in infections due to trauma and nosocomial exposure.

- Listeria causes up to 10% of infections, especially in newborns (probable GI source).

- Acute bacterial meningitis is nearly always fatal without treatment; there is a 10% mortality even with therapy.

PATHOPHYSIOLOGY

- Bacteria invade the central nervous system (CNS) due to the combination of aggressive organism $\pm$ host immunosuppression $\pm$ repetitive seeding.

- Bacteria invade the CNS

    - Hematogenous—mucosal colonization of the nasopharynx, or infections of the lung and skin result in seeding of the blood and transport to the meninges

- Contiguous—spreads directly to the meninges from otitis media or sinusitis

- Direct entry—trauma, lumbar puncture, or surgery can lead to direct inoculation of the CSF

- Encapsulated organisms are the most common—pneumococcus, meningococcus, *H. influenza*. They are usually from a respiratory or cranial source and they multiply rapidly in the CSF.

- Once in the CSF, bacterial products (especially lipopolysaccharide [LPS] and peptidoglycan) stimulate the production of inflammatory cytokines from endothelial cells and astrocytes including TNFα, IL-1, IL-8, and nitrous oxide (NO).

- These cytokines are chemotactic for neutrophils and lymphocytes resulting in the adhesion of the leukocytes to the endothelium, and endothelial injury and disruption of the blood-brain barrier leading to protein and cellular accumulation in the CSF.

- Endothelial injury causes vasospasm, initiation of the coagulation cascade, and vasogenic edema.

- Increased intracranial pressure (ICP) due to edema and CSF outflow obstruction leads to reduced cerebral blood flow (CBF), leading to brain ischemia, and eventually death.

PATIENT PRESENTATION

- There are two types of onset:

    - Rapid (25%)—hospitalized within 24-hours of the onset of symptoms; high mortality rate

    - Slow (75%)—days to weeks of preceding prodromal symptoms

- History:

    Recent upper respiratory symptoms; exposure to other ill individuals; sinusitis or otitis media; recent neurosurgery; immunosuppression; sickle-cell disease

- Symptoms:

    Headache; fever; stiff neck; rash; somnolence or irritability; photophobia; vomiting; seizures; blurred vision; numbness or weakness

- Examination:

    Fever; decreased level of consciousness; nuchal rigidity; Brudzinski and Kernig signs; cranial nerve palsies; focal neurologic deficits; rashes

DIFFERENTIAL DIAGNOSIS

- Viral meningitis

- Subarachnoid hemorrhage

- Migraine

- Influenza

- Carcinomatous meningitis

- Parameningeal foci of infection

KEYS TO ASSESSMENT

- Lumbar puncture—CSF results in bacterial meningitis:
    - Pressure—increased (mean pressure = 30 cm H_2O)
    - Protein—increased (>150 mg/dl)
    - Leukocytes—polymorphonuclear neutrophils (PMNs) (>1000/μl)
    - Glucose—decreased (<40 mg/dl)
    - Lactate—increased
    - Lactic dehydrogenase (LDH)—increased
    - Gram stain—60% to 80% sensitive, >90% specific
    - Culture—70% to 85% sensitive
    - India ink—cryptococcus
- CSF studies are being used in experimental trials:
    - C-reactive protein is elevated in over 97% of bacterial meningitis, but is nonspecific.
    - TNFα, IL-1, IL-6, complement, and endothelins are all being evaluated.
    - Immunology—counter immunoelectrophoresis (CIE), latex agglutination; polymerase chain reactions (PCR) for *S. pneumoniae*, *N. meningitidis*, *H. influenza*, *S. agalactiae*, HSV, enterovirus, and Listeria
- Serum with increased white blood cells (WBC); possible electrolyte disturbances, especially if the patient develops the syndrome of inappropriate antidiuretic hormone (SIADH) resulting in hyponatremia
- Computed tomography (CT) or magnetic resonance imaging (MRI) if there is evidence of increased intracranial pressure, equivocal CSF results, or focal neurologic findings on the physical examination

KEYS TO MANAGEMENT

- Early recognition, early identification, and rapid initiation
- The delay of antibiotics is a serious problem in all hospitals—cultures will not be decreased in diagnostic sensitivity if antibiotics are begin 1 to 2 hours before lumbar puncture.
- Isolation of the patient until the organism has been identified.
- Antibiotics—empiric often necessary
    - They should cover likely organisms—use gram stain results or broad empiric coverage.
    - They must penetrate the blood-brain barrier and be bactericidal—leukocyte phagocytosis is inefficient in CSF due to deficiency of complement and specific antibodies.
    - The choice of empiric antibiotics include the following:
        1) Ceftriaxone plus vancomycin
        2) Meropenem plus vancomycin
    - Tailor therapy to the gram stain, polymerase chain reaction (PCR), or culture results

- Dexamethasone
    - Used in children over 6 weeks of age with the first dose of antibiotics; it reduces the risk of complications such as hearing loss
    - It is still debated in adults; it it may be useful if there is clear evidence of increased intracranial pressure
- Monitoring and managing sequelae
    - ICP pressure bolt and management of increased ICP
    - Anticonvulsants for recurrent seizures
    - Support for sepsis
    - Shunt for refractory hydrocephalus
    - Support for disseminated intravascular coagulation (DIC) or syndrome of inappropriate antidiuretic hormone (SIADH)
- Reassess for long-term sequela—up to 25% of children have prolonged complications such as deafness, mental retardation, seizure disorder, spasticity, or paresis
- Prevention
    - Vaccination
        1) *H. influenza*—vaccinate all children >2 months of age
        2) *N. meningitidis*—vaccinate asplenic, immunocompromised, travelers to endemic areas, community and college outbreaks, and household contacts
        3) *S. pneumoniae*—vaccinate adults >65 years of age; those with chronic cardiovascular, pulmonary, hepatic, or renal disease; diabetics; alcoholism; CSF leak; immunocompromised; asplenia; lymphoma; HIV; nephrotic syndrome; or multiple myeloma. Administer booster every 6 years.

    - Chemoprophylaxis
        1) Contacts of cases of meningococcal disease—rifampin, minocycline, ciprofloxacin
        2) Contacts of cases of *H. influenza* meningitis—rifampin

Pathophysiology

What is going on in the disease process that influences how the patient presents and how he or she should be managed?

→

Clinical Link

What should you do now that you understand the underlying pathophysiology?

Pathophysiology	Clinical Link
Encapsulated organisms are common pathogens in bacterial meningitis, and the immune defenses in the CSF are relatively weak, so these organisms can multiply quickly.	Meningitis can progress rapidly to significant neurologic injury and must be treated with antibiotics that are bactericidal, not just bacteristatic, and for which the organism is not resistant.
The first step in host response to CSF bacterial invasion is via the production of inflammatory cytokines from endothelial cells and astrocytes (TNFα, IL-1, NO).	Meningitis is characterized by intense inflammation of the meninges and underlying brain tissue; drugs that block the various cytokines are being tested and steroids are used in children (still controversial in adults).
Increased intracranial pressure is the most ominous sequelae of meningitis and can result in decreased cerebral blood flow, brain ischemia, and herniation.	Patients must be monitored for deteriorating mental status, changes in vital signs, and papilledema; pressure monitoring and treatment with hydroventilation and osmotic agents may be necessary.
Meningitis and subarachnoid hemorrhage can occur in otherwise young and healthy people, and both present with headache, change in mental status, meningismus, and focal neurological deficits, particularly cranial nerve palsies.	Subarachnoid hemorrhage must be ruled out in a patient who does not describe the usual infectious prodromal symptoms and who has clinical evidence of increased intracranial pressure with MRI or (CT) scanning.
Bacteria in the CSF cause changes in the blood-brain barrier that allow cells (usually neutrophils) and protein into the CSF, use up the glucose, and produce lactate with their metabolism, and can often be seen on gram stain or cultured and be tested for with polymerase chain reaction (PCR).	Diagnosis of meningitis is usually made by lumbar puncture with CSF analysis indicating increased protein, neutrophils, and lactate, decreased glucose, and positive stains, cultures, and PCR testing.

BIBLIOGRAPHY

Ahmed, A. (1997). A critical evaluation of vancomycin for treatment of bacterial meningitis [review, 53 refs]. *Pediatric Infectious Disease Journal, 16*(9), 895-903.

Ashwal, S. (1995). Neurologic evaluation of the patient with acute bacterial meningitis [review, 105 refs]. *Neurologic Clinics, 13*(3), 549-577.

Azuma, H., Tsuda, N., Sasaki, K., & Okuno, A. (1997). Clinical significance of cytokine measurement for detection of meningitis. *Journal of Pediatrics, 131*(3), 463-465.

Bergemann, A., & Karstaedt, A. S. (1996). The spectrum of meningitis in a population with high prevalence of HIV disease. *QJM, 89*(7), 499-504.

Bonadio, W. A. (1996). Adjunctive dexamethasone therapy for pediatric bacterial meningitis [review, 40 refs]. *Journal of Emergency Medicine, 14*(2), 165-172.

Bradley, J. S., & Scheld, W. M. (1997). The challenge of penicillin-resistant *Streptococcus pneumoniae* meningitis: Current antibiotic therapy in the 1990s [review, 58 refs]. *Clinical Infectious Diseases, 24*(Suppl 2), S213-S221.

Davies, D. (1996). The causes of meningitis and meningococcal disease. *Nursing Times, 92*(6), 25-27.

Denning, D. W. (1997). Corticosteroids in pneumococcal meningitis [letter; comment]. *Journal of Antimicrobial Chemotherapy, 39*(4), 557-558.

Dorta-Contreras, A., & Miete, F. A. (1996). Dysfunction of the blood-cerebrospinal fluid barrier in bacterial meningitis [letter]. *Journal of Tropical Pediatrics, 42*(6), 372-373.

Duke, T., South, M., & Stewart, A. (1997). Cerebrospinal fluid nitric oxide metabolites and discrimination of bacterial meningitis from other causes of encephalopathy [letter]. *Archives of Disease in Childhood, 76*(3), 290.

Enting, R. H., Spanjaard, L., van de Beek, D., Hensen, E. F., de Gans, J., & Dankert, J. (1996). Antimicrobial susceptibility of Haemophilus influenzae, Neisseria meningitidis and Streptococcus pneumoniae isolates causing meningitis in The Netherlands, 1993-1994. *Journal of Antimicrobial Chemotherapy, 38*(5), 777-786.

Fassbender, K., Schminke, U., Ries, S., Ragoschke, A., Kischka, U., Fatar, M., & Hennerici, M. (1997). Endothelial-derived adhesion molecules in bacterial meningitis: Association to cytokine release and intrathecal leukocyte-recruitment. *Journal of Neuroimmunology, 74*(1-2), 130-134.

Grimwood, K., Anderson, V. A., Bond, L., Catroppa, C., Hore, R. L., Keir, E. H., Nolan, T., & Roberton, D. M. (1995). Adverse outcomes of bacterial meningitis in school-age survivors. *Pediatrics, 95*(5), 646-656.

Hall, L. M., Duke, B., & Urwin, G. (1995). An approach to the identification of the pathogens of bacterial meningitis by the polymerase chain reaction. *European Journal of Clinical Microbiology & Infectious Diseases, 14*(12), 1090-1094.

Hashim, I. A., Walsh, A., Hart, C. A., & Shenkin, A. (1995). Cerebrospinal fluid interleukin-6 and its diagnostic value in the investigation of meningitis. *Annals of Clinical Biochemistry, 32*(Pt 3), 289-296.

Hosoglu, S., Ayaz, C., Ceviz, A., Cumen, B., Geyik, M. F., & Kokoglu, O. F. (1997). Recurrent bacterial meningitis: A 6-year experience in adult patients. *Journal of Infection, 35*(1), 55-62.

Ichiyama, T., Hayashi, T., Nishikawa, M., & Furukawa, S. (1997). Levels of transforming growth factor beta 1, tumor necrosis factor alpha, and interleukin 6 in cerebrospinal fluid: Association with clinical outcome for children with bacterial meningitis. *Clinical Infectious Diseases, 25*(2), 328-329.

Johnson, A. P., & Speller, D. C. (1997). Antibiotic resistance. Epidemiology of antibiotic resistance: Blood and cerebrospinal fluid (CSF). *Journal of Medical Microbiology, 46*(6), 445-447.

Kaplan, S. L. (1997). Prevention of hearing loss from meningitis. *Lancet, #19;350*(9072), 158-159.

Koedel, U., Gorriz, C., Lorenzl, S., & Pfister, H. W. (1997). Increased endothelin levels in cerebrospinal fluid samples from adults with bacterial meningitis. *Clinical Infectious Diseases, 25*(2), 329-330.

Lopez-Cortes, L. F., Cruz-Ruiz, M., Gomez-Mateos, J., Jimenez-Hernandez, D., Viciana-Fernandez, P., & Jimenez-Mejias, E. (1997). Interleukin 6 in cerebrospinal fluid of patients with meningitis is not a useful diagnostic marker in the differential diagnosis of meningitis. *Annals of Clinical Biochemistry, 34*(Pt 2), 165-169.

Lopez-Cortes, L. F., Cruz-Ruiz, M., Gomez-Mateos, J., Viciana-Fernandez, P., Martinez-Marcos, F. J., & Pachon, J. (1995). Interleukin-8 in cerebrospinal fluid from patients with meningitis of different etiologies: Its possible role as neutrophil chemotactic factor. *Journal of Infectious Diseases, 172*(2), 581-584.

McIntyre, P. B., Berkey, C. S., King, S. M., Schaad, U. B., Kilpi, T., Kanra, G. Y., & Perez, C. M. (1997). Dexamethasone as adjunctive therapy in bacterial meningitis. A meta-analysis of randomized clinical trials since 1988. *Journal of the American Medical Association, 278*(11), 925-931.

Meissner, J. E. (1995). Caring for patients with meningitis. *Nursing, 25*(7), 50-51.

Miller, L. G., & Choi, C. (1997). Meningitis in older patients: How to diagnose and treat a deadly infection [review, 21 refs]. *Geriatrics, 52*(8), 43-44.

Ossege, L. M., Sindern, E., Voss, B., & Malin, J. P. (1996). Expression of tumor necrosis factor-alpha and transforming growth factor-beta 1 in cerebrospinal fluid cells in meningitis. *Journal of the Neurological Sciences, 144*(1-2), 1-13.

Papastamelos, A. G., & Tunkel, A. R. (1995). Antibacterial agents in infections of the central nervous system and eye [review, 81 refs]. *Infectious Disease Clinics of North America, 9*(3), 615-637.

Pfister, H. W., & Scheld, W. M. (1997). Brain injury in bacterial meningitis: Therapeutic implications [review, 44 refs]. *Current Opinion in Neurology, 10*(3), 254-259.

Quagliarello, V. J., & Scheld, W. M. (1997). Treatment of bacterial meningitis [review, 96 refs]. *New England Journal of Medicine, 336*(10), 708-716.

Richardson, M. P., Reid, A., Tarlow, M. J., & Rudd, P. T. (1997). Hearing loss during bacterial meningitis [published erratum appears in *Archives of Disease in Childhood, 76*(4), 386 1997]. *Archives of Disease in Childhood, 76*(2), 134-138.

Ries, S., Schminke, U., Fassbender, K., Daffertshofer, M., Steinke, W., & Hennerici, M. (1997). Cerebrovascular involvement in the acute phase of bacterial meningitis. *Journal of Neurology, 244*(1), 51-55.

Rockowitz, J., & Tunkel, A. R. (1995). Bacterial meningitis. Practical guidelines for management [review, 98 refs]. *Drugs, 50*(5), 838-853.

Roos, K. L. (1995). The use of adjunctive therapy to alter the pathophysiology of bacterial meningitis [review, 25 refs]. *Clinical Neuropharmacology, 18*(2), 138-147.

Schneeberger, P. M., Janssen, M., & Voss, A. (1996). Alpha-hemolytic streptococci: A major pathogen of iatrogenic meningitis following lumbar puncture. Case reports and a review of the literature [review, 38 refs]. *Infection, 24*(1), 29-33.

Schuchat, A., Robinson, K., Wenger, J. D., Harrison, L. H., Farley, M., Reingold, A. L., Lefkowitz, L., & Perkins, B. A. (1997). Bacterial meningitis in the United States in 1995. Active Surveillance Team. *New England Journal of Medicine, 337*(14), 970-976.

Spranger, M., Krempien, S., Schwab, S., Maiwald, M., Bruno, K., & Hacke, W. (1996). Excess glutamate in the cerebrospinal fluid in bacterial meningitis. *Journal of the Neurological Sciences, 143*(1-2), 126-131.

Sprenger, H., Rosler, A., Tonn, P., Braune, H. J., Huffmann, G., & Gemsa, D. (1996). Chemokines in the cerebrospinal fluid of patients with meningitis. *Clinical Immunology and Immunopathology, 80*(2), 155-161.

Strawser, D. (1997). Pediatric bacterial meningitis in the emergency department [review, 15 refs]. *Journal of Emergency Nursing, 23*(4), 310-315.

Torre, D., Zeroli, C., Martegani, R., & Speranza, F. (1996). Levels of interleukin-10 and tumor necrosis factor alpha in patients with bacterial meningitis [letter]. *Clinical Infectious Diseases, 22*(5), 883-885.

Townsend, G. C., & Scheld, W. M. (1996). The use of corticosteroids in the management of bacterial meningitis in adults [review, 31 refs]. *Journal of Antimicrobial Chemotherapy, 37*(6), 1051-1061.

van Furth, A. M., Roord, J. J., & van Furth, R. (1996). Roles of proinflammatory and anti-inflammatory cytokines in pathophysiology of bacterial meningitis and effect of adjunctive therapy [review, 165 refs]. *Infection and Immunity, 64*(12), 4883-4890.

van Furth, A. M., Seijmonsbergen, E. M., Groeneveld, P. H., van Furth, R., & Langermans, J. A. (1996). Levels of nitric oxide correlate with high levels of tumor necrosis factor alpha in cerebrospinal fluid samples from children with bacterial meningitis. *Clinical Infectious Diseases, 22*(5), 876-878.

Wilks, D., & Lever, A. M. (1996). Reasons for delay in administration of antibiotics to patients with meningitis and meningococcaemia. *Journal of Infection, 32*(1), 49-51.

CASE STUDY

MENINGITIS

INITIAL HISTORY:
- 22-year-old female college student who just completed winter exams
- Felt well until about 1 week ago when she developed an upper respiratory infection
- Improved slowly, but over the past 2 days has developed increasing cough production of rusty sputum, fever, myalgias, and now a bitemporal headache

Question 1.
What other questions about her symptoms would you like to ask this patient?

ADDITIONAL HISTORY:
- She states that her neck feels stiff and sore.
- She feels tired and is having trouble concentrating.
- Bright lights make her eyes hurt and her vision is slightly blurry; she denies double vision.
- She has had no rashes, vomiting, or diarrhea.
- She has had some shaking chills.
- She does not recall any of her recent contacts being ill.
- She denies dyspnea or chest pain.

Question 2.
What other questions about her history would you like to ask?

PAST MEDICAL HISTORY:
- She denies any past history of meningitis, head trauma, or neurological disease, pneumonia, immunodeficiency, or severe infections.
- She has never been hospitalized.
- She was tested for HIV last year and was negative; she has not been sexually active in 13 months.
- She is on no medications and has no allergies.
- She has a 10-pack/year smoking history.
- She had the usual childhood immunizations but has received none in recent years.

PHYSICAL EXAMINATION:
- Well-built, well-nourished female appearing tired but in no acute distress; coughing occasionally
- T = 38° orally; P = 85 and regular; RR = 20; BP = 95/75 right arm sitting

Skin
- Warm and moist
- No rashes on careful inspection
- No cyanosis

HEENT, Neck
- PERRLA, difficult to visualize fundi due to photophobia but no papilledema seen
- Ears and throat clear without lesions or exudates
- Neck stiff and painful with flexion
- Positive Kernig and Brudzinski signs

Lungs
- No chest deformity; chest expansion symmetrical
- Dullness to percussion over the right posterior inferior lung field
- Inspiratory crackles with egophony in the right posterior lung field

Cardiac, Extremities
- Apical impulse at the 5th intercostal space at the midclavicular line
- Regular rate and rhythm without murmurs or gallops
- Pulses full and symmetrical in all extremities
- No cyanosis, clubbing, rashes, or edema

Abdomen, Neurological
- Nondistended; no tenderness; no masses or organomegaly
- Bowel sounds heard in all four quadrants
- Oriented x 4 but mildly lethargic
- Cranial nerves all intact including ocular movements
- Strength 5/5 and symmetrical throughout
- Sensory intact and symmetrical
- DTR 2+ and symmetrical
- Gait steady

Question 3.
What are the pertinent positive and negative findings on exam and what might they mean?

Question 4.
What is your differential diagnosis at this time?

Question 5.
What laboratory tests and therapeutic interventions would be indicated at this time?

LABORATORY:
- Serum chemistries normal
- WBC = 12,000/mm^3 (90% PMNs); HCT = 40%; platelets = 280,000/mm^3
- Sputum gram stain = numerous PMNs with numerous gram-positive diplococci
- Chest x-ray = dense right lower lobe infiltrate with air bronchograms

LUMBAR PUNCTURE/CEREBROSPINAL FLUID RESULTS:
- Opening pressure = 30 cm water
- Increased protein; decreased glucose; increased lactate
- 120 WBC/mm^3, all PMNs
- Gram stain positive for gram-positive diplococci
- India ink negative for fungi

Question 6.
How would you interpret these lab findings?

Question 7.
What antibiotics would be indicated?

HOSPITAL COURSE:
- Patient is admitted.
- Her fever gradually resolves.
- She experiences decreasing headache and lethargy.

Question 8.
For what complications should this patient be monitored?

CHAPTER 23

MENOPAUSAL OSTEOPOROSIS

DEFINITION

- The disease is characterized by low bone mass and microarchitectural deterioration of bone tissue, leading to enhanced bone fragility and a consequent increase in fracture risk. It is age-related, and it is associated with decreases in stature and kyphosis. Type I = menopausal osteoporosis; type II = senile osteoporosis.

- A value of bone mineral density 2.5 standard deviations or more below the young adult mean.

EPIDEMIOLOGY

- The lifetime risk for osteoporotic fracture in Caucasian women in 40%.

- Osteoporosis causes 1.5 million fractures per year in the United States.

- 25% of women over 60 have spinal compression; 40% of women will develop vertebral fractures by age 75; and 20% of women will develop hip fractures by age 90.

- Peak bone mass is critical to the risk of osteoporotic fracture.

- 15% of young adults in the United States have osteopenia.

- Bone loss rises rapidly after menopause.

- 40% to 80% of risk is due to heredity.

- Risk factors:

    - Late menarche

    - Family history

    - European or Asian ancestry

    - Anorexia

    - Low body weight

    - Renal disease

    - Hyperthyroidism

    - Multiple pregnancies

    - Smoking, heavy caffeine intake

    - Low calcium or high phosphate intake

    - High-protein, high-fat diet

- High salt intake

- Low sun exposure

- Sedentary lifestyle

- Medications (steroids, thyroid hormone, phenytoin, heparin, diuretics, laxatives, benzodiazepines)

PATHOPHYSIOLOGY

- Maximum bone mass is achieved at age 35.

- Bone remodeling occurs constantly in the healthy adult at maturity with no net change in bone mass.

- Turnover is more rapid in trabecular (cancellous) bone (vertebral column, distal radium, proximal femur) than in cortical bone.

- Osteoclasts excavate erosion cavities on bone surfaces, and osteoblasts fill in the cavities with new bone giving it greater strength and repairing microfractures.

- Gonadal insufficiency (estrogen loss) accelerates bone turnover with increasing osteoclast activity and progressively greater surface of the bone being occupied by remodeling events.

- The total skeletal bone mineral content decreases by 7% over time, and 20% in trabecular bone.

- A new steady state is established after several years.

- Estrogens limit the activity of the osteoclasts such that infilling of the erosion sites by osteoblasts is increased with an increase in skeletal mass for several years until a new steady state is achieved.

- The removal of estrogen replacement results in a rapid decline in bone mass.

- Dietary calcium deficiency increases bone resorption and increases osteopenia. Calcium replacement induces transient increases in bone mass over 1 to 2 years; thereafter bone loss occurs at a rate slower than untreated patients.

- Osteoporosis of trabecular bone increases the risk of vertebral compression fracture, fractures of the distal forearm, and hip fracture.

PATIENT PRESENTATION

- History:

  Postmenopausal or surgical oophrectomy, elderly; housebound; late menarche; family history; thin; Caucasian or Asian; poor diet (low in calcium, high in phosphates); smoking; history of fractures.

- Symptoms:

  Loss of height; back pain; pain at fracture sites.

- Examination:

  Reduced height for weight; thin; "dowager hump;" evidence of fracture.

DIFFERENTIAL DIAGNOSIS

- Senile osteoporosis
- Iatrogenic osteoporosis (drugs)
- Hyperthyroidism
- Multiple myeloma
- Hyperparathyroidism
- Malignancy, metastatic carcinoma
- Osteomalacia
- Pagets disease
- Vitamin D deficiency
- Alcoholism
- Diabetes
- Rheumatoid arthritis

KEYS TO ASSESSMENT

- Identify at-risk patients.
- Yearly heights, lose 0.5 cm/yr.
- Follicle-stimulating hormone (FSH) levels if perimenopausal.
- Laboratory to rule out other causes of osteopenia:
    - Glucose (diabetes)
    - Blood urea nitrogen (BUN) and creatinine (Cr) (renal disease)
    - Calcium, phosphorous (hyperparathyroidism)
    - T_3, T_4 (hyperthyroidism), parathyroid hormone
    - Alkaline phosphatase (high in malignancy, multiple myeloma, Pagets)
    - Serum protein electrophoresis (multiple myeloma)
    - others PRN
- Laboratory to confirm osteoporosis:
    - Urinary type I collagen
    - Cross-linked N-telopeptide (NTX)
- Diagnostics:
    - X-rays
        1) Compression fractures of spine
        2) Osteopenia evident only after 30% of bone lost
        3) Phalangeal bone density (predicts hip fracture risk)

- Dual energy x-ray densitometry

- Quantitative ultrasound

- Photon absorptiometry

- Quantitative computed tomography (CT) scanning

KEYS TO MANAGEMENT

- Prevention

    - Maintain adequate calcium intake:
        1) 1000 mg/day if on estrogens; 1500 mg/day if not.
        2) Begin replacement at age 35.
        3) Calcium carbonate, gluconate, phosphate; calcium citrate is most bioavailable.

    - Reduce phosphorous intake (soft drinks, prepared foods).

    - Supplement vitamin D if not getting adequate sun exposure or dietary insufficiency (50,000 units twice a month).

    - Exercise both pre- and postmenopausally:
        1) Exercise should be begun in youth to maximize bone density.
        2) Weight-bearing and exercise increases total body calcium as well as vertebral bone density in postmenopausal women.

    - Smoking cessation

    - Balanced diet with moderation of protein and fat

    - Avoid caffeine

    - Avoid osteopenic medications (steroids, thyroxine) if possible

    - Oral contraceptives for anorexia or extreme exercise resulting in secondary amenorrhea

- Pharmacologic treatment

    - **Hormone replacement therapy (HRT)**
        1) Estrogen is the most effective therapy available; it results in >20% more bone density than in untreated women.
        2) It prevents bone loss, increases bone density, and decreases fracture risk.
        3) 0.625 mg orally or 0.3 mg combined with calcium replacement is the minimal effective dose.
        4) Oral or transdermal administration is equally effective.
        5) Treatment should be continuous for a minimum of 10 years.
        6) Treatment should be begun soon after menopause to maximize bone density.
        7) The benefits must be weighed against the increase in breast cancer risk (see Chapter 9).

    - **Biphosphonates**
        1) Alendronate reduces hip and spinal fractures by about 50% and increases bone mineral density significantly within 2 to 3 years; other biphosphonates include etidronate and pamidronate.
        2) They work by suppressing bone turnover by blocking osteoclasts.
        3) They are well tolerated with few side effects.

- **Calcitonin**
    1) It can be given SQ or via nasal spray.
    2) It increases bone mass and decreases fracture rate (less than HRT or biphosphonates).
    3) It has GI and skin toxicity.
    4) It has an analgesic effect on bone pain.

- **Estrogen analogues/receptor antagonists**
    1) Tamoxifen, toremifene, droloxifene, raloxifene—used as antiestrogens for breast cancer treatment but act like estrogen for increasing bone density
    2) Risk of endometrial cancer; increase hot flashes

- **Flourides**
    1) Reduces fractures but less so than estrogen
    2) A low dose has tolerable side effects but can cause significant toxicity in some patients.

- Monitoring therapy

    - Follow heights

    - Follow serum calcium and phosphate

    - Obtain careful breast, pelvic, pap, and maturation index yearly if on HRT

Pathophysiology

What is going on in the disease process that influences how the patient presents and how he or she should be managed?

→

Clinical Link

What should you do now that you understand the underlying pathophysiology?

Pathophysiology	Clinical Link
The risk of osteoporosis in postmenopausal women is related to the peak bone density achieved at age 35.	Adequate calcium intake, weight-bearing exercise, and oral contraceptives for secondary amenorrhea in young women can reduce the risk of osteoporosis later in life.
Osteoporosis affects trabecular bone more than cortical bone, so that the vertebrae, femoral necks, ribs, and distal radius are most often significantly involved.	Patients may present first with fractures of the hip, wrist, or rib, or may complain of acute back pain with a history of no or little trauma.
Estrogen limits the activity of osteoclasts such that the balance is shifted to the osteoblastic filling in of bone.	Gonadal insufficiency due to menopause results in increased osteoclast activity and weaker bones; estrogen HRT results in increased bone density and reduced risk of fracture.
Increased calcium in the diet results in decreased bone resorption and decreased osteopenia.	Adequate dietary calcium is an important component of prevention and treatment of osteoporosis.
Many other conditions can cause osteopenia including hyperthyroidism, hyperparathyroidism, malignancies, and many others.	The differential diagnosis of osteopenia requires testing for other potentially treatable conditions. A careful history, physical exam, and laboratory testing are necessary to establish the cause.
HRT with estrogen is the most effective treatment, but is associated with an increased risk for breast cancer.	HRT should be considered, but the benefit must weighed against the increased risk, especially in patients with other risks for breast cancer; some of the new estrogen analogues may provide safer alternatives.

BIBLIOGRAPHY

Abbott, T. A., Lawrence, B. J., & Wallach, S. (1996). Osteoporosis: The need for comprehensive treatment guidelines [review, 106 refs]. *Clinical Therapeutics, 18*(1), 127-149, discussion 126.

Abrahamsen, B., Bendtzen, K., & Beck-Nielsen, H. (1997). Cytokines and T-lymphocyte subsets in healthy post-menopausal women: Estrogen retards bone loss without effecting the release of ID-1 or IL-1ra. *Bone, 20*(3), 251-258.

Albala, C., Yanez, M., Devoto, E., Sostin, C. Zeballos, L., & Santos, J. L. (1996). Obesity as a protective factor for postmenopausal osteoporosis. *International Journal of Obesity and Related Metabolic Disorders, 20*(1), 1027-1032.

Berry, E., Truscott, J. G., Stewart, S. P., & Smith, M. A. (1996). Spatial distribution of femoral bone mineral in dual energy x-ray absorptionmetry images: A possible technique to improve discrimination between normal and osteoporotic patients. *British Journal of Radiology, 69*(824), 743-750.

Bowman, M. A., & Spangler, J. G. (1997). Osteoporosis in women [review, 63 refs]. *Primary Care, Clinics in Office Practice, (1), 27-36.

Carson, D. S. (1996). Menopause and osteoporosis: The role of HRT. *Journal of the American Pharmaceutical Association, NS36*(4), 234-242.

Cooper, G. S., & Sandler, D. P. (1997). Long-term effects of reproductive-age menstrual cycle patterns on peri- and postmenopausal fracture risk. *American Journal of Epidemiology, 145*(9), 804-809.

Cumming, R. G., Cummings, S. R., Nevitt, M. C., Scott, J., Ensrud, K. E., Vogt, T. M., & Fox, K. (1997). Calcium intake and fracture risk: Results from the study of osteoporotic fractures. *American Journal of epidemiology, 145*(1), 926-934.

Dargent-Molina, P., Favier, F., Grandjean, H., Baudoin, C., Schott, A. M., Hausherr, E., Meunier, P. J., & Breart, G. (1996). Fall-related factors and risk of hip fracture: The EPIDOS prospective study [published erratum appears in *Lancet, 348*(9024), 416, 1996 Aug 10]. *Lancet, 348*(9021), 145-149.

Davey, D. A. (1997). Calcium and the prevention and treatment of postmenopausal osteoporosis [editorial]. *South African Medical Journal, 87*(2), 132-133.

Delmas, P. D., Balena, R., Confravreaux, E., Hardouin, C., Hardy, P., & Bremond, A. (1997). Bisphosphonate risedronate prevents bone loss in women with artificial menopause due to chemotherapy of breast cancer: A double-blind, placebo-controlled study. *Journal of Clinical Oncology, 165*(3), 955-962.

Devogelaer, J. P., Broll, H., Correa-Rotter, R., Cumming, D. C., De Deuxchaisnes, C. N., Geusens, P., Hosking, D., Jaeger, P., Kaufman, J. M., Leite, M., Leon, J., Liberman, U., Menkes, C. J., Meunier, P. J., Reid, I., Rodriguez, J., Romanowicz, A., Seeman, E., Vermeulen, A., Hirsch, L. J., Lombardi, A., Plezia, K., Santora, A. C., Yates, A. J., & Yuan, W. (1996). Oral alendronate induces progressive increases in bone mass of the spine, hip, and total body over 3 years in postmenopausal women with osteoporosis. *Bone, 18*(2), 141-150.

Draper, M. W., Flowers, D. E., Huster, W. J., Neild, J. A., Harper, K. D., & Arnaud, C. (1996). A controlled trial of raloxifene (LY 139481) HCI: Impact on bone turnover and serum lipid profile in healthy postmenopausal women. *Journal of Bone and Mineral Research, 11*(6), 835-842.

Eiken, P., Kolthoff, N., & Nielsen, S. P. (1996). Effect of 10 years hormone replacement therapy on bone mineral content in postmenopausal women. *Bone, 19*(5 Suppl), 191S-193S.

Ensrud, K. E., Cauley, J., Lipschutz, R., & Cummings, S. R. (1997). Weight change and fractures in older women. Study of Osteoporotic Fractures research Group. *Archives of Internal Medicine, 157*(8), 857-863.

Eriksen, E. F., Kassem, M., & Langdahl, B. (1996). European and North American experience for HRT for the prevention of osteoporosis [review, 46 refs]. *Bone, 19*(5 Suppl), 179S-183S.

Fogelman, I. (1996). The effects of oestrogen deficiency on the skeleton and its prevention [review, 55 refs]. *British Journal of obstetrics and Gynaecology, 103*(Suppl 140, 5-9.

Fraser, W. D. (1997). Bone preservation and the menopause [review, 20 refs]. *British Journal of Hospital Medicine, 57*(5), 212-214.

Gonnelli, S., Cepollaro, C., Montomoli, M., Gennari, L., Montagnani, A., Plamieri, R., & Gennari, C. (1997). Treatment of post-menopausal osteoporosis with recombinant human growth hormone and salmon calcitonin: A placebo-controlled study. *Clinical Endocrinology, 46*(1), 55-61.

Hodsman, A. B., Fraher, L. J., Watson, P. H., Ostbye, T., Stitt, L. W., Adachi, J. D., Taves, D. H., & Drost, D. (1997). A randomized controlled trial to compare the efficacy of cyclical parathyroid hormone versus cyclical parathyroid hormone and sequential calcitonin to inprove bone mass in postmenopausal women with osteoporosis. *Journal of Clinical Endocrinology and Metabolism, 82*(2), 620-628.

Isenbarger, D. W., & Chapin, B. L. (1997). Osteoporosis. Current pharmacologic options for prevention and treatment [review, 21 refs]. *Postgraduate Medicine, 101*(1), 129-132.

Jeal, W., Barradell, L. B., & McTavish, D. (1997). Alendronate. A review of its pharmacological properties and therapeutic efficacy in postmenopausal osteoporosis [review, 70 refs]. *Drugs, 53*(3), 415-434.

Kanis, J. A. (1996). Estrogens, the menopause, and osteoporosis [review, 26 refs]. *Bone, 19*(5 Suppl), 185S-190S.

Karpf, D. B., Shapiro, D. R., Seeman, E., Ensrud, K. E., Johnson, C. C. J., Adami, S. Harris, S. T., Santora, A. C., Hirsch, L. J., Oppenheimer, L., & Thompson, D. (1997). Prevention of nonvertebral fractures by alendronate. A meta-analysis. Alendronate Osteoporosis Treatment Study Groups. *Journal of the American Medical Association, 277*(14), 1159-1164.

Kirk, J. K., & Spangler, J. G. (1996). Alendronate: A bisphosphonate for treatment of osteoporosis [see comments]. *American Family Physician, 54*(6), 2053-2060.

Koster, J. C, Hackeng, W. H., & Mulder, H. (1996). Diminished effect of etidronate in vitamin D deficient osteopenic postmenopausal women. *European Journal of Clinical Pharmacology, 51*(2) 145-147.

Licata, A. A. (1997). Bisphosphonate therapy][see comments] [review, 70 refs]. *American Journal of the Medical Sciences, 313*(1), 17-22.

Maughan, K. L. (1997). Preventing osteoporotic fractures with alendronate. *Journal of Family Practice, 44*(4), 336.

McClung, M. R. (1996). Current bone mineral density data on bisphosphonates in postmenopausal osteoporosis [review, 35 refs]. *Bone, 19*(5 Suppl), 195S-198S.

Millard, P. S., Rosen, C. J., & Johnson, K. H. (1997). Osteoporotic vertebral fractures in postmenopausal women [review, 26 refs]. *American Family Physician, 55*(4), 1315-1322.

Myers, A. (1997). Osteoporosis and low back pain. *Comprehensive Therapy, 23*(1), 57-59.

Nordin, B. E., Chatterton, B. E., Schultz, C. G., Need, A. G., & Horowitz, M. (1996). Regional bone mineral density interrelatioships in normal and osteoporotic postmenopausal women. *Journal of Bone and Mineral Research, 11*(6), 849-856.

Notelovitz, M. (1997). Estrogen therapy and osteoporosis: Principles and practice [see comments] [review, 121 refs]. *American Journal of the Medical Sciences, 313*(1), 2-12.

Orr-Walker, B., Wattie, D. J., Evans, M. C., & Reid, I. R. (1997). Effects of prolonged bisphosphonate therapy and its discontinuation on bone mineral density in post-menopausal osteoporosis. *Clinical Endocrinology, 46*(1), 87-92.

Pacifici, R. (1996). Estrogen, cytokines, and pathogenesis of postmenopausal osteoporosis [review, 99 refs]. *Journal of Bone and Mineral Research, 11*(8), 1043-1051.

Pak, C. Y., Adams-Huet, B., Sakhaee, K., Bell, N. H., Licata, A., Johnston, C., Rubin, B., Bonnick, S., Piziak, V., Graham, H., Ballard, J., Berger, R., Fears, W., Breslau, N., & Rubin, C. (1996). Comparison of nonrandomized trials with slow-release sodium fluoride with a randomized placebo-controlled trial in postmenopausal obsteoporosis. *Journal of Bone and Mineral Research, 11*(2), 160-168.

Pak, C. Y., Sakhaee, K., Rubin, C. D., & Zerwekh, J. E. (1997). Sustained-release sodium fluoride in the management of established postmenopausal osteoporosis [review, 30 refs]. *American Journal of the Medical Sciences, 313*(1), 23-32.

Pak, C. Y., Zerwekh, J. E., Antich, P. P., Bell, N. H., & Singer, F. R. (1996). Slow-release sodium fluoride in osteoporosis [review, 16 refs]. *Journal of Bone and Mineral Research, 11*(5), 561-564.

Persson, I., Bergkvist, L., Lindgren, C., & Yuen, J. (1997). Hormone replacement therapy and major risk factors for reproductive cancers, osteoporosis, and cardiovascular diseases: Evidence of confounding by exposure characteristics. *Journal of Clinical Epidemiology, 50*(5), 611-618.

Phillips, A. (1997). The Fracture Intervention Trial [letter; comment]. *Lancet, 349*(9050), 505-506.

Preisinger, E., Alacamlioglu, Y., Pils, K., Bosina, E., Metka, M., Schneider, B., & Ernst, E. (1996). Exercise therapy for osteoporosis: Results of a randomised controlled trial. *British Journal of Sports Medicine, 30*(3), 209-212.

Prince, R. L., Dick, I. M., Lemmon, J., & Randell, D. (1997). The pathogenesis of age-related osteoporotic fracture: Effects of dietary calcium deprivation. *Journal of Clinical Endocrinology and Metabolism, 82*(1), 260-264.

Rand, T., Seidl, G., Kainberger, F., Resch, A., Hittmair, K., Schneider, B., Gluer, C. C., & Imhof, H. (1997). Impact of spinal degenerative changes on the evaluation of bone mineral density with dual energy x-ray absorptiometry (DXA). *Calcified Tissue International, 60*(5), 430-433.

Ravn, P., Rix, M., Andreassen, H., Clemmensen, B., Bidstrup, M., & Gunnes, M. (1997). High bone turnover is associated with low bone mass and spinal fracture in postmenopausal women. *Calcified Tissue International, 60*(3), 255-260.

Reginster, J. Y., Deroisy, R. Collette, J., Albert, A., & Zegels, B. (1997). Prediction of bone loss rate in healthy postmenopausal women. *Calcified Tissue International, 60*(3), 261-264.

Riggs, B. L. (1996). Tibolone as an alternative to estrogen for the prevention of postmenopausal osteoporosis in selected postmenopausal women [editorial; comment] [published erratum appears in *Journal of Clinical Endocrinology and Metabolism 82*(1), 181, 1997 Jan]. *Journal of Clinical Endocrinology and Metabolism, 81*(7), 2417-2418.

Silverman, S. L. (1997). Calcitonin [review, 26 refs]. *American Journal of the Medical Sciences, 313*(1), 13-16.

Storm, T., Kollerup, G., Thamsborg, G., Genant, H. K., & Sorensen, O. H. (1996). Five years of clinical experience with intermittent cyclical etidronate for postmenopausal osteoporosis. *Journal of Rheumatology, 23*(9), 1560-1564.

Takada, M., Engelke, K., Hagiwara, S., Grampp, S., Jergas, M., Gluer, C. C., & Genant, H. K. (1997). Assessment of osteoporosis: Comparison of radiographic absorptiometry of the phalanges and dual x-ray absorptiometry of the radius and lumbar spine. *Radiology, 202*(3), 759-764.

Thamsborg, G., Jensen, J. E., Kollerup, G., Hauge, E. M., Melsen, F., & Sorensen, O. H. (1996). Effect of nasal salmon calcitonin on bone remodeling and bone mass in postmenopausal osteoporosis. *Bone, 18*(2), 207-212.

Torgerson, D. J., Donaldson, C., & Reid, D. M. (1996). Bone mineral density measurements: Are they worth while? [see comments]. *Journal of the Royal Society of Medicine, 89*(8), 457-461.

Vandevyver, C., Wylin, T., Cassiman, J. J., Raus, J., & Geusens, P. (1997). Influence of the vitamin D receptor gene alleles on bone mineral density in postmenopausal and osteoporotic women. *Journal of Bone and Mineral Research, 12*(2), 241-247.

Vecht-Hart, C. M., Zwamborn, A. W., Peeters, P. H., & Collette, J. H. (1997). Prediction of peripheral fracture risk by quantitative microdensitometry. *Preventive Medicine, 26*(1), 86-91.

Vedi, S., & Compston, J. E. (1996). The effects of long-term hormone replacement therapy on bone remodeling in postmenopausal women. *Bone, 19*(5), 535-539.

Watts, N. B. (1997). Introduction: Management of osteoporosis, 1997 [comment]. *American Journal of the Medical Sciences, 313*(1), 1.

Yildiz, A. Sahin, I., Gol, K., Taner, Z., Uluturk, A., & Biberoglu, K. (1996). Bone loss rate in the lumbar spine: A comparison between natural and surgically induced menopause. *International Journal of Gynaecology and Obstetrics, 5*592), 153-159.

CASE STUDY[*]

OSTEOPOROSIS

INITIAL HISTORY:
- 66-year-old female
- Back pain for 6 to 8 weeks
- Pain is constant and aggravated by activity
- Ibuprofen provides temporary relief

Question 1.
What is the differential diagnosis at this time?

Question 2.
What additional questions would you like to ask her about her symptoms?

ADDITIONAL HISTORY:
- Patient denies any acute or distant injury to her back.
- She states she has had a slight reduction in height.
- She denies change in weight.
- She denies any unusual bleeding.
- She denies fever or chills.
- She denies heat or cold intolerance or changes in her hair, skin, or nails.

[*] **Leslie Buchanan, RN, MSN, ENP, contributed this case study.**

Question 2.
What would you like to ask her about her past medical history?

PAST MEDICAL HISTORY:
- Patient has a history of mild hypertension for which she takes hydrochlorothiazide.
- She has never taken any other medications long-term.
- She has been postmenopausal since age 48 but does not take hormones at the advice of her nurse practitioner.
- She denies endocrine or renal disease.
- She denies a personal history of breast cancer but has a family history in both her mother and sister.
- Her mammogram last year was negative.

Question 4.
What would you like to ask her about her lifestyle?

LIFESTYLE HISTORY:
- Eats three "meat and potatoes" meals per day
- Gets very little exercise, mostly light housework
- Rarely gets outdoors
- 20 pack/year smoking history
- Drinks an occasional glass of wine
- Drinks 4 to 5 caffeinated beverages per day
- Does not take calcium or vitamin D supplements

PHYSICAL EXAMINATION:
- 66-year-old white female of slight stature, walking with normal gait in no acute distress
- Height = 5' 3.5"; weight = 120 lbs
- T = 37 orally; P = 84 regular; RR = 20 and unlabored; BP = 154/88 sitting

Skin, HEENT
- Dry skin; nails cracking
- No areas of tenderness, slight hair thinning
- Tympanic membranes pearly without bulging or retraction
- Conjunctiva clear, PERRL, funduscopic without lesions
- Clear without drainage or erythema

Neck
- Moderate cervical lordosis
- No bony tenderness
- Full range of motion without pain elicited
- Thyroid nontender without thyromegaly, no masses palpable
- No adenopathy

Chest
- Normal chest excursion, clear to auscultation and percussion
- Cardiac exam with regular rate and rhythm without murmurs or gallops

Abdomen, Neurologic
- Bowel sounds present throughout
- No tenderness; no organomegaly; no masses
- Alert and oriented x 3, recent and remote memory intact
- Cranial nerves intact
- No focal motor deficits; no gross sensory deficits
- DTRs 1+ and symmetrical throughout
- Negative Kernig and Brudzinski signs

Muscoloskeletal
- Tenderness with palpation of the bony prominences of L1 and L2
- Limited flexion and extension of the back
- Lateral bending unlimited and nonpainful
- No dorsal kyphosis (dowager hump)
- No deformity or swelling of joints

Question 5.
What are the pertinent positive and negative findings on physical exam?

Question 6.
What initial diagnostic testing is indicated?

LUMBOSACRAL SPINE X-RAY RESULTS:
- Osteopenia
- Compression fracture of L2

Question 7.
Based on this result, what further diagnostic resting is now indicated?

LABORATORY RESULTS:
- Chemistries including phosphate and calcium, normal
- CBC normal
- Thyroid function tests normal
- Rheumatoid factor negative
- Serum and 24-hour urine alkaline phosphates normal
- Erythrocyte sedimentation rate and serum protein electrophoresis normal
- Dual energy x-ray densitometry consistent with significant osteopenia

Question 8.
Now what is your diagnosis?

Question 9.

What is your treatment plan?

Question 10.

What further care would you recommend?

CHAPTER 24

OSTEOARTHRITIS

DEFINITION

- Osteoarthritis (OA) is defined as a heterogeneous group of conditions that leads to joint symptoms and signs which are associated with defective integrity of articular cartilage in addition to related changes in the underlying bone.

- Primary osteoarthritis is idiopathic.

- Secondary osteoarthritis occurs due to an identifiable risk factor or cause such as joint trauma, anatomic abnormalities, infection, neuropathy, metabolic alterations in cartilage (hemochromatosis), or subchondral bone alteration (acromegaly, Paget disease).

EPIDEMIOLOGY

- OA is the most common form of joint disease in the world.

- It affects approximately 7% of the United States population; it affects 60% to 70% of people over age 65.

- There is an increasing risk with increasing age; prevalence is rising rapidly as the population ages.

- Autosomal dominant hereditary patterns have been identified in certain subgroups of osteoarthritis:

    - Primary generalized OA associated with human lymphocyte antigen (HLA) A1 B8 haplotype

    - Familial chondrocalcinosis (crystal deposition in joints)

    - Chondrodysplasias

- Several genes have been linked to various changes in cartilage components (e.g., mutation on chromosome 12 [COL2A1] linked to abnormal type II collagen).

- The risk factors for primary OA include increasing age, obesity, repetitive joint overuse, immobilization, and increased bone density (less "shock absorption"—see below).

PATHOPHYSIOLOGY

- Cartilage components become disorganized and degraded in OA.

    - Mechanical factors result in the release of enzymes (collagenase and stromelysin) resulting in proteoglycan depletion and type II collagen disordering.

    - There is a loss of the cartilage matrix, especially at the medial cartilage surface.

- Inflammatory cytokines (interleukin-1 [IL-1], prostaglandin E2 [PGE 2], tumor necrosis factor α [TNF α], interleukin-6 [IL-6]) promote joint inflammation and cartilage degradation.

- Chondrocytes become unresponsive to growth factors such as transforming growth factor-β and insulin-like growth factor, and cannot fully compensate for matrix loss.

- An imbalance of cartilage synthesis and degradation develops with abrasions, pitting, and fissuring of the articular surface.

- The articular cartilage becomes overhydrated and swollen.

- Matrix degradation and overhydration lead to a loss in compressive stiffness and elasticity with transmission of greater mechanical stress to the subchondral bone.

- The subchondral trabecular bone is damaged and loses its normal hydraulic "shock absorption;" bone cysts may form from this excess subchondral bone stress.

- Repair mechanisms at the edge of the articular surface (cartilage-bone interface) result in increased synthesis of cartilage and bone forming overgrowths called osteophytes.

- Some patients are found to have various forms of calcium crystals concentrated in the damaged articular cartilage. The pathogenesis of this crystal deposition is unclear but is correlated with a more rapid disease progression in these patients.

- Articular cartilage requires physiologic weight loading and motion to allow adequate penetration of nutrients from the synovial fluid into the cartilage; nonphysiologic loads (either in excess or insufficient) result in poor cartilage nutrition.

- Human joints require maximal mobility while avoiding articular tissue injury. One hypothesis is that there is a "protective muscular reflex" that prevents the joint from exceeding its normal range of excursion; it has been postulated that disordered neuromuscular activity may play a role in the pathogenesis of OA.

- Joint instability is correlated with a high risk of OA. Increasing the strength of the "bridging" muscles across a joint can improve joint stability, decrease joint loading, and reduce mechanical stress. Thus exercise can improve symptoms and joint function, even though there may be little radiologic improvement.

- The pain of OA is believed to be due to three major causes: pain with movement from mechanical factors, pain at rest from synovial inflammation, and night pain from intraosseous hypertension.

PATIENT PRESENTATION

- <u>History</u>:

  Family history of OA; history of joint trauma; weight gain; occupation that includes repetitive movements, especially of the knees (squatting), elbows and back (heavy lifting), and hands (assembly line and mill work).

- <u>Symptoms</u>:

  Nagging pain that has been present for years in one or more joints, and waxes and wanes in intensity according to the weather and exertion; stiffness after prolonged inactivity that "loosens up" with activity (may become permanent in late stages); swelling and deformity, especially of the knees and fingers, with development of "knobby" joints at the distal and proximal interphalangeal joints (DIP and PIP); inability to grip with the hands or comb the hair; restricted walking and fatigue.

- Examination:

  Limping gait; Heberdens nodes (DIP osteophytes) and Bouchard nodes (PIP osteophytes); flexor and lateral deviations of the distal phalanx; decreased range of motion and crepitus with passive motion; swelling, warmth, and tenderness (inflammation) during "flares."

DIFFERENTIAL DIAGNOSIS

- Secondary osteoarthritis
- Rheumatoid arthritis
- Gout
- Systemic lupus erythematosus
- Rheumatic fever
- Septic arthritis

KEYS TO ASSESSMENT

- Carefully assess all joints; assess for deformity, creptitus, and decreasing range of motion.

- Examine the eyes, skin, and organs for evidence of systemic rheumatic disease.

- In a patient with (1) a classic history for OA; (2) a joint exam revealing Heberdens nodes and decreased range of motion without evidence of significant joint deformity or inflammation; and (3) a general physical exam without evidence of systemic disease, consideration should be given for empiric treatment without further diagnostic testing.

- Specific joint involvement is frequently assessed with x-ray (weight bearing for the knee), looking for joint space narrowing, subchondral bone cysts, and sclerosis, and osteophytes.

- Serum markers for evidence of articular cartilage destruction are being used experimentally as a means of detecting OA before there is radiologic evidence. These include keratin sulfate and cartilage oligomeric matrix protein; these are not yet indicated for routine evaluation.

- Technetium 99 m scintigraphy and magnetic resonance imaging (MRI) are sensitive indicators of OA, but they contribute little to the general clinical evaluation of OA.

- In a patient with severe disease or suspicious aspects to the history and physical, further diagnostic testing is indicated:

  - Chemistries including blood urea nitrogen (BUN) and creatinine (Cr)

  - Erythrocyte sedimentation rate (ESR) and rheumatoid factors

  - Other specific tests for rheumatologic disease such as anti-deoxyribonucleic acid (anti-DNA), HLA-B27, and uric acid

  - Arthrocentesis with chemistries, cell counts, cultures and stain, and rheumatoid factor

KEYS TO MANAGEMENT

- There is increasing evidence that exercise is beneficial in the management of OA. Recent short-term studies suggest that exercise improves symptoms and quality of life in patients with mild to moderate OA.

- Physical therapy including passive range of motion and water exercises can be helpful.

- Diet for weight loss if appropriate.

- Increased intake of vitamin C has been correlated with decreased knee OA progression and pain.

- Use of capsaicin as a topical analgesic (decreases neuronal substance P, a neurotransmitter implicated in arthritis pain).

- Iontophoresis to deliver topical steroids deeply into the tissues has been used for years, but there is little evidence that tissue penetration is greater than with passive diffusion alone.

- Diathermy with ultrasound can facilitate tendon extensibility and muscle relaxation with decreased pain.

- Acetaminophen has been shown in many studies to be as effective in reducing pain with OA as nonsteroidal antiinflammatory drugs (NSAIDs).

- Although OA is now known to have an inflammatory component, the use of long-term NSAIDs remains controversial.

    - The risk of side effects (upper gastrointestinal [GI] ulceration and bleeding) are of particular risk in the elderly.

    - NSAIDs have not been shown to slow disease progression.

    - There is evidence that NSAIDs may actually inhibit cartilage synthesis and repair; they have even been associated with acceleration of disease progression.

    - Some patients will have greater analgesia with NSAIDs than acetaminophen; usually they will respond at low doses thus reducing the risk of side effects.

    - New nonsteroidals such as meloxicam are being studied that have a more selective ability to block inflammatory cytokine synthesis (COX-2 > COX-1), thus maximizing the antiinflammatory and analgesic effects while minimizing GI side effects.

- Oral tetracycline derivatives have been found to be chondroprotective and are undergoing extensive investigation.

- Tidal irrigation of large joints such as the knee improves symptoms dramatically in selected patients.

- Intraarticular injection of steroids during acute inflammatory "flares" can provide rapid symptom relief; frequency of injections greater than 3 to 4 times per year may be associated with decreased cartilage repair.

- Chondroprotective drugs that are undergoing extensive research include glucosamine polysulfate, chondroitin sulfate, sodium pentosan polysulfate, and glycosaminoglycan peptide complex orally, and intraarticular hyaluronic acid injection.

- Autologous chondrocyte implantation has been used in some patients with severe disease; early studies are encouraging.

- Orthopedic surgery, including joint debridement, abrasion arthroplasty, chondral shaving, and joint replacement, can successfully be used with selected patients.

Pathophysiology →

What is going on in the disease process that influences how the patient presents and how he or she should be managed?

Clinical Link

What should you do now that you understand the underlying pathophysiology?

Mechanical factors contribute to enzyme release that can cause articular cartilage degradation, and joint instability is correlated with a high risk of OA.	Overuse and trauma to joints are risk factors for OA.
The articular cartilage requires some joint "loading" to receive maximal supply of synovial fluid nutrients; exercise that improves muscle strength can improve joint function.	Exercise is beneficial to the health and healing of the articular cartilage.
Inflammatory cytokines have been found to play a significant role in the pathophysiology of OA, but their inhibition with antiinflammatory drugs has not resulted in an improvement in disease progression.	OA is no longer considered a purely noninflammatory joint disease, but the role of antiinflammatory medications in the long-term management of OA is highly controversial.
Unresponsiveness of chondrocytes to growth factors and the loss of "chondroprotection" have been implicated in the pathogenesis of OA.	New treatments for OA include chondroprotective drugs that may prevent cartilage degradation and improve healing.
Bone is laid down at the perimeter of the articular cartilage, forming growth of bone called osteophytes.	OA is characterized by bony protuberances in the joints, especially at the distal interphalangeal joints (Heberdens nodes) and at the vertebral disc spaces that can limit range of motion.

BIBLIOGRAPHY

Balint, G., & Szebenyi, B. (1996). Diagnosis of osteoarthritis. Guidelines and current pitfalls [review, 113 refs]. *Drugs, 52*(Suppl 3), 1-13.

Barner, A. (1996). Review of clinical trials and benefit/risk ratio of meloxicam [review, 15 refs]. *Scandinavian Journal of Rheumatology,* (Suppl 102), 29-37.

Bellamy, N., Kirwan, J., Boers, M., Brooks, P., Strand, V., Tugwell, P., Altman, R., Brandt, K., Dougados, M., & Lequesne, M. (1997). Recommendations for a core set of outcome measures for future phase III clinical trials in knee, hip, and hand osteoarthritis. Consensus development at OMERACT III [review, 6 refs]. *Journal of Rheumatology, 24*(4), 799-802.

Blackburn, W. D. (1996). Management of osteoarthritis and rheumatoid arthritis: prospects and possibilities [review, 47 refs]. *American Journal of Medicine, 100*(2A), 24S-30S.

Blackburn, W. D. J., Chivers, S., & Bernreuter, W. (1996). Cartilage imaging in osteoarthritis [review, 65 refs]. *Seminars in Arthritis and Rheumatism, 25*(4), 273-281.

Block, J. A., & Schnitzer, T. J. (1997). Therapeutic approaches to osteoarthritis [review, 6 refs]. *Hospital Practice, 32*(Office Edition), 159-164.

Cicuttini, F. M., & Spector, T. D. (1996). Genetics of osteoarthritis [review, 46 refs]. *Annals of the Rheumatic Diseases, 55*(9), 665-667.

Higgs, P. E., & Young, V. L. (1996). Cumulative trauma disorders [review, 34 refs]. *Clinics in Plastic Surgery, 23*(3), 421-433.

Hochberg, M. C. (1996). Development and progression of osteoarthritis [editorial] [review, 23 refs]. *Journal of Rheumatology, 23*(9), 1497-1499.

Hochberg, M. C. (1996). Prognosis of osteoarthritis [review, 37 refs]. *Annals of the Rheumatic Diseases, 55*(9), 685-688.

Hodler, J., & Resnick, D. (1996). Current status of imaging of articular cartilage [review, 41 refs]. *Skeletal Radiology, 25*(8), 703-709.

Huch, K., Kuettner, K. E., & Dieppe, P. (1997). Osteoarthritis in ankle and knee joints [review, 67 refs]. *Seminars in Arthritis and Rheumatism, 26*(4), 667-674.

Kang, R., Ghivizzani, S. C., Herndon, J. H., Robbins, P. D., & Evans, C. H. (1997). Gene therapy for arthritis: principles and clinical practice [review, 37 refs]. *Biochemical Society Transactions, 25*(2), 533-537.

Katz, W. A. (1996). Pharmacology and clinical experience with tramadol in osteoarthritis [review, 49 refs]. *Drugs, 52*(Suppl 3), 39-47.

Kraus, V. B. (1997). Pathogenesis and treatment of osteoarthritis [review, 170 refs]. *Medical Clinics of North America, 81*(1), 85-112.

Lahr, D. D. (1996). Does running exercise cause osteoarthritis? [review, 18 refs]. *Maryland Medical Journal, 45*(8), 641-644.

Lane, N. E. (1996). Physical activity at leisure and risk of osteoarthritis [review, 23 refs]. *Annals of the Rheumatic Diseases, 55*(9), 682-684.

Lane, N. E. (1997). Pain management in osteoarthritis: the role of COX-2 inhibitors [review, 30 refs]. *Journal of Rheumatology, 24*(Suppl 49), 20-24.

March, L. M., & Brooks, P. M. (1996). Clinical trials in osteoarthritis [editorial] [review, 27 refs]. *Annals of the Rheumatic Diseases, 55*(8), 491-493.

Marshall, K. W. (1996). The case for a simple method of grading osteoarthritis severity at arthroscopy [editorial; comment] [review, 24 refs]. *Journal of Rheumatology, 23*(4), 582-585.

Messner, K., & Gillquist, J. (1996). Cartilage repair. A critical review [see comments] [review, 58 refs]. *Acta Orthopaedica Scandinavica, 67*(5), 523-529.

Nevitt, M. C., & Felson, D. T. (1996). Sex hormones and the risk of osteoarthritis in women: epidemiological evidence [review, 47 refs]. *Annals of the Rheumatic Diseases, 55*(9), 673-676.

Noble, S., & Balfour, J. A. (1996). Meloxicam [review, 43 refs]. *Drugs, 51*(3), 424-430, discussion 431-432.

Perrot, S., & Menkes, C. J. (1996). Nonpharmacological approaches to pain in osteoarthritis. Available options [review, 97 refs]. *Drugs, 52*(Suppl 3), 21-26.

Preidler, K. W., Brossmann, J., & Resnick, D. (1996). Osteoarthritis [review, 73 refs]. *Seminars in Roentgenology, 31*(3), 208-219.

Preidler, K. W., & Resnick, D. (1996). Imaging of osteoarthritis [review, 63 refs]. *Radiologic Clinics of North America, 34*(2), 259-271.

Rothschild, B. M. (1996). Cartilage as a target organ in arthritis: new approaches [review, 18 refs]. *Comprehensive Therapy, 22*(11), 727-730.

Ryan, M. E., Greenwald, R. A., & Golub, L. M. (1996). Potential of tetracyclines to modify cartilage breakdown in osteoarthritis [see comments] [review, 76 refs]. *Current Opinion in Rheumatology, 8*(3), 238-247.

Sun, Y., Gunther, K. P., & Brenner, H. (1997). Reliability of radiographic grading of osteoarthritis of the hip and knee [review, 38 refs]. *Scandinavian Journal of Rheumatology, 26*(3), 155-165.

Towheed, T. E., & Hochberg, M. C. (1997). A systematic review of randomized controlled trials of pharmacological therapy in osteoarthritis of the knee, with an emphasis on trial methodology [review, 103 refs]. *Seminars in Arthritis and Rheumatism, 26*(5), 755-770.

Westacott, C. I., & Sharif, M. (1996). Cytokines in osteoarthritis: mediators or markers of joint destruction? [review, 140 refs]. *Seminars in Arthritis & Rheumatism, 25*(4), 254-272.

Williams, M. H. (1996). Challenges for clinical decision making in the management of osteoarthritis of the knee [editorial; comment] [review, 63 refs]. *Journal of Rheumatology, 23*(4), 586-589.

Wollheim, F. A. (1996). Current pharmacological treatment of osteoarthritis [review, 97 refs]. *Drugs, 52*(Suppl 3), 27-38.

CASE STUDY

OSTEOARTHRITIS

INITIAL HISTORY:
- 74-year-old woman complaining of a several-year history of aching in her knees, right greater than left, that is worse when it rains
- Now she is having difficulty going up the stairs in her home.
- She has also had low back pain for many years.
- Suffered a broken right hip 3 years ago when she fell on an icy sidewalk

Question 1.
What questions would you like to ask this patient about her symptoms?

ADDITIONAL HISTORY:
- Her knees started to get significantly more painful after she gained 15 pounds over the past 6 months.
- She denies any swollen, red, hot, or deformed joints.
- She played field hockey in college and had a right knee injury at that time, but never needed surgery.
- Her joints are the most stiff after she has been sitting or lying still, they "loosen up" with activity.
- Her back pain doesn't seem to be getting any worse, and her hip seems to have healed well.
- She denies any numbness, weakness, or shooting pains in her legs.
- She takes ibuprofen 400 mg QID with some relief, but it gives her indigestion.

Question 2.
What would you like to ask this patient about her medical history?

YET MORE HISTORY:
- She denies ever having been told she has arthritis.
- She has been worried about osteoporosis, but has never been diagnosed as having it.
- She has had mild hypertension for many years and was once hospitalized for diverticulitis.
- She denies cardiac, lung, or renal diseases; she has never had blood in her stool or an ulcer.
- She had a hysterectomy without oophrectomy 20 years ago; she has never taken hormones.
- She is taking no prescribed medications and has no allergies.

Question 3.
Are there any important things to ask her about her lifestyle and social history?

LIFESTYLE AND SOCIAL HISTORY:
- She exercises regularly in the pool; but can no longer walk daily as she has in the past.
- She has a well-balanced diet, but it is high in prepared foods and soft drinks and low in calcium.
- She does not smoke and drinks 1 to 2 mixed drinks each evening.
- She lives with her 80-year-old sister in a 2-story home on the outskirts of town.

Question 4.
Based on the history alone, what is the differential diagnosis of this patient's musculoskeletal complaints?

PHYSICAL EXAMINATION:
- Alert, obese white female in no distress
- T = 37 orally; P = 70 and regular; RR = 12 and unlabored; BP = 155/88 right arm, sitting

HEENT, Skin, Neck
- PERRL, fundi without vascular changes, pharynx clear
- Skin without rashes or ecchymoses
- No thyromegaly, adenopathy, or bruits

Lungs, Cardiac
- Good chest excursion; lungs clear to auscultation and percussion
- RRR without murmurs or gallops

Abdomen, Neurological

- Abdomen without tenderness or organomegaly; stool heme negative
- Cranial nerves intact; sensory exam normal and symmetrical
- Strength 5/5 in both upper extremities; 4/5 in lower extremities
- Gait slow but without specific deficits

Musculoskeletal

- Full passive and active range of motion at shoulders and elbows
- Decreased range of motion, and Bouchards and Heberdens nodes in bilateral hand exam
- Back with decreased flexion and extension with mild scoliosis
- Both knees enlarged with decreased range of motion and crepitus, right greater than left
- Right hip with decreased external and internal rotation but without pain
- No joint heat, tenderness, or erythema

Question 5.

What are the pertinent positives and negatives in this patient's exam?

Question 6.

What laboratory studies are indicated now?

LABORATORY RESULTS:
- Chemistries including BUN, Cr, calcium, and phosphate normal
- CBC including HCT normal
- Thyroid functions normal
- X-ray of right knee reveals joint space narrowing, subchondral sclerosis, and bone cysts; no radiographic evidence of osteoporosis
- X-ray of lumbosacral spine reveals disc space narrowing and osteophyte formation especially at L3-L4 and L4-L5 without evidence of compression fracture

Question 7.
What is the diagnosis?

Question 8.
How should this patient be managed?

CHAPTER 25

ALTERATIONS DURING MENOPAUSE

DEFINITION

- Menopause is defined by the World Health Organization as the permanent cessation of menstruation resulting from the loss of ovarian follicular activity. After 1 year of amenorrhea, the final menstrual period is retrospectively designated as the time of menopause.

- Postmenopause is defined as commencing from the time of the final menstrual period.

- Perimenopause (climacteric) or menopause transition is defined as the physiologic antecedents associated with the transition from premenopausal to postmenopausal follicular function and comprises the period of time (2 to 8 years) preceding the menopause and one year following the final menses. (Thus the last year of the perimenopause coincides with the first year of the postmenopause.)

EPIDEMIOLOGY

- Women in the United States can now expect to spend ⅓ of their lives postmenopausal.

- The average age of menopause is between 48 and 52 years (age 51 is most often quoted) but anytime between age 40 and 60 is normal.

- The factors associated with early menopause include smoking (average 1 to 2 years younger), menstrual cycles shorter than 26 days, gynecologic surgery (without oophorectomy), and cancer chemotherapy or radiotherapy (ovarian failure in 40% to 85% especially if age over 40 during treatment).

- The factors associated with late menopause are controversial but may include early menarche and high parity.

- Although this is a natural process of aging, 90% of women are symptomatic, and there are clear health implications.

PATHOPHYSIOLOGY

- Early perimenopause

  - There are fewer oocytes by the time of the perimenopause (ovary contains 380,000 oocytes at menarche, but there is significant oocyte atresia and one is used per cycle).

  - The cycle length is slightly shortened because of a shortened follicular phase (first clinical indication of the perimenopause).

- Follicle stimulating hormone (FSH) levels begin to rise (first laboratory indication of the perimenopause).
- Ovarian gonadotropin receptors diminish.

- Middle menopause

  - There are changes in the menstrual pattern with unpredictable variations in cycle length. Women often experience long intermenstrual intervals interspersed with short cycles.
  - The unpredicted variations are probably due to erratic maturation of the remaining ovarian follicles with some ovulatory cycles (estrogen rise followed by leutinizing hormone [LH] and progesterone secretion) mixed with other cycles that are anovulatory (no LH and progesterone surge).
  - Follicle stimulating hormone (FSH) levels rise significantly (>25 mIU/mL).
  - Beginning symptoms include hot flashes, breast tenderness, and dysfunctional uterine bleeding.

- Late perimenopause and postmenopause

  - There is no ovulation; estradiol levels fall.
  - Ovarian stroma continues to produce androgens (androstenedione and testosterone).
  - Androstenedione is converted to estrone and estradiol in peripheral fat cells so that there is some protective estrogen effect until late in life, especially in obese women.
  - A small amount of progesterone is made by the adrenal gland.

PATIENT PRESENTATION

- History:

  Woman in her late 40s or early 50s; menstrual cycle changes with shortened cycles followed by erratic cycles; smoking; chemotherapy; surgery; hormone use.

- Symptoms:

  - Perimenopausal symptomatology involves three interacting factors:
    1) Loss of estrogen
    2) Sociologic changes in aging
    3) Psychologic changes in aging

  - Perimenopausal symptomatology:
    1) Hot flashes/perspiration
    2) Atrophic vaginitis/vaginal discharge/dyspareunia
    3) Uterovaginal prolapse/urethritis/stress incontinence
    4) Decreased cognitive ability/memory loss
    5) Fatigue/insomnia/anxiety/mood lability
    6) Decreased muscle strength
    7) Osteoporosis/fractures
    8) Alopecia/hirsutism
    9) Skin dryness/pruritus/wrinkles

  - Hot flash (vasomotor instability)
    1) It is a specific thermoregulatory disorder triggered by a neuroendocrine imbalance from the hypothalamus that is believed to be initiated by estrogen deficiency.

2) Prevalence is 50% to 85% in perimenopausal women in the United States; it declines as the time since the last menstrual period increases.

3) It is characterized by low level surges in LH occurring every hour; LH centers in the hypothalamus are near areas that regulate body temperature.

4) 70% of these LH surges result in an increase in skin temperature of up to 4°C with associated symptoms.

5) An increased frequency of symptomatic episodes has been associated with stress. It may be mediated in part by the lack of estrogen regulation of catecholamines; exercise appears to help this aspect.

6) Peripheral vasodilation is followed by vasoconstriction and shiver.

7) There are episodes of flushing of the skin, perspiration, palpitations, nausea, and dizziness.

8) It may disrupt sleep cycles.

9) The presence of hot flashes may be associated with an increased risk for osteoporosis and other metabolic abnormalities, such as hyperglycemia, but this is controversial.

- <u>Examination</u>:

  - Dry skin, alopecia; hirsutism; loss of height; vaginal dryness and discharge; uterine prolapse.

KEYS TO ASSESSMENT

- If patient is younger than 40 years of age, evaluate for possible causes of premature menopause (gynecologic surgery especially with oophrectomy, chemotherapy, congenital abnormalities [Turners syndrome]).

- Obtain a careful menstrual history including menarche, premenopause, perimenopause, and postmenopausal bleeding.

- Carefully review symptoms; ask about sleep, fatigue, and mood.

- Assess for medical contraindications for hormone replacement (breast or endometrial cancer, active thrombotic disease, undiagnosed uterine bleeding, hepatic failure).

- Perform a careful physical exam with special attention to the cardiovascular and gynecologic exams.

- Possible laboratory evaluation for osteoporosis (see Chapter 23).

- Measure serum FSH levels.

- Assess the patient's symptoms and risk for cardiovascular disease and osteoporosis.

- Assess the patient's understanding and perceptions of hormone replacement therapy.

KEYS TO MANAGEMENT

- Nonpharmacologic

  - Exercise has been shown to result in improvement in hot flashes, mood, muscle strength, bone mineral density, and overall quality of life, while decreasing postmenopausal cardiac risk.

  - Smoking cessation can result in improved estrogen effects and decreased cardiovascular risk.

  - Help the patient identify and avoid stimuli that trigger vasomotor flashes including hot weather, alcohol, caffeine, and hot spicy foods; layered clothing may help with temperature control.

- Modify diet to include soy; vitamins B, C, and E; and milk (contains calcium and L-tryptophan to promote sleep).

- Educate the patient about using vaginal lubricants.

- Create a safe and caring environment for patients so that open discussion can occur about symptoms, aging, and relationship concerns—reassurance that all women experience some difficulties in making the transition to older life can be very helpful.

- Hormone replacement therapy (HRT)

  - Risks and benefits of HRT have been extensively studied, and there remains some controversy over several issues.

  - Risks:
    1) A possible risk for breast cancer (see Chapter 9).
    2) A definite risk for endometrial cancer if HRT is given without adequate progesterone ("unopposed estrogen") in patients who have not undergone hysterectomy.
    3) HRT increases risk of thromboembolic disease.
    4) It may increase migraines.
    5) It may worsen hepatic failure.

  - Benefits of HRT are numerous:
    1) Prevention and treatment of osteoporosis (see Chapter 23)
    2) Improve cardiovascular risk
       - Improved lipid profile (decreases low density lipoprotein [LDL] and lipoprotein [a] [Lp(a)] and increases high density lipoprotein [HDL])
       - Reduced risk of atherosclerosis (decreases LDL oxidation and its incorporation into vessel walls and may promote endothelial repair)
       - Decreased risk of myocardial infarction (MI) (by as much as 50%) (improves red blood cell [RBC] deformability; decreases fibrinogen; increases coronary vasodilation)
    3) Reduce clinically unsuspected cerebral ischemic events
    4) Reduce blood pressure (improves arterial compliance)
    5) Improve carbohydrate metabolism (improves insulin sensitivity and diabetic control)
    6) Reduce risk of Alzheimer's disease (by as much as 60%)
    7) Improve cognitive function and memory
    8) Improve self-image and mood
    9) Increase muscle strength
    10) Reduce hot flashes
    11) Improve sleep
    12) Prevent and treat urogenital atrophy (vaginitis, urethritis, uterine prolapse)
    13) Reduce wrinkles

  - Decisions about HRT should be collaborative with the patient and should be made after careful patient education. A discussion of the risks versus the benefits in that individual should be discussed.

  - The type of hormone replacement and the mode of administration should be tailored to the individual patient.
    1) Oral estrogen comes as conjugated (Premarin), esterified (Ogen) or micronized (Estrace).
    2) Transdermal estrogen is also effective; it may cause localized bruising.

3) Estrogen should be given daily. The common dose of Premarin is 0.625 mg/day; new studies suggest that 0.3 mg/day results in positive bone and lipid changes without inducing endometrial hyperplasia (more study is needed).

4) Progesterone should be given to all women who receive estrogen and still have a uterus. Controversy continues, but recent evidence refutes previous studies that suggested that progesterone may antagonize some of the cardiac benefits of HRT.
   - Progesterone can be given daily—results in up to a year of unpredictable vaginal spotting but complete amenorrhea occurs in 90% of women at 12 months.
   - Progesterone can be given monthly—results in predictable monthly withdrawal bleeding.
   - If given every 3 months, it results in predictable heavy bleeding every 3 months.

5) The duration of HRT remains highly controversial. Bone mineralization will reverse rapidly with cessation of estrogen, and cardiovascular risk also rises; however the risk of breast cancer is greatest in those taking estrogens for 10 years or more.

- Nonestrogen pharmacologic treatment

  - Progestins alone can help reduce hot flashes, but they are associated with dysfunctional uterine bleeding, mood changes, worsening of vaginal atrophy, and adverse serum lipid changes.

  - Androgens are used with estrogen in some women to increase libido, decrease breast tenderness, and decrease migraines; there is no approved indication for androgens alone.

  - Phytoestrogens are estrogen-like compounds created by the intestinal bacterial conversion of isoflavonoids (found in soybean products) and ligands (found in cereals, seeds, and nuts); they may have an antiestrogenic (and possibly anticancer) effect on breast tissue while reducing hot flashes. Ginseng also contains some plant estrogens with similar effects.

  - Selective estrogen receptor modulators (SERMs)
    1) SERMs are synthetic estrogen agonist/antagonists with differing effects on estrogen receptors in breast, bone, liver, hypothalamus, urogenitalia, endometrium, and other organs.
    2) All are antiestrogenic in the breast.
    3) Tibolone prevents bone loss, relieves vaginal dryness, and causes endometrial atrophy; negative effects include a reduction in HDL.
    4) Tamoxifen analogs such as tormeifene, droloxifene, and raloxifene reduce bone loss and may be useful in the treatment of osteoporosis, but these drugs increase hot flashes. Most cause a decrease in LDL and have variable effects on HDL; some prevent endometrial hyperplasia and others cause it.

  - A variety of other drugs have been used for vasomotor symptoms with variable effectiveness and considerable side effects including clonidine, methyldopa, veralipride, bellergal, propranolol, and naloxone.

Pathophysiology   →   ## Clinical Link

What is going on in the disease process that influences how the patient presents and how he or she should be managed?

What should you do now that you understand the underlying pathophysiology?

Perimenopause is characterized by fewer oocytes with decreased follicular estradiol production.	Premenopausal causes of increased oocyte loss (e.g., chemotherapy) can result in early onset menopause.
Decreased estradiol levels, increased FSH, erratic ovulation, and decreased ovarian gonadotropin receptors are associated with perimenopoause.	The perimenopausal period can be diagnosed by increasing FSH levels and changes in the menstrual cycle such as shortened intermenstrual periods.
Estrogen is important to maintaining normal functioning of the skin, neurons, blood vessels, bones, muscles, and the urogenital epithelium.	Perimenopausal estrogen deficiency is characterized by thin, dry skin, decreased cognitive ability, increased cardiovascular risk, osteoporosis, decreased muscle strength, and atrophic vaginitis.
In the last perimenopause, LH levels demonstrate low-level frequent, episodic surges associated with hypothalamic-induced changes in body temperature. These LH surges are inhibited by exogenous estrogen replacement.	Vasomotor instability (hot flashes) occurs frequently in perimenopausal women and is associated with a feeling of heat and sweating that can be effectively treated with HRT.
Hot flashes cause sleep cycle disturbance.	HRT improves sleep.
Estrogen decreases LDL and Lp(a), increases HDL, improves vascular compliance and dilation, decreases fibrinogen, and decreases LDL oxidation and its incorporation into the vessel.	HRT reduces cardiovascular risk by as much as 50%.

Pathophysiology   →   **Clinical Link**

Pathophysiology	Clinical Link
Estrogen causes a possible increase in breast cancer risk, a definite increase in endometrial hyperplasia and endometrial cancer risk, and an increase in the risk of thromboembolism.	Patients should be well-educated about their individual risk-benefit profile for HRT, and treatment discussions should be made collaboratively with the patient and tailored to her individual needs.
New estrogen agonists/antagonisis have antiestrogen effects in the breast, but they have variable effects on estrogen receptors in bone, heart, liver, and endometrium.	New options for HRT may reduce the risk of breast cancer but must be selected based on their effects on hot flashes, osteoporosis, heart disease, and endometrium.

BIBLIOGRAPHY

Abernathy, K. (1997). Hormone replacement therapy [review, 18 refs]. *Professional Nurse, 12*(10), 717-719.

Abernethy, K. (1997). The menopause and hormone replacement therapy [review, 24 refs]. *Nursing Standard, 11*(31), 49-53, quiz 55-56.

Akahoshi, M., Soda, M., Nakashima, E., Shimaoka, K., Seto, S., & Yano, K. (1996). Effects of menopause on trends of serum cholesterol, blood pressure, and body mass index. *Circulation, 94*(1), 61-66.

Andersson, B., Mattsson, L. A., Hahn, L., Marin, P., Lapidus, L., Holm, G., Bengtsson, B. A., & Bjorntorp, P. (1997). Estrogen replacement therapy decreases hyperandrogenicity and improves glucose homeostasis and plasma lipids in postmenopausal women with noninsulin-dependent diabetes mellitus. *Journal of Clinical Endocrinology and Metabolism, 82*(2), 638-643.

Armstrong, A. L., Oborne, J., Coupland, C. A., Macpherson, M. B., Bassey, E. J., & Wallace, W. A. (1996). Effects of hormone replacement therapy on muscle performance and balance in post-menopausal women. *Clinical Science, 91*(6), 685-690.

Arpels, J. C. (1996). The female brain hypoestrogenic continuum from the premenstrual syndrome to menopause. A hypothesis and review of supporting data, [review, 87 refs]. *Journal of Reproductive Medicine, 41*(9), 633-639.

Bastian, L. A., Couchman, G. M., Rimer, B. K., McBride, C. M., Feaganes, J. R., & Siegler, I. C. (1997). Perceptions of menopausal stage and patterns of hormone replacement therapy use. *Journal of Womens Health, 6*(4), 467-475.

Beresford, S. A., Weiss, N. S., Voigt, L. F., & McKnight, B. (1997). Risk of endometrial cancer in relation to use of estrogen combined with cyclic progestagen therapy in postmenopausal women. *Lancet, 349*(9050), 458-461.

Bergkvist, L., & Persson, I. (1996). Hormone replacement therapy and breast cancer. A review of current knowledge [review, 79 refs]. *Drug Safety, 15*(5), 360-370.

Binder, E. F., Birge, S. J., & Kohrt, W. M. (1996). Effects of endurance exercise and hormone replacement therapy on serum lipids in older women [see comments]. *Journal of the American Geriatrics Society, 44*(3), 231-236.

Blumberg, G., Kaplan, B., Rabinerson, D., Goldman, G. A., Kitai, E., & Neri, A. (1996). Women's attitudes towards menopause and hormone replacement therapy. *International Journal of Gynaecology & Obstetrics, 54*(3), 271-277.

Brooks, E. M., Morgan, A. L., Pierzga, J. M., Wladkowski, S. L., O'Gorman, J. T., Derr, J. A., & Kenney, W. L. (1997). Chronic hormone replacement therapy alters thermoregulatory and vasomotor function in postmenopausal women. *Journal of Applied Physiology, 83*(2), 477-484.

Callens, A., Vaillant, L., Lecomte, P., Berson, M., Gall, Y., & Lorette, G. (1996). Does hormonal skin aging exist? A study of the influence of different hormone therapy regimens on the skin of postmenopausal women using non-invasive measurement techniques [see comments]. *Dermatology, 193*(4), 289-294.

Clemente, C., Caruso, M. G., Berloco, P., Buonsante, A., Giannandrea, B., & Di, L. A. (1996). alpha-Tocopherol and beta-carotene serum levels in post-menopausal women treated with transdermal estradiol and oral medroxyprogesterone acetate. *Hormone and Metabolic Research, 28*(10), 558-561.

Connell, E. B. (1997). Transdermal estrogen therapy. *Postgraduate Medicine, 101*(6), 115-116.

Crandall, S. G. (1997). Menopause made easier. *RN, 60*(7), 46-50, quiz 51.

Davis, S. R., & Burger, H. G. (1996). Clinical review 82: Androgens and the postmenopausal woman, [review, 59 refs]. *Journal of Clinical Endocrinology & Metabolism, 81*(8), 2759-2763.

Disaia, P. J. (1997). Estrogen replacement therapy for the breast cancer survivor: a reappraisal [editorial] [review, 35 refs]. *Journal of Surgical Oncology, 64*(3), 175-180.

Doren, M., & Schneider, H. P. (1996). The impact of different HRT regimens on compliance [review, 49 refs]. *International Journal of Fertility and Menopausal Studies, 41*(1), 29-39.

Douketis, J. D., Ginsberg, J. S., Holbrook, A., Crowther, M., Duku, E. K., & Burrows, R. F. (1997). A reevaluation of the risk for venous thromboembolism with the use of oral contraceptives and hormone replacement therapy [review, 95 refs]. *Archives of Internal Medicine, 157*(14), 1522-1530.

Folsom, A. R., McGovern, P. G., Nabulsi, A. A., Shahar, E., Kahn, E. S., Winkhart, S. P., & White, A. D. (1996). Changes in plasma lipids and lipoproteins associated with starting or stopping postmenopausal hormone replacement therapy. Atherosclerosis Risk in Communities Study. *American Heart Journal, 132*(5), 952-958.

Freedman, R. R., & Woodward, S. (1996). Core body temperature during menopausal hot flashes. *Fertility and Sterility, 65*(6), 1141-1144.

Gelfand, M. M., & Wiita, B. (1997). Androgen and estrogen-androgen hormone replacement therapy: a review of the safety literature, 1941 to 1996 [review, 107 refs]. *Clinical Therapeutics, 19*(3), 383-404, discussion 367-368.

Gibaldi, M. (1996). Hormone replacement therapy: Estrogen after menopause. *Pharmacotherapy, 16*(3), 366-375.

Graziottin, A. (1996). HRT: the woman's perspective. *International Journal of Gynaecology and Obstetrics, 52*(Suppl 1), S11-S6.

Greendale, G. A., & Sowers, M. (1997). The menopause transition [review, 121 refs]. *Endocrinology and Metabolism Clinics of North America, 26*(2), 261-277.

Griesmacher, A., Peichl, P., Pointinger, P., Mateau, R., Broll, H., Hartl, W., & Gruber, W. (1997). Biochemical markers in menopausal women. *Scandinavian Journal of Clinical & Laboratory Investigation, 227*(Suppl), 64-72.

Grodstein, F., Stampfer, M. J., Manson, J. E., Colditz, G. A., Willett, W. C., Rosner, B., Speizer, F. E., & Hennekens, C. H. (1996). Postmenopausal estrogen and progestin use and the risk of cardiovascular disease [see comments] [published erratum appears in *New England Journal of Medicine,* 1996 Oct 31, 335(18), 1406]. *New England Journal of Medicine, 335*(7), 453-461.

Haj-Ahmad, J. A. (1996). Menopause update: change is good [review, 6 refs]. *Journal of Practical Nursing, 46*(1), 9-12.

Hammond, C. B. (1997). Management of menopause [review, 38 refs]. *American Family Physician, 55*(5), 1667-1674.

Hampson, S. E., & Hibbard, J. H. (1996). Cross-talk about the menopause: Enhancing provider-patient interactions about the menopause and hormone therapy [review, 44 refs]. *Patient Education and Counseling, 27*(2), 177-184.

Handa, V. L., Landerman, R., Hanlon, J. T., Harris, T., & Cohen, H. J. (1996). Do older women use estrogen replacement? Data from the Duke Established Populations for Epidemiologic Studies of the Elderly (EPESE) [see comments]. *Journal of the American Geriatrics Society, 44*(1), 1-6.

Hartmann, B. W., & Huber, J. C. (1997). The mythology of hormone replacement therapy [review, 98 refs]. *British Journal of Obstetrics and Gynaecology, 104*(2), 163-168.

Hemminki, E., & McPherson, K. (1997). Impact of postmenopausal hormone therapy on cardiovascular events and cancer: pooled data from clinical trials. *British Medical Journal #19, 315*(7101), 149-153.

Hendrix, S. L. (1997). Nonestrogen management of menopausal symptoms [review, 53 refs]. *Endocrinology and Metabolism Clinics of North America, 26*(2), 379-390.

Holmes, S. (1996). Hormone replacement therapy and its role in the menopause [review, 19 refs]. *Nursing Times, 92*(28), 34-39.

Israel, D., & Youngkin, E. Q. (1997). Herbal therapies for perimenopausal and menopausal complaints [review, 74 refs]. *Pharmacotherapy, 17*(5), 970-984.

Jahnige, K., & Fiebach, N. (1997). Postmenopausal estrogen use among African American and white patients at an urban clinic. *Journal of Womens Health, 6*(1), 93-101.

Jeppesen, J., Schaaf, P., Jones, C., Zhou, M. Y., Chen, Y. D., & Reaven, G. M. (1997). Effects of low-fat, high-carbohydrate diets on risk factors for ischemic heart disease in postmenopausal women. *American Journal of Clinical Nutrition, 65*(4), 1027-1033.

Kaunitz, A. M. (1997). The role of androgens in menopausal hormonal replacement [review, 19 refs]. *Endocrinology and Metabolism Clinics of North America, 26*(2), 391-397.

King, K., & Thorne, R. (1996). Matching HRT to the patient. *Practitioner, 240*(1568), 650-654.

King, K. M. (1996). Estrogen replacement therapy and coronary heart disease in postmenopausal women [review, 20 refs]. *Health Care for Women International, 17*(3), 247-254.

King, K. M., & Kerr, J. R. (1996). The women's health agenda: evolution of hormone replacement therapy as treatment and prophylaxis for coronary artery disease [review, 39 refs]. *Journal of Advanced Nursing, 23*(5), 984-991.

Kuh, D. L., Wadsworth, M., & Hardy, R. (1997). Women's health in midlife: The influence of the menopause, social factors and health in earlier life. *British Journal of Obstetrics and Gynaecology, 104*(8), 923-933.

Liang, Y. L., Teede, H., Shiel, L. M., Thomas, A., Craven, R., Sachithanandan, N., McNeil, J. J., Cameron, J. D., Dart, A., & McGrath, B. P. (1997). Effects of estrogen and progesterone on age-related changes in arteries of postmenopausal women. *Clinical and Experimental Pharmacology and Physiology, 24*(6), 457-459.

Lichtman, R. (1996). Perimenopausal and postmenopausal hormone replacement therapy. Part 1. An update of the literature on benefits and risks [review, 269 refs]. *Journal of Nurse-Midwifery, 41*(1), 3-28.

Lichtman, R. (1996). Perimenopausal and postmenopausal hormone replacement therapy. Part 2. Hormonal regimens and complementary and alternative therapies [review, 109 refs]. *Journal of Nurse-Midwifery, 41*(3), 195-210.

Lip, G. Y., Blann, A. D., Jones, A. F., & Beevers, D. G. (1997). Effects of hormone-replacement therapy on hemostatic factors, lipid factors, and endothelial function in women undergoing surgical menopause: Implications for prevention of atherosclerosis. *American Heart Journal, 134*(4), 764-771.

Lucerno, M. A., & McCloskey, W. W. (1997). Alternatives to estrogen for the treatment of hot flashes. *Annals of Pharmacotherapy, 31*(7-8), 915-917.

Miller, K. L. (1996). Hormone replacement therapy in the elderly [review, 66 refs]. *Clinical Obstetrics and Gynecology, 39*(4), 912-932.

Moore, A. A., & Noonan, M. D. (1996). A nurse's guide to hormone replacement therapy [review, 43 refs]. *Journal of Obstetric, Gynecologic, and Neonatal Nursing, 25*(1), 24-31.

Mosinger, B. J. (1997). Human low-density lipoproteins: Oxidative modification and its relation to age, gender, menopausal status and cholesterol concentrations. *European Journal of Clinical Chemistry and Clinical Biochemistry, 35*(3), 207-214.

Nenseter, M. S., Volden, V., Berg, T., Drevon, C. A., Ose, L., & Tonstad, S. (1996). Effect of hormone replacement therapy on the susceptibility of low-density lipoprotein to oxidation among postmenopausal hypercholesterolaemic women. *European Journal of Clinical Investigation, 26*(12), 1062-1068.

Pearlstein, T., Rosen, K., & Stone, A. B. (1997). Mood disorders and menopause [review, 137 refs]. *Endocrinology and Metabolism Clinics of North America, 26*(2), 279-294.

Perz, J. M. (1997). Development of the menopause symptom list: a factor analytic study of menopause associated symptoms. *Women and Health, 25*(1), 53-69.

Porter, M., Penney, G. C., Russell, D., Russell, E., & Templeton, A. (1996). A population based survey of women's experience of the menopause. *British Journal of Obstetrics and Gynaecology, 103*(10), 1025-1028.

Rajkumar, C., Kingwell, B. A., Cameron, J. D., Waddell, T., Mehra, R., Christophidis, N., Komesaroff, P. A., McGrath, B., Jennings, G. L., Sudhir, K., & Dart, A. M. (1997). Hormonal therapy increases arterial compliance in postmenopausal women. *Journal of the American College of Cardiology, 30*(2), 350-356.

Robinson, G. (1996). Cross-cultural perspectives on menopause [review, 23 refs]. *Journal of Nervous and Mental Disease, 184*(8), 453-458.

Rothert, M. L., Holmes-Rovner, M., Rovner, D., Kroll, J., Breer, L., Talarczyk, G., Schmitt, N., Padonu, G., & Wills, C. (1997). An educational intervention as decision support for menopausal women. *Research in Nursing and Health, 20*(5), 377-387.

Rousseau, M. E., & McCool, W. F. (1997). The menopausal experience of African American women: Overview and suggestions for research [review, 66 refs]. *Health Care for Women International, 18*(3), 233-250.

Sarrel, P. M. (1997). Hormone replacement therapy in the menopause [review, 23 refs]. *International Journal of Fertility and Womens Medicine, 42*(2), 78-84.

Scanlon, C. (1997). Estrogen replacement: are the benefits worth the risks? *Hospital Practice (Office Edition), 32*, 67-68.

Scharf, M. B., McDannold, M. D., Stover, R., Zaretsky, N., & Berkowitz, D. V. (1997). Effects of estrogen replacement therapy on rates of cyclic alternating patterns and hot-flash events during sleep in postmenopausal women: A pilot study. *Clinical Therapeutics, 19*(2), 304-311.

Schunkert, H., Danser, A. H., Hense, H. W., Derkx, F. H., Kurzinger, S., & Riegger, G. A. (1997). Effects of estrogen replacement therapy on the renin-angiotensin system in postmenopausal women. *Circulation, 95*(1), 39-45.

Seals, D. R., Silverman, H. G., Reiling, M. J., & Davy, K. P. (1997). Effect of regular aerobic exercise on elevated blood pressure in postmenopausal women. *American Journal of Cardiology, 80*(1), 49-55.

Shaw, C. R. (1997). The perimenopausal hot flash: Epidemiology, physiology, and treatment [review, 52 refs]. *Nurse Practitioner, 22*(3), 55-56.

Sherwin, B. B. (1996). Hormones, mood, and cognitive functioning in postmenopausal women. *Obstetrics and Gynecology, 87*(2 Suppl), 20S-26S.

Sherwin, B. B. (1997). Estrogen effects on cognition in menopausal women [review, 36 refs]. *Neurology, 48*(5 Suppl 7), S21-S6.

Slaven, L., & Lee, C. (1997). Mood and symptom reporting among middle-aged women: The relationship between menopausal status, hormone replacement therapy, and exercise participation. *Health Psychology, 16*(3), 203-208.

Smigel, K. (1997). Next generation of SERMs being seen in clinic [news]. *Journal of the National Cancer Institute, 89*(13), 913

Sotelo, M. M., & Johnson, S. R. (1997). The effects of hormone replacement therapy on coronary heart disease [review, 70 refs]. *Endocrinology and Metabolism Clinics of North America, 26*(2), 313-328.

Stafford, R. S., Saglam, D., Causino, N., & Blumenthal, D. (1997). Low rates of hormone replacement in visits to United States primary care physicians. *American Journal of Obstetrics and Gynecology, 177*(2), 381-387.

Stevenson, E. T., Davy, K. P., Jones, P. P., Desouza, C. A., & Seals, D. R. (1997). Blood pressure risk factors in healthy postmenopausal women: Physical activity and hormone replacement. *Journal of Applied Physiology, 82*(2), 652-660.

Sulak, P. J. (1997). Endometrial cancer and hormone replacement therapy. Appropriate use of progestins to oppose endogenous and exogenous estrogen [review, 41 refs]. *Endocrinology and Metabolism Clinics of North America, 26*(2), 399-412.

Taddei, S., Virdis, A., Ghiadoni, L., Mattei, P., Sudano, I., Bernini, G., Pinto, S., & Salvetti, A. (1996). Menopause is associated with endothelial dysfunction in women. *Hypertension, 28*(4), 576-582.

Taskinen, M. R., Puolakka, J., Pyorala, T., Luotola, H., Bjaorn, M., Kaarianen, J., Lahdenpera, S., & Ehnholm, C. (1996). Hormone replacement therapy lowers plasma Lp(a) concentrations. Comparison of cyclic transdermal and continuous estrogen-progestin regimens. *Arteriosclerosis, Thrombosis and Vascular Biology, 16*(10), 1215-1221.

Taylor, M. (1997). Alternatives to conventional hormone replacement therapy [review, 88 refs]. *Comprehensive Therapy, 23*(8), 514-532.

Thacker, H. L. (1997). Menopause [review, 46 refs]. *Primary Care, Clinics in Office Practice* (1), 205-221.

Theriault, R. L. (1996). Hormone replacement therapy and breast cancer: An overview [review, 17 refs]. *British Journal of Obstetrics and Gynaecology, 103*(Suppl 13), 87-90, discussion 90-91.

Tilly-Kiesi, M., Kahri, J., Pyorala, T., Puolakka, J., Luotola, H., Lappi, M., Lahdenpera, S., & Taskinen, M. R. (1997). Responses of HDL subclasses, Lp(A-I) and Lp(A-I:A-II) levels and lipolytic enzyme activities to continuous oral estrogen-progestin and transdermal estrogen with cyclic progestin regimens in postmenopausal women. *Atherosclerosis, 129*(2), 249-259.

Tonetti, D. A., & Jordan, V. C. (1996). Design of an ideal hormone replacement therapy for women [review, 21 refs]. *Molecular Carcinogenesis, 17*(3), 108-111.

van, N. P. A., Dubas, J. S., Dorland, M., Boersma, H., & te, V. E. (1997). Age at natural menopause in a population-based screening cohort: The role of menarche, fecundity, and lifestyle factors. *Fertility and Sterility, 68*(1), 95-102.

Vassilopoulou-Sellin, R., & Klein, M. J. (1996). Estrogen replacement therapy after treatment for localized breast carcinoma. Patient responses and opinions. *Cancer, 78*(5), 1043-1048.

Vassilopoulou-Sellin, R., Theriault, R., & Klein, M. J. (1997). Estrogen replacement therapy in women with prior diagnosis and treatment for breast cancer. *Gynecologic Oncology, 65*(1), 89-93.

Wilmoth, M. C. (1996). The middle years: women, sexuality, and the self [review, 34 refs]. *Journal of Obstetric, Gynecologic, and Neonatal Nursing, 25*(7), 615-621.

CASE STUDY

ALTERATIONS DURING MENOPAUSE

INITIAL HISTORY:
- 54-year old white female
- Complaining of fatigue, hot flashes, perivaginal itching, dyspareunia, and vaginal discharge
- Periods stopped 1 year ago after several months of erratic cycles
- She has had no vaginal bleeding in the past year.

Question 1.
What would you like to ask this patient about her symptoms?

ADDITIONAL HISTORY:
- Her fatigue has increased gradually over the past 2 years.
- She has hot flashes many times during the day and is frequently awakened at night.
- Her vaginal symptoms have occurred gradually and are not accompanied by abdominal pain or dysuria.
- She denies any history of vaginal infections.
- She has had one sexual partner for 20 years.

Question 2.
What would you like to ask about her past medical history?

PAST MEDICAL HISTORY:
- No history of migraines, gallbladder disease, deep venous thrombosis, or hepatic disease
- Has a long history of hypercholesterolemia but has never had chest pain or been diagnosed with heart or cerebrovascular disease
- No personal or family history of breast cancer
- Normal mammogram last year
- Is on no medications and has no allergies

Question 3.
What would you like to ask her about her lifestyle?

LIFESTYLE HISTORY:
- She eats a low-fat diet and tries to watch her weight and cholesterol, but she admits her diet is low in calcium and high in phosphate.
- She used to walk regularly but got "out of the habit."
- She does not smoke or drink alcohol.

PHYSICAL EXAMINATION:
- Alert thin female with no acute distress; mild kyphosis especially at the upper thoracic spine
- T = 37 orally; P = 80 and regular; RR = 15 and unlabored; BP = 142/75 right arm

HEENT, Skin:
- Skin is thin and dry without rashes
- PERRL, fundi without hemorrhages or exudates
- Pharynx clear

Lungs, Cardiac:
- Good chest excursion; lungs clear to auscultation and percussion
- Cardiac with RRR without murmurs or gallops

Abdomen, Extremities:
- Abdomen soft, nontender, without organomegaly or masses
- Extremities with full pulses without edema

Breasts, Pelvic:
- Breasts symmetrical without masses, tenderness, or nipple discharge; axillae without adenopathy
- Pelvic with dry perivaginal and vaginal tissues; decreased estrogen effect; pap pending; no uterine or adnexal masses

Neurological:
- Oriented x 4
- Strength and sensation normal and symmetrical
- DTR 2+ and symmetrical
- Gait normal

Question 4.
What are the pertinent positives and negatives on exam?

Question 5.
What laboratories would you order?

LABORATORY RESULTS:

- FSH increased
- Chemistries including calcium and phosphate normal
- CBC including HCT normal
- Liver function tests normal
- Lipid profile shows increased LDL and decreased HDL.
- Mammogram consistent with postmenopause without masses or abnormal calcifications
- Dual energy x-ray densitometry consistent with decreased bone mineral density

Question 6.

What recommendations for management should be made for this patient?

SUGGESTED SOLUTIONS
AND RATIONALES

CHAPTER 1

QUESTION #1

SUGGESTED SOLUTIONS

- Do you remember how high the blood pressure was?
- Have you ever had an elevated blood pressure in the past?
- Do you have any other health problems?
- Is there any family history of hypertension?
- Do you have a history of chest pain, shortness or breath, numbness or weakness, syncope?

RATIONALE

Getting some idea of the severity and duration of the patient's blood pressure abnormality and the presence of a family history influences the likelihood that this one measurement is indicative of true hypertension. Underlying health problems can increase the risk of hypertension, and elevated blood pressures can worsen many other diseases. Symptoms of cardiac and neurologic disease might suggest end organ damage from sustained hypertension.

QUESTION #2

SUGGESTED SOLUTIONS

- What is your diet like, do you eat much fatty food and/or salt?
- Do you smoke or drink alcohol?
- Do you exercise?
- Have you gained any weight recently?
- Have you ever had your cholesterol checked?

RATIONALE

Assessment of risk factors provides more information about the likelihood that this patient indeed does have hypertension or is at risk for it in the future. In addition, this history provides the basis for lifestyle modification in this patient that would be indicated whether he has hypertension or not.

QUESTION #3

SUGGESTED SOLUTIONS

- Age and gender
- African American
- Family history
- Alcohol intake
- Weight gain
- Probable high-fat, high-salt, low-fiber diet
- Hypercholesterolemia

RATIONALE

Known risk factors for hypertension include increasing age, African American race, family history, obesity, alcohol, smoking, high sodium intake, and low potassium intake. Hypercholesterolemia not only puts the patient at increased risk for end-organ disease but could be a contributor to renal vascular disease as a cause of secondary hypertension.

QUESTION #4

SUGGESTED SOLUTIONS

- Obesity $\rightarrow$ risk factor
- BP elevated in both arms
- Fundi possibly suggestive of early hypertensive changes
- S_4 $\rightarrow$ myocardial stiffening
- No bruits to suggest renal vascular disease or advanced carotid or peripheral atherosclerotic disease.
- No abdominal masses suggestive of adrenal tumor.
- No edema to indicate CHF.
- No evidence of neurologic disease.

RATIONALE

The patient's exam confirms a persistent elevation in his blood pressure. Obesity is confirmed as an additional risk factor. His fundal changes are consistent with mild hypertensive changes but show no evidence of advanced damage. The S_4 most likely indicates a thick walled myocardium that may be stiff due to hypertrophic changes in response to sustained work-load for the heart. There is no other evidence of end-organ damage or secondary causes of hypertension.

QUESTION #5

SUGGESTED SOLUTIONS

- Obtain previous medical records.
- Suggest that the patient returns another day.

RATIONALE

The diagnosis of hypertension requires accurate measurement of an elevated blood pressure on at least three different occasions. Obtaining past records may indicate a longer history of blood pressure elevation.

QUESTION #6

SUGGESTED SOLUTIONS

- He should avoid caffeine and alcohol prior to his next visit.
- Once he arrives, he will need to rest for at least 5 minutes before his blood pressure is obtained.
- During the measurement, he should be seated with his arm at heart level.
- He should have his pressure checked twice, 2 minutes apart and averaged.

RATIONALE

A patient should not consume alcohol, caffeine (or tobacco) for at least 4 hours prior to getting his blood pressure checked. He should be as relaxed as possible and positioned comfortably with his arm in a pressure-neutral position. Accurate measurement requires averaging two pressures taken at least two minutes apart for each of the three diagnostic visits.

QUESTION #7

SUGGESTED SOLUTIONS

- Patient asked to return for a third visit.

RATIONALE

The diagnosis is not yet established, one more confirmatory measurement on another day is indicated.

QUESTION #8

SUGGESTED SOLUTIONS	RATIONALE
• The diagnosis of hypertension is confirmed. • Urinalysis • Chemistries including BUN and Cr and fasting glucose • Calcium and magnesium • Complete blood count • Lipid profile • Electrocardiogram	*The diagnosis is confirmed on the third visit. Consideration could be given to 24 hour blood pressure monitoring, but the advantages of this over conventional methods has not been established for all patients. The lab studies listed here are those recommended by JNC VI to rule out secondary causes of hypertension and to evaluate for cardiac risk and left ventricular hypertrophy. Other more specialized studies such as for adrenomedullary dysfunction are not indicated unless the patient's hypertension becomes more severe or is refractory to conventional therapy.*

QUESTION #9

SUGGESTED SOLUTIONS	RATIONALE
• No evidence of renal disease • No evidence of adrenocortical tumor • No evidence of other underlying disease • Hypercholesterolemia—increased risk for atherosclerotic disease • Left ventricular hypertrophy on ECG	*Normal sodium and potassium makes adrenocortical disease unlikely, and the normal urinalysis, BUN and Cr make renal parenchymal disease also unlikely. The increase in total cholesterol and LDL with a low HDL puts this patient in a significant risk category for atherosclerosis, especially coronary disease given his now established risk factor of HTN. Left ventricular hypertrophy signifies long-standing significant blood pressure elevations and increased myocardial work. This adds to his coronary risk as well as increases his risk for congestive heart failure.*

QUESTION #10

SUGGESTED SOLUTIONS	RATIONALE
• Weight reduction and exercise • Low-fat, low-salt diet • Decrease alcohol intake to less than 2 beers per day • Increase potassium calcium, and magnesium intake • Begin diuretic—careful patient teaching about side effects is important • Schedule echocardiogram • Follow up carefully	*The first step in hypertension management is lifestyle modification as described here. Weight reduction, exercise, decreased fat and salt intake, and increased potassium, calcium, and magnesium intake have all been associated with blood pressure improvement. Although his blood pressure is not dangerously high at this time, his evidence of retinal and myocardial end-organ damage indicate the need for pharmacologic intervention. Given their established safety and association with decreased risk for ischemic heart disease, diuretics make an excellent first choice. An echocardiogram is now indicated for further evaluation of left ventricular function. He must be monitored for blood pressure response and for side effects, another agent such as an angiotensin converting enzyme inhibitor or calcium channel blocker may need to be tried instead. If lifestyle modification is successful, it may be possible to taper him off of the medications after one year of good blood pressure control. Future evidence of regression of the left ventricular hypertrophy on ECG and echocardiogram indicates significant physiologic response to blood pressure modification and lowered cardiac risk.*

CHAPTER 2

QUESTION #1

SUGGESTED SOLUTIONS

- Have you ever had chest pain or neurologic symptom such as numbness, weakness, or difficulty speaking?
- Do you have any medical history?
- Have you ever been diagnosed with hypertension, diabetes, or cholesterol problems?
- Do you smoke or use alcohol?
- Are you on any medications?
- Do you have any allergies?
- What illnesses have there been in your family?
- Who do you live with? Are you working? What are your hobbies?
- How do you feel about your overall health?

RATIONALE

Further history should include questions about his overall health. Even with only this brief initial history, atherothrombotic obstruction of his leg artery must be considered so further history of risk factors for atherosclerosis or heart disease will help determine the likelihood of this diagnosis.

QUESTION #2

SUGGESTED SOLUTIONS

- Acute left lower extremity arterial occlusion

RATIONALE

Acute pain is caused by tissue ischemia. The sudden onset of ischemic pain is consistent with an acute occlusion rather than progressively worsening vascular disease. The asymmetric distribution of both the pain and physical signs indicate an arterial occlusion in the leg rather than the abdominal aorta.

QUESTION #3

SUGGESTED SOLUTIONS

- Femoral artery thrombus secondary to peripheral arterial-occlusive disease
- Thromboembolism of cardiac origin
- Femoral arterial aneurysm occluding arterial flow

RATIONALE

The distribution of the skin color and temperature changes, as well as diminished distal pulses, indicate an occlusion to blood flow in the distal left femoral artery. Although the immediate problem is the acute arterial occlusion, other potential causes of the occlusion will need to be explored. Patients with cardiac valve disease, endocarditis, and dysrhythmias are at risk for embolic phenomenon of cardiac origin. Patients with a history significant for hypertension, atherosclerotic vascular disease, prior vascular surgery, or prior history of aneurysms are at increased risk for anatomic changes in the structure of their arteries.

QUESTION #4

SUGGESTED SOLUTIONS

- Distal tissue ischemia/cellular death
- Potential loss of limb
- Potential infection and sepsis

RATIONALE

Persistent ischemia contributes to pain and necrosis of the affected tissue. The margin of necrotic tissue bordering perfused tissue can potentially lead to skin ulceration, infection, and sepsis.

QUESTION #5

SUGGESTED SOLUTIONS

- Conservative medical management with anticoagulant therapy
- Intra-arterial thrombolytic therapy in a specialized angiography setting
- Surgical embolectomy

RATIONALE

Anticoagulant therapy is indicated in this case in order to prevent further thrombus formation with in the arterial lumen but it will be insufficient in reversing the obvious tissue ischemia. Immediate anticoagulant therapy includes continuous heparin infusion titrating to a therapeutic heparin PTT. Intra-arterial thrombolytic therapy is most appropriate as the patient demonstrates some degree of circulation. Thrombolytic therapy is less invasive, does not require surgery, and can effectively restore baseline circulation to the affected area. This procedure involves arterial cannulation and flouroscopic visualization of the arterial perfusion using contrast dye. The thrombolytic agent is infused directly into the affected artery. In the event thrombolytic therapy does not restore full circulation, or if perfusion acutely deteriorates, a surgical embolectomy could be performed.

QUESTION #6

SUGGESTED SOLUTIONS

- CBC, PLT, PT, PTT, FBG
- Electrolytes, BUN, Cr
- Urine for myoglobin
- Rectal exam
- 12-lead ECG
- Type and screen to blood bank
- Lipid profile, glucose

RATIONALE

Since this patient will receive anticoagulant therapy and thrombolytic therapy, a baseline assessment of coagulation, HGB, HCT, and PLT values is necessary. These values will be monitored frequently during the course of therapy to assess the degree of anticoagulation and potential blood loss. Baseline renal function assessment is essential prior to any angiography procedure involving the use of contrast dye. Urine should be tested for myoglobin to obtain baseline data for evidence of muscle destruction. A rectal exam is necessary to rule out occult gastric blood loss in preparation for anticoagulant and thrombolytic therapy. An electrocardiogram is needed to rule out cardiac dysrhythmias or other abnormalities. It is essential to have blood ready for transfusion ion the event surgery becomes necessary. Although not integral to this patient's immediate medical needs, there should be a high index of suspicion that this man suffers from vascular disease; thus, the lipid profile and glucose will assist in analysis of his risk factors for atherosclerotic vascular disease.

QUESTION #7

SUGGESTED SOLUTIONS	RATIONALE

SUGGESTED SOLUTIONS

- Nonmodifiable:
  - Male, over age 50
- Modifiable/controllable:
  - Rule-out hypertension
  - Rule-out adult onset diabetes mellitus
  - Hyperlipidemia
  - Smoking
  - Mild obesity

RATIONALE

This patient's age, gender, lipid profile, smoking history, and mild obesity put him at risk for atherosclerotic peripheral vascular disease. His current evaluation reveals a blood pressure and glucose highly suggestive of the risk factors of hypertension and type 2 diabetes, and he should be evaluated further for these possibilities.

QUESTION #8

SUGGESTED SOLUTIONS

- Persistent extremity ischemia
- Compartment syndrome

RATIONALE

Although these signs are all consistent with persistent ischemia, the increased calf edema, diminished distal pulses, myoglobinuria, and neurosensory changes can also indicate probable left calf compartment syndrome. Compartment syndrome, in this instance, is most likely related to the combination of prolonged tissue ischemia and subsequent reperfusion injury. Due to cellular ischemia, necrosis, and resulting edema, pressure will continue to develop within the muscle compartments and eventually impinge the muscle's own blood and nerve supply. Treatment for compartment syndrome in this case would consist of releasing compartmental pressure by opening the muscle fascia with a 2 to 8 cm incision. In addition, myoglobinuria warrants aggressive intravenous hydration to prevent renal damage.

QUESTION #9

SUGGESTED SOLUTIONS

- Anticoagulation therapy:
  - Begin warfarin therapy
  - Continue intravenous therapy heparin until PT/INR is therapeutic
  - After 3 to 6 months, change anticoagulation regimen to aspirin or other antiplatelet agent
- Control hypertension
- Control blood glucose levels
- Arrange/ensure postdischarge follow-up with a primary provider

RATIONALE

Anticoagulation therapy is essential to prevent clotting and restenosis of the lesion. This usually involves heparin IV followed by institution of warfarin therapy. Once the PT or INR is therapeutic, the heparin can be discontinued. The warfarin should be continued for 3 to 6 months with subsequent antiplatelet therapy with aspirin or other antiplatelet agent. If the patient is found to have hypertension or diabetes, he should be treated to reduce the risk of further atherothrombotic disease. Finally, the patient will need close follow-up after discharge to manage his anticoagulation therapy and to evaluate for further complications.

QUESTION #10

SUGGESTED SOLUTIONS

- Smoking cessation counseling
- Dietary changes, including a low-fat, low-cholesterol, American Diabetes Association (ADA) diet
- Optimize body weight with diet and exercise
- Exercise regimen to improve vascular tone and maintain effective circulation.
- Medication instructions: coumadin therapy
- Incision care and effective wound healing measures after fasciotomy
- Further evaluation of his hyperglycemia and appropriate management should be instituted as soon as possible.

RATIONALE

Continued care of this patient should include atherosclerotic risk reduction and exercise. In addition, the patient should receive careful instructions about warfarin and its possible adverse effects. Incision care can often be accomplished successfully at home with proper instruction. Further management of the hyperglycemia should include full evaluation for type 2 diabetes and subsequent appropriate intervention (see Chapter 15).

CHAPTER 3

QUESTION #1

SUGGESTED SOLUTIONS

- Myocardial infarction
- Angina
- Costochondritis
- Pericarditis
- Aortic dissection
- Peptic ulcer or gastroesophageal reflux
- Pulmonary embolus
- Pneumonia
- Pneumothorax

RATIONALE

The differential diagnosis of chest pain is broad and includes cardiac, great vessel, pulmonary, and gastrointestinal sources for the pain. The character of the pain helps to narrow the most likely causes, but it is difficult to rule any of these out based on the history or even the physical exam alone.

QUESTION #2

SUGGESTED SOLUTIONS

- Does the pain radiate?
- Did it begin with exercise, stress, or cold exposure?
- Are you short of breath?
- Are you nauseated?
- Do you feel sweaty?
- Have you been coughing?
- Have you had a fever?
- Is the pain worse when you take a deep breath or cough?
- Is there anything that makes the pain better?

RATIONALE

Obtaining a detailed description of the pain and the associated symptoms helps to decide how likely it is that this patient is having cardiac pain. The symptoms associated with a high risk of myocardial infarction include pressure-like chest pain and radiation to the left arm that have been present for more than 1 hour but less than 48 hours. Fever and pleuritic pain suggests a pulmonary source of the symptoms.

QUESTION #3

SUGGESTED SOLUTIONS

- Do you smoke?
- Do you have high blood pressure?
- What is your diet like? Do you have cholesterol problems?
- Does anyone in your family have heart disease?
- Do you have diabetes?
- Do you exercise?
- Have you gained any weight?

RATIONALE

An assessment of the cardiac risk factors provides more evidence for the likelihood that the current episode represents cardiac pain, and provides the basis for future interventions regardless of the current diagnosis. Risk factors that can be obtained from the usual history include smoking, hypertension, dyslipidemia, family history, diabetes, sedentary lifestyle, and obesity.

QUESTION #4

SUGGESTED SOLUTIONS

- Have you had any pain like this before?
- Do you ever get short of breath?
- Do you get heartburn or blood in your stools?
- Have you ever passed out?
- Do you have any lung disease?
- Have you ever been hospitalized?
- Are you taking any medications or do you have any allergies?

RATIONALE

Further past medical history can help detect previous episodes likely to represent angina, peptic disease, neurologic events suggestive of cerebrovascular disease or sudden loss of cardiac function (arrhythmias), or lung disease.

QUESTION #5

SUGGESTED SOLUTIONS

- The differential diagnosis has not changed.
- His risk factors and past medical history make myocardial infarction or angina most likely.

RATIONALE

As stated in Question #1 above, the differential diagnosis remains broad. Although myocardial infarction or angina are now the most likely based on his history of multiple risk factors and possible previous ischemic events (while jogging), the others cannot be ruled out by history.

QUESTION #6

SUGGESTED SOLUTIONS

- Tachycardic, hypertensive, and diaphoretic
- No decrease in pulse pressure or pericardial rubs
- Occasional ectopy
- No mentioned corneal arcus or xanthelasma
- Tachypneic and using accessory muscles with basilar crackles and a soft S_3 but no significant jugular venous distention, hepatosplenic congestion, or edema
- No murmurs of S_4
- No abdominal or neurologic findings
- Bruit suggestive of peripheral vascular atherosclerosis

RATIONALE

His hyperdynamic state could be the result of almost any anxiety-inducing state, or they could be the direct result of myocardial injury. There is no evidence of pericardial disease (narrowing of the pulse pressure with a pericardial rub and an S_4 might indicate pericardial effusion or constriction). Occasional premature beats are common, but in the setting of possible ischemic heart disease, cardiac monitoring would be essential in all patients. He has no obvious evidence of severe dyslipidemia. He has evidence of mild pulmonary congestion and minimal cardiac enlargement, but no severe heart failure and no evidence of pleural disease. There is no evidence of valvular disease or evidence of abdominal or neurologic disease. Peripheral bruit is suggestive that there is some atherosclerosis present, increasing the likelihood that he might have coronary involvement.

QUESTION #7

SUGGESTED SOLUTIONS

- ECG
- Oximetry
- Chest x-ray
- Draw blood for CBC, troponin I, electrolytes, CPK-MB

RATIONALE

The electrocardiogram is the basic diagnostic test in suspected myocardial ischemia. Oximetry is to assess for adequate oxygenation. The chest x-ray evaluates for aortic and pulmonary disease as well as for CHF. Cardiac enzymes will confirm the diagnosis of myocardial infarction versus transient ischemia.

QUESTION #8

SUGGESTED SOLUTIONS

- ST elevation of ≥ 2 mm with T wave inversion in the precordial leads is classic for acute anterior myocardial ischemia.
- Arterial blood gases show a mild respiratory alkalosis and an increase in the A-a gradient.
- Chest x-ray confirms mild pulmonary congestion without evidence of other pulmonary or pleural disease.

RATIONALE

The ECG is diagnostic for myocardial ischemia and suggests infarction but this could still represent angina, and a follow-up ECG after the cessation of pain is important. The arterial blood gases suggest mild hyperventilation and hypoxemia consistent with mild pulmonary congestion. The chest x-ray confirms the pulmonary congestion and helps to rule out underlying pulmonary parenchymal or pleural disease. The lack of widening of the mediastinum helps to reassure that this is not aortic dissection but is not a very sensitive test for the diagnosis.

QUESTION #9

SUGGESTED SOLUTIONS

- Oxygen administration and getting IV access for quick medication administration
- Aspirin
- Topical nitrates, IV furosemide, and morphine
- Patient reassurance

RATIONALE

Oxygen administration will maximize coronary oxygen delivery. IV access is essential for administering medications promptly. The diagnosis of myocardial ischemia is now established; aspirin has been shown to decrease MI mortality when given acutely. Nitrates provide coronary vasodilation to improve perfusion, morphine for pain, and furosemide for the pulmonary congestion. Reducing anxiety will improve patient outcome and reduce catecholamine output.

QUESTION #10

SUGGESTED SOLUTIONS

- The normal CPK-MB and troponin I are not helpful in diagnosing infarction versus transient ischemia since less than 3 to 4 hours have passed since his pain began.
- Frequent re-evaluation of the patient is essential.

RATIONALE

The cardiac isoenzymes may not be diagnostic for several more hours. Reevaluation reveals improved pulmonary congestion and the ECG confirms the diagnosis of MI. Of concern is that he continues to have some pain and his LV function is not known.

QUESTION #11

SUGGESTED SOLUTIONS

- Additional morphine given to relieve pain
- Echocardiography to assess LV function
- Assess if patient is a candidate for thrombolysis

RATIONALE

Complete pain relief is the goal. Echocardiography is a rapid and safe way to assess LV function which will influence therapy and prognosis (LV function is the most important determinant of prognosis in ischemic heart disease). Thrombolysis or PTCA should be offered to this patient to reduce infarct size and improve prognosis.

QUESTION #12

SUGGESTED SOLUTIONS

- Accelerated tPa, reteplace, or PTCA followed by heparin
- IV beta-blocker
- Consider ACE inhibitor

RATIONALE

These three options have similar effects on limiting infarct size and improving LV function and prognosis. IV beta-blockers improve mortality and prevent MI recurrence. ACE inhibitors are controversial in patients with an ejection fraction (EF) >40%, but many centers use them in all post-MI patients to prevent ventricular remodeling.

QUESTION #13

SUGGESTED SOLUTIONS

- Patient is counseled on how to limit his activities and when to begin cardiac rehab classes, and to stop smoking.
- Psychosocial therapies are recommended such as group therapy, relaxation training, and possible individual counseling.
- He is given diet instructions including salt restriction, low cholesterol, low fat; consider vitamin E and folate supplementation.
- He is to take 80 to 325 mg aspirin/day, to continue on beta-blockers, consider ACE inhibitors if he remains hypersensitive, and sublingual nitrates PRN.
- He is to follow up with his nurse practitioner closely and to return to the emergency room for symptoms of chest pain or dyspnea.

RATIONALE

Risk reduction, especially smoking cessation, exercise, and diet modification can greatly reduce the recurrence of MI and sudden death. Patients need reassurance and careful instructions on how to safely increase their activity over time; cardiac rehab centers provide important support. Aspirin and beta-blockers clearly reduce MI recurrence; the continued use of ACE inhibitors is controversial but might be the best choice in this patient with hypertension.

CHAPTER 4

QUESTION #1

SUGGESTED SOLUTIONS

- Heart failure
- Myocardial infarction
- Unstable angina
- Chronic lung disease with cor pulmonale
- Large pleural effusions
- Pneumonia
- Pericarditis

RATIONALE

We know this patient has many of the cardinal symptoms suggestive of heart failure, such as paroxysmal nocturnal dyspnea, dyspnea on exertion, lower extremity edema, and decreased exercise tolerance. However, in elderly persons an acute MI or unstable angina may be exhibited by symptoms of left ventricular failure. Chronic lung disease with right ventricular failure or large pleural effusions may result in peripheral edema and dyspnea. Pneumonia and pericarditis can cause the symptoms of dyspnea and chest pain.

QUESTION #2

SUGGESTED SOLUTIONS

- Do you have any heart problems?
- Do you have high blood pressure?
- Do you have diabetes?
- Do you smoke cigarettes?
- How much alcohol do you drink?
- Do you have a cough?
- Is the cough productive?
- Have you had any palpitations?
- Do you have a history of lung disease?
- Have you had any episodes of fainting or near fainting?

RATIONALE

Additional questions should look for cardiac risk factors, potential causes of heart failure, evidence of lung disease, or recent upper respiratory infection.

QUESTION #3

SUGGESTED SOLUTIONS

- History of coronary artery disease
- Multiple risk factors for heart failure
- History of cigarette smoking remote but lung disease remains in the differential

RATIONALE

The historical evidence strongly suggests heart failure with potentially an ischemic origin at this time.

QUESTION #4

SUGGESTED SOLUTIONS	RATIONALE
• + jugular venous distension (JVD) • + hepatojugular reflex (HJR) • Bibasilar crackles • Right base dull to percussion • Point of maximal impulse (PMI) displaced laterally • + S_3 • Holosytolic murmur at apex • Bilateral edema in lower extremities	*The physical examination revealed several findings consistent with the diagnosis of heart failure. A third heart sound and a + HJR are very sensitive physical findings. Elevated JVD, although helpful in identifying elevated right atrial pressures are not independently specific for heart failure. Although the presence of pulmonary crackles suggests failure, many patients with pulmonary capillary wedge pressures greater than 18 do not have this physical finding. A laterally displaced PMI suggests left ventricular enlargement. Mitral regurgitation, identified by a soft blowing systolic murmur at the apex, is frequently found in patients with dilated left ventricles. Peripheral edema due to heart failure is bilateral and seen in patients with evidence of right-sided failure. In the absence of elevated JVD, paroxysmal nocturnal dyspnea, or orthopnea, and other causes of peripheral edema such as venous insufficiency should be explored. Bilateral pleural effusions may be found in patients with heart failure and elevated venous pressures. If unilateral, the pleural effusion is generally right sided. The rapid heart rate is due to a compensatory sympathetic response to the diminished cardiac output and also suggests that the patient either was not adequately medicated with the beta-blocker or that he did not take the prescribed medication.*

QUESTION #5

SUGGESTED SOLUTIONS	RATIONALE
• Arterial blood bases • Cardiac isoenzymes • CBC • Serum albumin, Cr, electrolytes • BUN • T_4, thyroid-stimulating hormone (TSH) • Liver function tests • Urinalysis • Electrocardiogram (ECG) • Chest x-ray	*It is essential to establish whether the patient is able to ventilate and oxygenate adequately. Cardiac isoenzymes will be helpful in determining recent myocardial ischemia or injury. Routine chemistries and measures to evaluate renal and hepatic function are helpful to establish current status and to guide future therapies. T_4 and TSH should be obtained on all persons over the age of 65; persons with new onset heart failure; or persons with new onset atrial fibrillation to evaluate for the presence of thyroid disease. Heart failure may be aggravated by hematocrits less than 35%. Low serum albumin may exacerbate heart failure. A chest x-ray is a valuable tool in the diagnosis of heart failure. Pulmonary congestion, cardiomegaly, and calcified heart valves can be evident on a PA and lateral chest x-ray. The ECG may be helpful if acute ischemia or a dysrhythmia has precipitated the heart failure.*

QUESTION #6

SUGGESTED SOLUTIONS

- IV loop diuretic
- O$_2$
- Initiate ACE inhibitor

RATIONALE

The patient's symptoms of paroxysmal nocturnal dyspnea, dyspnea on exertion, and peripheral edema suggest moderate volume overload. Use of an IV loop diuretic will initiate rapid diuresis and an improvement in symptoms. Thiazide diuretics result in a more gradual diuresis and can be used in cases of less severe volume overload. A short-acting ACE inhibitor should be administered to evaluate the patient's response to therapy. The use of digoxin is premature at this point. Digoxin may be added if the patient remains symptomatic after optimal management with diuretics and ACE inhibitors. Digoxin is indicated in cases of severe heart failure.

QUESTION #7

SUGGESTED SOLUTIONS

- CLCR (ml/min) = [(140-age) x weight (kg)/72 x serum Cr (mg/dl)] x (0.85 for women)
- CLCR = 140-66) x 82/72 x 1.9
- CLCR = 159.4 ml/min
- Normal = 70-130 ml/min

RATIONALE

This formula is helpful in determining the estimated glomerular filtration rate and in adjusting drug dosages in renal impairment. A 24-hour urine specimen for Cr clearance is necessary for a more accurate evaluation of renal function.

QUESTION #8

SUGGESTED SOLUTIONS

- Potassium replacement
- SaO$_2$ monitoring

RATIONALE

Patients with heart failure frequently have ventricular dysrhythmias. Potassium supplementation may be necessary to maintain serum potassium levels around 4. The slight respiratory acidosis may be improved as the patient diuresis and improves oxygenation. The increased BUN and Cr reflect the reduced cardiac output.

QUESTION #9

SUGGESTED SOLUTIONS

- ACE inhibitor
- Diuretic

RATIONALE

If the patient tolerates the test dose of a short-acting ACE inhibitor while in the emergency room, a longer acting ACE inhibitor should be prescribed. Caution should be used in prescribing ACE inhibitors in patients with severe renal insufficiency or failure. Because this patient is volume overloaded, he will require a diuretic. In general, a single daily dose of a loop or thiazide diuretic is recommended. Potassium sparing diuretics should be used with caution when ACE inhibitors are prescribed. As the patient is followed on an outpatient basis, the clinician may consider changing the current beta blocking agent to an agent with nonselective beta blocking and alpha blocking properties.

QUESTION #10

SUGGESTED SOLUTIONS	RATIONALE
• Evaluation of left ventricular function • Evaluation of coronary graft status • Lipid profile evaluation	*Heart failure due to an ischemic process may be reversible and efforts should be made for revascularization if appropriate. Because the patient has a history of coronary artery disease and bypass surgery, cardiac catheterization may be the best diagnostic test to evaluate graft patency and left ventricular function. Aggressive management of elevated cholesterol and triglyceride levels is recommended to slow the progression of atherosclerosis.*

QUESTION #11

SUGGESTED SOLUTIONS	RATIONALE
• Dietary restrictions • Signs and symptoms of worsening failure • Daily weights • Exercise plan • Medication teaching	*Patient education is an essential component of managing patients with heart failure. Instructions on low-sodium diets (2000 to 3000 mg) and fluid restrictions will help minimize fluid accumulation. The patient should be instructed to weigh himself first thing every morning after urinating. Weight gains of 2 to 3 pounds in 2 days or 5 pounds in 1 week should be promptly reported to the health care provider. Unless patients demonstrate severe NYHA class IV symptoms, a daily exercise plan, such as walking, is recommended. Weight lifting exercises are discouraged. Patients should be instructed to notify the health care provider if they have increased shortness of breath from their baseline, persistent nausea or vomiting, weight gain as described above, excessive fatigue, prolonged episodes of palpitations, an increase in the number of pillows they sleep on, sudden shortness of breath at night, or an increasing cough.*

CHAPTER 5

QUESTION #1

SUGGESTED SOLUTIONS

- Asthma
- Anaphylaxis
- Cystic fibrosis
- Foreign body
- Pulmonary embolus
- Bronchitis
- Mitral valve prolapse
- Arrhythmia

RATIONALE

We know that the patient is young and developed symptoms while being exposed to potential allergens while mowing. Her prodromal symptoms sound like allergic rhinitis, and chest tightness is characteristic of asthma. We still have no past medical history so we cannot rule out an underlying lung disorder or an infectious etiology. Finally, cardiac abnormalities can also be a source of acute dyspnea even in a young person.

QUESTION #2

SUGGESTED SOLUTIONS

- Do you have a history of asthma or other lung diseases?
- Are you allergic to anything?
- Could you have inhaled some foreign object?
- Have you had a recent cough or cold?
- Do you have any chest pain or hemoptysis?
- Do you have any heart problems?

RATIONALE

Additional questions should include a history of underlying lung diseases, aspiration, infectious symptoms, evidence for pulmonary embolism, or history of heart disease.

QUESTION #3

SUGGESTED SOLUTIONS

- Asthma history with positive family history.
- Atopic history c/w extrinsic asthma, now with exposure to grass while mowing.
- Increasing frequency of symptoms suggests move from mild intermittent to moderate persistent.
- No history to suggest other pulmonary or cardiac disease.

RATIONALE

The historical evidence points strongly at extrinsic asthma. As discussed in the chapter, the old categories of asthma overlap in their pathophysiology and are not used in the United States to identify types of asthma patients. In the author's opinion however, the categories do suggest useful insights into special issues of diagnosis and management among the various patient presentations. Much of the world's literature continues to use these categories. Her severity classification has changed from mild intermittent to moderate persistent in that they are occurring daily and requiring the daily use of a β-agonist inhaler.

QUESTION #4

SUGGESTED SOLUTIONS	RATIONALE
• Oximetry—if saturation <91% then do arterial blood gases • Peak flow • Electrolytes • HCT and CBC • ECG • Chest x-ray	*A rapid assessment of her ability to oxygenate with oximetry should be followed by arterial blood gas measurement if her oxygen saturation is low. Studies have shown that early measurement of peak flow can prevent underestimation of the severity of airway obstruction and positively influence management outcomes. Electrolyte and blood count evaluation helps to rule out acidosis and signs of underlying infection. A chest x-ray would only be indicated if there is evidence of pneumonia or pneumothorax on examination.*

QUESTION #5

SUGGESTED SOLUTIONS	RATIONALE
• Oxygen via mask • IV D_5W at KVO • Heart monitor • Pulse oximeter • Nebulized $beta_2$ agonist • Prednisone 60 mg PO	*As with any patient in acute distress, maintenance of adequate ventilation and oxygenation is of immediate concern. In addition, hypoxemia and/or hypercapnia as well as β-agonists can result in arrhythmias, so a heart monitor is indicated. Finally, β-agonists remain the safest and most effective first-line therapy for acute asthma attacks. In a severe attack such as this, oral steroids should be begun immediately.*

QUESTION #6

SUGGESTED SOLUTIONS	RATIONALE
• $PaO_2 = (760 - 47) \times FIO_2 - PaCO_2/0.8$ • $PaO_2 = 713 \times 0.21 - 30/0.8$ • $PaO_2 = 150 - 38$ • $PaO_2 = 112$ • A-a gradient = 112 - 65 = 47 (normal = <10)	*The alveolar gas equation is used to determine the extent of lung dysfunction based on how much oxygen is able to diffuse from the alveoli to the arterial blood. The equation calculates the amount of alveolar oxygen (PaO_2) using the barometric pressure (760 mmHg), a constant for water vapor (47 mmHg), the fraction of inspired oxygen ($FIO_2 = 0.21$ in room air), the $PaCO_2$ from the arterial blood gas (in this case 30 mmHg), and the respiratory quotient (0.8). The result is compared to the PaO_2 from the blood gas, the difference between the two (A-a gradient) should be less than 10 (in this case the difference is 47 which is abnormal).*

QUESTION #7

SUGGESTED SOLUTIONS	**RATIONALE**

- Worsening of bronchospasm
- Increased respiratory rate and wheezing—patient is deteriorating
- Peripheral vasoconstriction from hypoxemia → cool extremities
- Cyanosis due to hypoxemia and peripheral vasoconstriction
- Hypoxemia with poor cerebral oxygenation leading to confusion
- Worsening hypoxia **plus**
- Normalization of CO_2 despite increased respiratory rate = decreased ventilation (ominous sign)

It is clear from her exam and repeat blood gases that the patient is developing increasing bronchospasm and hypoxemia. What is not so obvious is that the normalization of her CO_2 is an ominous sign of impending respiratory failure. Given her increased respiratory rate, her CO_2 would be expected to decrease further. Instead, it is rising indicating a reduction in minute volume due to a decrease in tidal volume (MV=RR x TV). This inability to ventilate adequately is the result of increasing air-trapping and fatigue, and, if not treated, will progress rapidly to respiratory failure.

QUESTION #8

SUGGESTED SOLUTIONS	**RATIONALE**

- Increase FIO_2
- Repeat beta$_2$ agonist
- Ipratropium 0.5 mg
- Consider steroids IV
- Consider intubation
- Consider aminophylline

Increasing her oxygen should be accompanied by increased efforts to relieve bronchospasm. β_2-agonists can be used safely in repeated doses, or even as a continuous nebulizer. Ipratropium may work synergistically to relieve the bronchospasm and does not increase side effects. High dose IV steroids have been shown to be safe and effective in acute asthma. Intubation may be necessary if the $PaCO_2$ continues to rise. Aminophylline IV in acute asthma is controversial and is usually used only in patients already on oral theophylline who come in with subtherapeutic serum levels; however, her peak flow and severe clinical status may serve as indications for aminophylline therapy.

QUESTION #9

SUGGESTED SOLUTIONS	**RATIONALE**

- Admit to the hospital.
- Monitor closely through the night with repeat ABG and peak flow measurements.
- Repeat beta$_2$ agonists, ipratropium Q 4 hours
- Continue steroids
- Monitor for worsening symptoms at 4 to 8 hours.

Despite the obvious improvement in her exam, this was clearly a life-threatening episode and she should be observed in the hospital. Although her ABG seem improved, calculation of her A-a gradient reveals significant continued pulmonary dysfunction (A-a = 298). In addition she may experience a recurrence of her symptoms in association with the Late Asthmatic Response (LAR) so she should be monitored closely with repeated doses of bronchodilators and antiinflammatory medications.

QUESTION #10

SUGGESTED SOLUTIONS

- Beta inhaler Q 4 to 6 hours
- Ipratropium Q 6 hours
- Prednisone 40 mg QD
- Avoid allergen exposure
- Return immediately if symptoms recur.
- See primary provider for steroid inhaler, allergy shots, and close follow-up.

RATIONALE

Although this patient should be seen soon after discharge by her primary care provider, it is important to continue her medications to reduce residual inflammation and prevent recurrence. She should avoid repeat allergen exposure if possible and return to the ER without delay if she worsens again. Her long-term care should include daily inhaled antiinflammatory medication (steroids or the new leukotriene inhibitors) and evaluation for desensitization therapy.

QUESTION #11

SUGGESTED SOLUTIONS

- Reduce amount of allergen in the home environment (remove carpeting, stuffed animals).
- Home peak flow monitoring
- Treat respiratory infections promptly.
- Get influenza and pneumococcal vaccine when available.
- Obtain evaluation for chronic sinusitis and gastroesophageal reflux.

RATIONALE

Allergens in the environment can continuously sensitize the asthma patient and increase the severity of their disease, simple household modifications can result in significant symptomatic improvement over time. A home peak flow monitor helps patients follow their responses to medication and better assess a need for more aggressive intervention. Respiratory infections are a common cause of asthma exacerbations and should be treated before a severe attack occurs. Vaccination can prevent many potentially serious infections. Finally, exacerbations in asthma have been associated with chronic sinusitis and gastroesophageal reflux disease, treatment of these conditions can result in significant improvement in asthma symptoms.

CHAPTER 6

QUESTION #1

SUGGESTED SOLUTIONS

- Do you smoke?
- What color is your sputum?
- Is there any blood in it?
- Do you have any fever, chills, or chest pain?
- Do you normally have a cough or any other chronic symptoms?
- Have you lost any weight?
- Do you have any heart disease?

RATIONALE

A patient with a long history of progressive dyspnea who now presents with new symptoms of increasing dyspnea, cough and edema probably is experiencing an acute respiratory deterioration superimposed on chronic lung disease. One would want to decide whether the new symptoms represent an infection while also characterizing the likely underlying chronic disease. Pedal edema could represent either left heart disease (congestive heart failure [CHF]) or right heart disease due to pulmonary vasoconstriction (cor pulmonale).

QUESTION #2

SUGGESTED SOLUTIONS

- How is your general health?
- Have you had any previous lung infections?
- Do you have any occupational exposures?
- Have you ever had similar symptoms before?
- Do you have any family history of lung disease?

RATIONALE

Delineation of the patient's past medical history will help characterize the current problem. A previous history of lung infection such as tuberculosis or of occupational exposures such as asbestos contribute to the differential diagnosis. It is important to ask about the severity of this episode and whether it is a repetitive exacerbation. A family history of lung disease might point to a genetic cause such as alpha 1-antitrypsin deficiency.

QUESTION #3

SUGGESTED SOLUTIONS

- COPD
- Acute bronchitis
- Pneumonia
- Asthma
- Bronchiectasis
- Pulmonary fibrosis
- Recurrent pulmonary emboli
- Heart disease

RATIONALE

In a smoker with these symptoms and no other pertinent medical history, COPD tops the list. The patient may have a superimposed infectious bronchitis or pneumonia. The age of onset, lack of atopic history, and lack of family history argues against asthma but it is still in the differential. The normally small amount of sputum production argues against bronchiectasis. Fibrosis, emboli, and primary heart disease are still possible but unlikely.

QUESTION #4

SUGGESTED SOLUTIONS

- Using accessory muscles of respiration, pursed lip breathing, tachypnea
- Barrel chest, decreased diaphragmatic excursion, decreased breath sounds, expiratory wheezes and rhonchi
- Precordial heave and loud S_2, hepatosplenomegaly, and pedal edema

RATIONALE

Use of accessory muscles with pursed lips and tachypnea indicate increased work of breathing. This is most likely from the hyperinflation that is evidenced by the barrel chest, poor diaphragm movement, and decreased breath sounds. Expiratory wheezes suggest that there is expiratory airway obstruction and airtrapping. A heave with a loud S_2 suggests right ventricular enlargement due to pulmonary hypertension with congestion of the systemic venous circulation.

QUESTION #5

SUGGESTED SOLUTIONS

- Serum chemistries including calcium
- CBC
- Liver function tests
- Sputum stain
- Arterial blood gases
- Chest x-ray
- Spirometry

RATIONALE

The probability of chronic lung disease with possible respiratory acidosis makes assessment of serum electrolytes important, especially the bicarbonate. In this patient with a long smoking history, a calcium level and careful review of a chest x-ray is necessary to evaluate for possible carcinoma. A CBC will evaluate for polycythemia (increased HCT) or leukocytosis (indicating infection). Liver function tests can help determine if her hepatomegaly is due to hepatic disease or a result of her chronic lung disease. Sputum stain would be indicated to assess for acute infection or hemoptysis. Arterial blood gases will establish her level of hypoxemia and hypercapnia to determine her baseline values, and to be certain she does not have an element of acute CO_2 retention at this time. Chest x-ray will evaluate for infectious exacerbations, and neoplastic lesions, and may show evidence of emphysema if her disease is advanced. Spirometry can confirm obstructive lung disease and quantify its severity.

QUESTION #6

SUGGESTED SOLUTIONS

- A high bicarbonate may indicate metabolic compensation for chronic respiratory acidosis.
- Elevated HCT indicates chronic hypoxemia.
- No evidence of other systemic complications.
- Sputum is mildly infected with probable pneumococcus.

RATIONALE

Acute hypoventilation with associated decrease in minute volume and increase in serum CO_2 would result in acidosis; in this patient the hypercapnia is chronic and the kidney is retaining bicarbonate to buffer the retained CO_2. Polycythemia is a compensatory response to chronic hypoxemia. Sputum with polymorphonucleocytes and bacteria indicates infection; in this case, gram-positive diplococci are seen which are most often S. pneumoniae *(pneumococcus) in smokers.*

QUESTION #7

SUGGESTED SOLUTIONS

- Normal pH with elevated CO_2 indicates chronic metabolically compensated hypercapnia
- $PaO_2 = (760 - 47) \times FIO_2 - PaCO_2/0.8$
- $PaO_2 = 713 \times 0.21 - 56/0.8$
- $PaO_2 = 150 - 70$
- $PaO_2 = 80$
- A-a gradient $= 80 - 54 = 26$ (normal $= <10$)
- A-a gradient $= 26$: abnormal but mild difficulty with oxygenation, most of the hypoxemia is due to the chronic hypercapnia.

RATIONALE

The arterial blood gas confirms the compensated chronic hypercapnia. The alveolar gas equation is used to determine the extent of lung dysfunction based on how much oxygen is able to diffuse from the alveoli to the arterial blood either because of lung damage or hypoventilation. The equation calculates the amount of alveolar oxygen (PaO_2) using the barometric pressure (760 mmHg), a constant for water vapor (47 mmHg), the fraction of inspired oxygen ($FIO_2 = 0.21$ in room air), the $PaCO_2$ from the arterial blood gas (in this case 56 mmHg), and the respiratory quotient (0.8). The result is compared to the PaO_2 from the blood. In this patient, the gradient is relatively small indicating that most of the hypoxemia is due to the hypoventilation and hypercapnia rather than actual parenchymal damage.

QUESTION #8

SUGGESTED SOLUTIONS

- Decreased forced expiratory volume on 1 second (FEV_1) indicates expiratory airflow obstruction.
- Decreased forced vital capacity (FVC) is consistent with COPD when the FEV_1/FVC ratio is also decreased as it is in this patient.

RATIONALE

Emphysema is characterized by expiratory airway collapse. On spirometry, this is evidenced by a decreased FEV_1, a somewhat decreased FVC, and a reduced FEV_1/FVC ratio. Air trapping results in an increased total lung capacity (TLC), but this does not benefit the patient. In fact, the increased TLC (hyperinflation) puts the respiratory muscles at a mechanical disadvantage resulting in an increased work of breathing and hypoventilation.

QUESTION #9

SUGGESTED SOLUTIONS

- Hyperinflation is evidenced on the x-ray by flattened diaphragms, increased A-P diameter, and increased retrosternal space, consistent with expiratory airway obstruction with air trapping.
- Scarring and bullae are evidence of destruction of airways and alveoli and are consistent with emphysema.
- Enlarged pulmonary vasculature suggests pulmonary hypertension due to diffuse pulmonary vasoconstrictive response to hypoxia and hypercapnia.

RATIONALE

In emphysema, unopposed elastase activity results in a loss of the normal elastic recoil of the small airways and expiratory airway obstruction. This air trapping can be worsened by intrabronchial mucus and infection. As the hyperinflation increases, the respiratory muscles (especially the diaphragm) are pushed out of their normal shape and develop a mechanical disadvantage that increases the work of breathing. These elastases also cause alveolar destruction and airspace enlargement seen on x-ray as scarring and bullae. Diffuse pulmonary vasoconstriction causes increased resistance in the pulmonary vasculature with resultant increased pulmonary artery pressure and enlarged pulmonary arteries that can be seen as large vascular shadows on chest x-ray.

QUESTION #10

SUGGESTED SOLUTIONS

Acute:
- Low-flow oxygen—follow ABG frequently
- Ipratropium 2 puffs
- Beta$_2$ agonist by nebulizer
- Antibiotics

RATIONALE

Given the lack of acute acidosis and evidence of pneumonia in this patient, it may be possible to improve her breathing enough as an outpatient as long as there will be close follow-up. Low-flow oxygen should be administered to raise her PaO$_2$ to at least 65, but careful attention must be paid to see if she develops hypoventilation and hypercapnia. Ipratropium can be given quickly and safely while a nebulizer is set up for the patient to use with a beta$_2$ agonist. With her infected sputum, an antibiotic should be prescribed; amoxicillin or sulfamethoxazole would be appropriate choices given her sputum stain, but modifications may be necessary if she has a resistant organism.

Chronic:
- Exercises
- Nutritional counseling
- Check oximetry at night for possible home oxygen therapy
- Ipratropium inhaler 4 to 6 times daily
- PRN beta$_2$ agonist
- If worsens, consider therapeutic trial of theophylline or steroids

Respiratory muscle exercise plus regular aerobic exercise will strengthen the patient and have been shown to improve dyspnea. Many patients with COPD have poor nutrition and require guidance to keep up their strength and weight. A PaO$_2$ of 54 while awake may not qualify this patient for insurance support of home O$_2$ even though some studies indicate that this level of hypoxia is associated with increased risk of death. A documented desaturation at night would qualify the patient, then she should be encouraged to wear the oxygen all night and most of the day. Ipratropium is the first line bronchodilator for COPD and is safe to use continuously, whereas beta$_2$ agonists should be used on an as-needed basis. If the patient worsens, a trial of theophylline or steroids may be indicated, but should be continued only if there is documented improvement in pulmonary function tests.

CHAPTER 7

QUESTION #1

SUGGESTED SOLUTIONS

- What other symptoms do you have?
- Do you have a history of lung disease?
- Do you smoke?
- Has anyone else around you been ill?
- Do you have any risk for immunocompromise?
- What is your general state of health?
- Are you on any medications?
- Have you had any immunizations?
- Have you traveled recently?
- Do you use drugs or alcohol?
- Do you have any allergies?

RATIONALE

The history should include information about other symptoms that might be suggestive of significant systemic illness as well as to identify any prodromal symptoms. Risk factors would include smoking, exposure to other potentially ill contacts, immunocompromise, and other underlying diseases, especially lung disease. Medications, immunizations, travel, alcohol and drug, and allergic history may also be very helpful.

QUESTION #2

SUGGESTED SOLUTIONS

- Acute bronchitis
- Viral pneumonia
- Sinusitis
- Bacterial pneumonia
- Influenza
- Asthma

RATIONALE

The history is now suggestive of either a viral or bacterial infection. The lack of prodrome makes influenza less likely, and the negative past medical history argues strongly against asthma, but neither possibility has been completely ruled out. Sinusitis with significant postnasal drainage can mimic a true productive cough, but in the absence of headache, bronchitis or pneumonia top the list.

QUESTION #3

SUGGESTED SOLUTIONS

- Febrile, tachypneic, and tachycardic without orthostatic blood pressure changes or skin dryness to suggest dehydration.
- Flushed skin is consistent with fever.
- HEENT findings are consistent with upper respiratory infection.
- Use of accessory muscles in a patient with moderate respiratory distress.
- Percussion and auscultation findings consistent with consolidation in the right middle lobe.
- Rest of the exam is normal.

RATIONALE

The fever and tachycardia are very nonspecific, but significant tachypnea is suggestive of pulmonary disease, especially with the chest findings. The lack of orthostatic blood pressure findings and moist skin and mucous membranes are reassuring that the patient is not dehydrated. The use of accessory muscles in an otherwise healthy patient is consistent with moderate respiratory distress. Crackles (rales), egophony, whispered pectoriloquy, and dullness to percussion are very suggestive of pneumonia, in this case in the area of the right middle lobe. There are no other findings to suggest disseminated infection or underlying illness.

QUESTION #4

SUGGESTED SOLUTIONS

- Arterial blood gases
- Chemistries
- CBC with differential
- Liver functions
- Sputum stain

RATIONALE

The use of accessory muscles and moderate respiratory distress in this patient would indicate a need for arterial blood gas measurement to better assess ventilation and oxygenation (may determine need for hospitalization). Blood chemistries, CBC, and liver functions may help identify a viral or bacterial cause (e.g., legionella pneumophila *causes liver function changes) and assess the general condition of the patient. Sputum stain may suggest the specific etiologic organism and thus influence choice of treatment.*

QUESTION #5

SUGGESTED SOLUTIONS

- A-a gradient:
  $A = (PB-47)FIO_2 - PaCO_2/0.8$
  $= (760-47)0.21 - 26/0.8$
  $= 150 - 33$
  $= 117$
- A-a gradient $= 117-90 = 27$.

RATIONALE

A PaO$_2$ of 90 mmHg would result in a normal O$_2$ saturation on oximetry, and, in the absence of arterial blood gas measurement and calculation of the A-a gradient, might lead the provider to underestimate the degree of pulmonary parenchymal disease. In the tachypneic patient, the PaO$_2$ should be considerably higher than what is found in this patient. The equation calculates the amount of alveolar oxygen (PaO$_2$) using the barometric pressure (760 mmHg), a constant for water vapor (47 mmHg), the fraction of inspired oxygen (FIO$_2$ =0.21 in room air), the PaCO$_2$ from the arterial blood gas (in this case 26 mmHg), and the respiratory quotient (0.8). The result is compared to the PaO$_2$ from the blood. In this patient, the gradient is abnormal (>10), indicating pulmonary parenchymal disease. Although her PaO$_2$ and PaCO$_2$ do not fit the criteria for admission and this information may not immediately alter therapy, the A-a gradient will be invaluable if the patient should require hospitalization and oxygen therapy as her disease progresses.

QUESTION #6

SUGGESTED SOLUTIONS

- Chemistries, HCT, and liver functions normal
- WBC elevated with left-shift consistent with bacterial infection
- Sputum with PMN indicating infection, GM+ diplococci most common *pneumococcus*

RATIONALE

No evidence of underlying disease. Liver functions are normal and do not suggest legionella. Elevated total white blood count with a predominance of PMNs is more consistent with bacterial rather than viral infection. Sputum PMN indicates respiratory infection, in this case the gram stain is suggestive of streptococcus pneumoniae.

QUESTION #7

SUGGESTED SOLUTIONS

- Dense infiltrate in the right middle lobe obscuring the right heart border
- Air bronchograms visible

RATIONALE

The infiltrate does not obscure the right diaphragm, but does obscure the right heart border on the PA film, this means it is anteriorly located. The lateral defines the major and minor fissure as the borders of the infiltrate, confirming the right middle lobe (RML) location. Air bronchograms indicate alveolar consolidation without atelectasis.

QUESTION #8

SUGGESTED SOLUTIONS

- RML pneumonia
- GM+ diplococci = possible *pneumococcus*
- Other possibilities: *H. influenza*, mycoplasma,, chlamydia, viral
- Immune compromise?

RATIONALE

As above, the x-ray and sputum stain are most consistent with pneumococcal pneumonia as it is the most common community acquired bacterial pneumonia and it often results in lobar consolidation. Other common infections have not been completely ruled out. Immune compromise would broaden the differential to include opportunistic infections.

QUESTION #9

SUGGESTED SOLUTIONS

- Possibly admit to hospital
- Oximetry; recheck ABG if condition changes
- Antibiotics empirically; erythromycin vs doxycycline vs amoxicillin vs ampicillin + clavulanate
- Deep breathing, cough
- Close follow-up; repeat chest x-ray when treatment is complete

RATIONALE

The patient's age is close to that which is commonly used as a criterion for admission (age 65) and her tachypnea also suggests the possible need for hospitalization. The decision would most likely rest on this patient's preference and whether she has an adequate living situation (reasonable proximity to emergency care, has support from family or friends, etc). Although the A-a gradient is abnormal, oxygenation and ventilation remain adequate but should be monitored closely. There are many antibiotic choices. Erythromycin or doxycycline are excellent choices for empiric outpatient coverage in an otherwise healthy patient. In this patient, her sputum gram stain is suggestive of pneumococcus and her underlying health is excellent, therefore consideration could be given to amoxicillin alone or ampicillin + clavulanate. Allergic history and tolerance to medications must be considered. A lack of prompt response to therapy would indicate the sure need for hospitalization as well as sputum cultures and modification of antibiotic choice.

CHAPTER 8

QUESTION #1

SUGGESTED SOLUTIONS

- Worsening COPD
- Bronchitis
- Pneumonia
- Allergy
- Pneumothorax
- Cancer
- Ischemic heart disease
- CHF
- Arrhythmia

RATIONALE

The nonspecific symptoms of increasing dyspnea and cough in a patient with known COPD raise many possibilities. Conditions that contribute to her underlying COPD such as infections, allergy, or pneumothorax must be considered. In any smoker, cancer is high on the list. It is important to consider primary cardiac disease in these patients. Smoking is a risk factor for ischemic heart disease and CHF. Cardiac or pulmonary disease predispose to arrhythmias; in this patient, atrial fibrillation is quite possible.

QUESTION #2

SUGGESTED SOLUTIONS

- How dyspneic are you?
- Does your dyspnea get worse when you lie down?
- Are you coughing up discolored sputum or have any fever?
- Are you coughing up any blood?
- Are you having any chest pain? If so, is it worse when you take a deep breath or cough?
- Are you having any edema or palpitations?
- Have you lost any weight?

RATIONALE

Quantitating the dyspnea helps to assess the urgency of the evaluation. Discolored sputum or fever might indicate pneumonia or bronchitis. Hemoptysis would be very worrisome for cancer. Pleuritic chest pain would suggest primary pulmonary or pleuritic disease, whereas substernal chest pain might indicate ischemic heart disease. Edema and palpitations could be the result of CHF or worsening COPD with hypoxia and cor pulmonale. Weight loss could indicate worsening COPD or cancer.

QUESTION #3

SUGGESTED SOLUTIONS

- How much do you smoke?
- How long have you had emphysema?
- Have you ever had pulmonary function testing?
- Have you ever had pneumonia or bronchitis?
- Have you ever had heart trouble?
- Do you have any allergies?
- Any recent vaccinations?

RATIONALE

The number of pack-years (number of packs smoked per day multiplied by the number of years smoked) provides some indication of the risk for lung cancer or emphysema. A history of diagnosed lung disease would help determine the cause of the dyspnea, as well as assess for risk of lung cancer. A history of heart disease might indicate a cardiac cause of her symptoms. An allergy and vaccination history further elucidate the likelihood of allergic or infectious pulmonary conditions

---

QUESTION #4

SUGGESTED SOLUTIONS

- Afebrile
- Tachypnea with mildly labored pursed lip breathing and use of accessory muscles
- No cyanosis or edema
- Increase in anteroposterior diameter, tympany, decreased excursions, and scattered wheezes
- Afebrile, no dullness, rubs, splinting, or crackles
- Heart normal size, no ectopy, murmurs, gallops, or bruits

RATIONALE

The tachypnea, use of accessory muscles, pursed lip breathing, increased anterioposterior diameter, low and poorly moving diaphragms, distant breath and heart sounds, and scattered wheezing are all characteristic of COPD. The lack of fever, crackles, or areas of consolidation makes pneumonia less likely. The lack of dullness or rubs makes pleural disease less likely. No cyanosis or edema makes cor pulmonale less likely. The cardiac exam is normal and not suggestive of CHF, and there is no evidence of atherosclerotic disease, peripherally.

QUESTION #5

SUGGESTED SOLUTIONS

- Cancer moves up the list.
- Worsening of COPD is still quite possible.
- Infectious pulmonary disease is much less likely.
- Cardiac disease is less likely; but has not been ruled out.

RATIONALE

The exam and history make cancer and COPD worsening the most likely possibilities. A 4-month bout of bronchitis or pneumonia without fever, sputum production, rhonchi, or rales seems quite unlikely. Cardiac disease cannot be ruled out, but the exam reveals no evidence of coronary or peripheral artery atherosclerosis.

QUESTION #6

SUGGESTED SOLUTIONS

- Arterial blood gases
- Electrocardiogram (ECG)
- Pulmonary function testing
- Chest x-ray
- Sputum cytology

RATIONALE

The patient's pulmonary status must be evaluated with arterial blood gases and pulmonary function testing. An ECG will help evaluate for ischemic heart disease. The chest x-ray will look for masses or infiltrates, and sputum cytology is an excellent screening tool.

QUESTION #7

SUGGESTED SOLUTIONS

- Compensated hypercapnia (no acidosis) and moderate hypoxemia
- ECG without evidence of cardiac disease
- Pulmonary function tests consistent with significant obstructive airway disease.
- Chest x-ray worrisome for a malignant mass.
- Sputum cytology not diagnostic

RATIONALE

The patient's pH is normal despite hypercapnia indicating renal compensation for chronic hypoventilation, and she is moderately hypoxic. These are all consistent with her emphysema. Baseline values would be very helpful. The normal ECG does not rule out ischemic heart disease. A decrease in forced expiratory volume in 1 second is characteristic of COPD. The noncalcified spiculated features of the mass make it much more likely that this is a malignant lesion. Sputum cytology is not diagnostic, but atypia is suggestive of possible malignancy.

QUESTION #8

SUGGESTED SOLUTIONS

- The patient needs referral for diagnosis and management.
- Further testing is likely to include CT scan, bronchoscopy, and/or fine needle aspiration.
- If malignancy is confirmed and the cell type is identified, then evaluation of resectability (staging), operability (functional status, ventilation/perfusion scanning) is warranted; evaluation for another primary tumor site.

RATIONALE

The patient now requires specialized care; a pulmonologist or thoracic surgeon are possibilities. CT scanning allows for more careful evaluation of the lesion and for mediastinal involvement for staging. Bronchoscopy may allow for direct visualization and biopsy, but is less sensitive for peripheral lesions where CT guided fine needle aspiration may have a higher yield. If a tumor is confirmed, resectability and operability must be evaluated. If the tumor is an adenocarcinoma, the possibility that this tumor is a metastasis from another primary tumor site (e.g., breast, colon) must be considered.

QUESTION #9

SUGGESTED SOLUTIONS

- She must stop smoking immediately.
- She should receive detailed information about her type of lung cancer and what her options are.
- Surgery has a good likelihood of cure since she is stage I.
- She should increase her calories maximally and receive instruction on optimizing her breathing techniques and medication.
- She should have her family come in with her to learn about how to help her before and after surgery.

RATIONALE

Stopping smoking now will improve her operative outcome, and smoking cessation efforts are often most successful after the diagnosis of a smoking-related illness. She needs to be fully informed and to have her options discussed. In her case, surgery offers her the best chance for cure. Optimizing nutrition status preoperatively will help with postoperative recovery. Her underlying COPD should be managed for optimization of her pulmonary function (see Chapter 6). Getting her family involved will be very helpful postoperatively as well. Overall, having a very open and accessible relationship with this type of patient is essential to providing optimal care during a very difficult time in his/her life.

QUESTION #10

SUGGESTED SOLUTIONS

- She should expect to remain weak for a while, but most patients return to a high quality of life by 3 to 6 months after surgery.
- She should continue with a high caloric intake and breathing exercises.
- She can use nonsteroidal antiinflammatories and alternative methods of pain control (therapeutic touch, transcutaneous electrical nerve stimulation [TENS], etc.), but should minimize narcotics if possible.
- She must never smoke.
- She must have close follow-up.

RATIONALE

Most patients who undergo surgery for early-stage lung cancer have an improved quality of life 3 to 6 months postoperatively. Given her significant preoperative lung disease, her recovery may be slower. Continuing to optimize nutrition and exercise will speed recovery. Narcotics may cause respiratory depression in patients with chronic hypoventilation; alternatives should be used if possible. Close, honest, caring follow-up will provide this patient with the best opportunity for rapid recovery and for continued success in smoking cessation.

CHAPTER 9

QUESTION #1

SUGGESTED SOLUTIONS

- Benign breast disease
- Cyst
- Breast cancer

RATIONALE

In this patient, her relatively young age and lack of associated breast changes make a benign process more likely, but in no way rules out the possibility of breast cancer.

QUESTION #2

SUGGESTED SOLUTIONS

- Do you practice breast self-examination?
- Have you noticed the lump before?
- Have you had previous mammograms and what were their findings?
- Do you have a family history of breast cancer or benign breast disease?
- Have you had a previous breast biopsy? What was the finding?
- What is your menstrual history (age of menarche, and where are you currently is in your cycle)?
- Do you have children? What are their ages? If so, did you breastfeed?
- Any significant past medical history?

RATIONALE

Further questions should try to establish whether the patient has a history of previous breast disease and evidence of any hereditary or endocrine risk factors for breast cancer.

QUESTION #3

SUGGESTED SOLUTIONS

- Increasing age
- Personal history of previous breast cancer
- First degree relative (mother, sister, or daughter) with breast cancer
- History of fibrocystic disease associated with hyperplastic lesions (i.e., atypical hyperplasia)

RATIONALE

Most (77%) breast cancers occur in women older than 50 years of age. A woman with a history of breast cancer is at an increased risk for subsequent breast cancer by 0.7% per year after the diagnosis of the initial cancer. Approximately 15% to 20% of breast cancers occur in women with a positive family history. Women with atypical hyperplasia plus a family history of breast cancer have an 11-fold greater breast cancer risk.

QUESTION #4

SUGGESTED SOLUTIONS

- High dietary fat intake
- Hormone use
- Excess alcohol consumption
- History of pregnancy termination before full-term
- Obesity
- Genetic testing (BRCA1 and BRCA2 gene)

RATIONALE

Although a causal relationship between dietary fat and the development of breast cancer has not been firmly established, until more data is available, it is reasonable to suggest a well-balanced diet with reduced fat intake. The use of exogenous hormones and breast cancer continues to be controversial. Although a few studies have suggested that the long-term use of oral contraceptives, especially prior to first pregnancy, may promote onset of breast cancer, most studies suggest that they may actually be protective. Postmenopausal hormone replacement therapy with estrogen is associated with some increase in breast cancer risk, but this potential risk must be weighed against the substantial benefits of HRT including reduced osteoporosis and heart disease. Abortion (especially in the first trimester) and the use of alcohol have been linked to breast cancer, but the correlation has been weak and the research results are often contradictory. Obesity and breast cancer risk may be related to estrogen metabolism; increased adipose tissue makes available an increased amount of androstenedione for conversion to estrone. Genetic testing for BRCA1 and BRCA2 genes is controversial. Women who are potentially at "genetic risk" must go through a formal genetic screening and counseling program to weigh the risks and benefits of genetic screening. If the woman tests negative, there is still no way to guarantee that breast cancer will not develop. If women test positive, there are no proven effective methods of prevention, but a more aggressive screening program initiated as early as age 25 has been suggested.

QUESTION #5

SUGGESTED SOLUTIONS

- The lesion within the left breast appears different from the diffuse cystic changes in both breasts.

RATIONALE

The lesion in the upper outer quadrant of the left breast is larger and more firm and nonmobile than the diffuse cystic nodules found in both her breasts. The lack of skin changes or nipple discharge is reassuring, but does not rule out the possibility that the palpable nodule is cancerous. She has no evidence of metastasis on exam, but the lack of palpable axillary nodes provides little information since the axillary exam is insensitive for detection of nodal involvement.

QUESTION #6

SUGGESTED SOLUTIONS

- Mammography
- Ultrasound

RATIONALE

Since the physical exam findings are new and the nodule feels different from the rest of her breast exam, further evaluation is indicated. In addition, her positive family history is a significant risk factor. A mammogram with a possible follow-up ultrasound is indicated.

QUESTION #7

SUGGESTED SOLUTIONS

- The patient should be thoroughly educated about her breast exam findings and the reasons for the diagnostic mammogram.
- The mammogram procedure includes the use of low-dose radiation.
- Stop drinking caffeinated beverages several days before the test.
- The mammogram should be obtained 1 week after menses so that breasts will be less tender.
- If the patient regularly experiences breast pain—take a pain reliever before the test (tylenol or motrin).
- Patient should discuss her fears or concerns with the technologist who is performing the exam.

RATIONALE

Of course, the patient should be made aware of all the potential risks of mammography including exposure to low-dose radiation and breast discomfort. Instructions to help ensure that the breasts are not unusually tender can spare the patient any undue pain with the mammogram.

QUESTION #8

SUGGESTED SOLUTIONS

- Provide emotional support and initial education as to treatment for the patient.
- CBC with differential, liver function studies
- Chest x-ray and bone scan (only if alkaline phosphastase is elevated or patient has been symptoms or pain)
- Refer to breast surgeon

RATIONALE

Now that the diagnosis of cancer has been established, the patient will require considerable support. A limited workup for possible metastases should be undertaken, with special attention to the most likely targets of lung and bone. Referral to a breast surgeon is indicated if the patient is interested in pursuing appropriate treatment.

QUESTION #9

SUGGESTED SOLUTIONS

- Survival is equivalent with surgical options; the choice is based on:
    - Location and size of lesion (multicentric or extensive multifocal should not elect breast-conserving surgery [BCT])
    - Breast size
    - Appearance of the mammogram (diffusely abnormal mammograms should not elect BCT)
    - Patient's desire for breast preservation
    - Pregnancy
- Prior radiation to the breast is a contraindication
- Social circumstances that would prevent a patient from receiving radiation therapy on a regular basis
- Primary advantage of lumpectomy plus radiation is cosmetic and normal sensation of the preserved breast

RATIONALE

In patients who meet the criteria for a small, localized lesion, the survival with lumpectomy is equivalent with any of the surgical options. The patient should be able to receive local radiation therapy to the region to reduce the risk of local recurrence. The primary advantage of lumpectomy plus radiation is cosmetic and normal sensation of the preserved breast.

QUESTION #10

SUGGESTED SOLUTIONS

- Yes

RATIONALE

Women who are premenopausal, have tumors greater than 1 cm, and have a high grade tumor (Grade III), should be referred even if they are node-negative.

QUESTION #11

SUGGESTED SOLUTIONS

- The patient would be recommended to one of three standard therapies:
    - CMF (cytoxan, methotrexate, and 5-FU)
    - AC (adriamycin and cytoxan)
    - CAF (cytoxan, adriamycin, and 5-FU)
- Note that CMF is standard adjuvant therapy. The use of an adriamycin-based regimen has not been proven to be "better" than standard CMF.
- CMF is given over 6 months intravenously (IV) (or oral cytoxan may be used day 1 to 4). The regimen consists of all three drugs day 1, MF only day 8, then a 2-week break. This is continued for 6 cycles of therapy.

RATIONALE

Adjuvant chemotherapy and has been found to impact disease-free interval and overall survival but decreases the risk of systemic recurrence by only 30% . (Hence, if our patient has a 25% chance of recurrence, her risk would be reduced by only 7.5% or to 17.5%.) This is an important educational point since only a small portion of women will benefit from chemotherapy and there are potential risks from therapy.

QUESTION #12

SUGGESTED SOLUTIONS

- All of these side effects are potential, including:
    - Nausea and vomiting, mucositis, diarrhea
    - Fatigue, hair loss
    - Myelosuppression, secondary neoplasms
    - Infertility, amenorrhea
    - Potential for infection related to myelosuppression, alterations in body image and sexuality

RATIONALE

Chemotherapy side effects primarily involve areas of the body where there are rapidly dividing cells including hair follicles, the GI and GU tracts, and the bone marrow. The suppression of the marrow results in pancytopenia with immune suppression and susceptibility to a wide variety of common and opportunistic infections. In addition, chemotherapy can increase the risk of secondary neoplasms occurring in the future; this would be of special concern to this young patient.

QUESTION #13

SUGGESTED SOLUTIONS

- Localized pain of the bone
- Progressive back pain
- Muscular weakness
- Headache
- Any new neurologic complaints
- Respiratory symptoms (cough, chest pain dyspnea)
- Nausea/vomiting, weight loss
- Jaundice
- RLQ abdominal pain or abdominal distention

RATIONALE

Two-thirds of patients diagnosed with breast cancer metastatic to bone have vertebral involvement. Progressive back pain, weakness, paresthesias, or bowel/bladder dysfunction suggest possible spinal cord compression and would be evaluated immediately. Approximately 9% to 25% of all patients with breast cancer develop brain metastases, 60% develop pulmonary metastases (including lung nodules, lymphangitic spread, and pleural effusions), and 60% develop liver metastases.

CHAPTER 10

QUESTION #1

SUGGESTED SOLUTIONS

- His entire history is suspect.

RATIONALE

*Other warning signs include: **a**symmetry, irregular **b**order, uneven **c**olor, and **d**iameter greater than 6 mm, (**abcd**); family history of melanoma; history of severe sun burning in childhood and adolescence; and history of acute and intermittent exposure to sun or ultraviolet radiation. Further, any lesion that has undergone a recent change or has begun to itch or bleed should be suspect.*

QUESTION #2

SUGGESTED SOLUTIONS

- A dysplastic nevus is a distinct melanocytic lesion that may be a precursor to melanoma.

RATIONALE

Clinically, dysplastic nevi tend to be larger than commonly acquired nevi, often measuring >5 mm. The skin lesion may have an irregular or fuzzy border, and the pigmentation is often an uneven pattern. The central nevus component is often a different color than the peripheral, giving it a "fried-egg" appearance. Patients often have dozens to hundreds of these nevi. There is a small probability that a single dysplastic nevus will evolve into a melanoma, however a person with dysplastic nevus syndrome and a positive family history of melanoma has close to a 100% chance of developing melanoma themselves.

QUESTION #3

SUGGESTED SOLUTIONS

- While the occupation of a P.E. teacher would generally be considered very healthy, it probably increases his exposure to sun.

RATIONALE

Natural sunlight is composed primarily of UVB radiation that damages the DNA of the skin cells, causing sunburn. It is thought to be a promoter of melanoma, especially in genetically susceptible individuals. Tanning beds emit mostly UVA radiation that penetrates more deeply into the dermis and causes sun-damage changes and wrinkling. Both UVA and UVB have been implicated as promoters in the carcinogenesis of melanoma. There is no such thing as a safe tan. The damaging effects of sunlight may occur many years before melanoma is diagnose;, therefore, sun protection during childhood and adolescence is very important. The strongest UVB radiation is between the hours of 10 a.m. and 2 p.m., the most likely hours this patient may be teaching classes.

QUESTION #4

SUGGESTED SOLUTIONS

- The majority of physical examination findings for this patient are encouraging.
- His skin exam is typical for many people diagnosed with melanoma.

RATIONALE

Aside from looking for other suspicious skin lesions near the primary and on the entire body, a complete physical exam is essential to rule out metastatic disease. A funduscopic look at the retina to rule out ocular involvement; complete evaluation of lymph nodes to rule out adenopathy; auscultation and percussion of lungs to rule out lung involvement; abdomen and liver palpation to rule out liver and/or abdominal involvement; and a neuro exam to rule out brain metastases is recommended.

QUESTION #5

SUGGESTED SOLUTIONS

- No

RATIONALE

Melanoma may originate in any area of the body that contains melanocytes, which are dendritic pigmented cells found usually within the epithelial surfaces. Unusual variants of melanoma include ocular melanoma (originating in the pigment cells of the choroid); conjunctival melanoma; and mucosal melanomas, such as nasopharyngeal, oral, vulvar, and anorectal melanomas, and even in lymph node capsules. About 4% of patients present with metastatic disease originating from an unknown primary site.

QUESTION #6

SUGGESTED SOLUTIONS

- Regional lymph nodal basins are the most common sites of first metastases, followed by regional skin, subcutaneous tissue, and lung.

RATIONALE

Melanoma can metastasize to virtually any organ of the body. Other common sites are the liver, brain, and bone. Although any cancer spread to the small bowel is uncommon, it does occur with melanoma. Ocular melanoma most frequently metastasizes to the liver.

QUESTION #7

SUGGESTED SOLUTIONS

- An excisional biopsy would be most appropriate for this lesion.

RATIONALE

Tumor thickness is the most important factor in determining prognosis and treatment. The biopsy therefore should be to level of subcutaneous tissue. A smaller skin lesion may be biopsied with a punch-type biopsy, and a larger lesion should be excised. Shave biopsies should be avoided. Depending on the initial depth of the lesion, a wider excision will be planned with a 0.5 cm to 2 cm margin.

QUESTION #8

SUGGESTED SOLUTIONS

- According to the TNM classification, a lesion of 2.2 mm thickness and Clark Level IV would be classified as a T3.
- Assuming he has no nodal involvement or distant metastases, he will be considered a stage II.
- The 5-year survival rate for stage II is 60% to 80% with surgery alone.

RATIONALE

The 5-year survival rate by stage is as follows:

I   >85%
II   60% to 80%
III 30% to 50% (inversely correlated with the number of positive lymph nodes)
IV   <10% (mean 14-month survival with only skin or node metastases; 4 months if visceral)

Other negative prognostic factors include ulceration, high mitotic rate, and microscopic satellite lesions.

QUESTION #9

SUGGESTED SOLUTIONS

- Superficial spreading (SSM) type of melanoma is the most common (70%) of histologic types, located on any body site; however, it is more common on the upper back of males and legs of females.
- It is characterized by horizontal or radial extension along the dermal-epidermal junction.
- Lesions usually arise in a flat nevus.
- It is increasingly common in young adults.

RATIONALE

There are three other major growth patterns of melanoma: nodular, lentigo maligna, and acral lentiginous melanoma. Nodular melanomas (NM) make up 15% to 30% of melanoma cases, occurring more commonly among older men, on any body site. They usually have vertical growth, frequently without a recognizing preexisting mole. Lentigo maligna melanoma (LMM) comprise 1% to 5% of melanomas and typically appear on the face and neck of severely sun-damaged elderly persons. They usually have radial growth, but usually this is associated with a good prognosis. Acral lentiginous melanomas (ALM) occur on the palms and soles or under nail beds or sublingually. They occur more commonly in darker pigmented (especially black) people. They have radial growth and comprise 5% to 10 % of melanomas diagnosed.

QUESTION #10

SUGGESTED SOLUTIONS

- Since this patient did not have any other suspicious physical exam findings, a chest x-ray and liver function blood profile would be the only tests indicated.

RATIONALE

After biopsy and pathologic interpretation, work-up of any suspicious physical examination findings are indicated for accurate staging. If the patient has a pathologic stage or clinical stage of III or IV, then they should have full staging work-up to include a computed tomography (CT) of the head, chest, and abdomen, and a bone scan because they are at higher risk for metastases. Persons with ocular melanoma should be particularly screened for liver involvement, because that is the primary metastatic site.

QUESTION #11

SUGGESTED SOLUTIONS

- Any patient with clinically positive lymph nodes should be offered a complete lymph node dissection (CLND).
- However, this patient did not have any palpable adenopathy, and the value of elective lymph node dissection (ELND) has been somewhat controversial in the past.
- Current literature suggests that anyone with a lesion over 1.5 mm would benefit from a sentinel lymph node biopsy (SLNBX). The greater the depth of the lesion, the more likely it has spread to regional lymph nodes. If regional lymph nodes are involved, the patient would be offered adjuvant treatment.
- Therefore, SLNBX should be offered to this patient for a 2.2 mm melanoma as a staging tool.

RATIONALE

The first or "sentinel" lymph node that drains a melanoma is determined by using the technique of lymphoscintigraphy. Technetium-99 and/or isosulfan blue dye are injected subdermally around the primary lesion. This drains into the lymphatics, and, with the aid of a gamma counter and visualization of a blue node, the sentinel lymph node is identified and biopsied. If the sentinel lymph node is not involved, there is a less than 5% chance that any lymph nodes are involved. The procedure offers a good method for staging, has very low morbidity compared to CLND, and is also helpful in more accurately identifying the drainage basin for lesions that are on the upper back, close to midline (sometimes they drain to both axilla and the neck).

QUESTION #12

SUGGESTED SOLUTIONS

- Currently no adjuvant treatment would be offered to this patient with stage II disease.
- He has an approximately 6% chance of developing a local recurrence and a 20% chance of harboring distant metastases.

RATIONALE

Recombinant alpha-interferon is currently indicated for adjuvant therapy for patients with stage III disease (melanomas >4 mm in thickness or with positive lymph node involvement). It is commonly used alone or in combination for treatment of metastatic disease, producing up to a 22% response rate. Severe side effects and high cost are other factors that contribute to the decision making for patients with more advanced melanomas.

QUESTION #13

SUGGESTED SOLUTION

- Patient education should focus on surveillance for recurrent local disease, metastatic disease, and prevention of new melanomas.
- Preventive measures include avoiding peak times of sun exposure, using sunscreen with a sun protection factor (SPF) of 15 or greater, wearing protective clothing while outdoors, avoiding artificial sun lamps, and performing regular self-examination.
- Any new constitutional symptoms should be reported to the practitioner for evaluation.

RATIONALE

A patient with a melanoma has a higher risk for developing a second primary melanoma than an individual in the general population without melanoma. The risk of developing a second primary melanoma is 5% in 10 years.

QUESTION #14

SUGGESTED SOLUTION

- Follow-up should include a thorough physical exam focusing on skin and lymph nodes.
- During the first 3 years, follow-up should be every 3 to 4 months; for years 4 and 5, it should be every 6 months; and it should be annually thereafter.
- A chest x-ray and liver function test should be performed periodically.
- Any systemic complaint should be evaluated.
- Photographs of the skin may help document changes over time.

RATIONALE

Most experts agree that lifetime follow-up is indicated to rule out local recurrence and metastases.

CHAPTER 11

QUESTION #1

SUGGESTED SOLUTIONS	RATIONALE

- When did you notice the foot weakness and what is it like?
- Have you had any other weakness, numbness, difficulty walking or speaking, passing out spells, seizures, or blurring of your vision?
- Have you had an increase in thirst, appetite, or need to urinate?
- How long have you had the rash? Does anything make it worse or better?
- Have you had any chest pain, shortness of breath, swelling of your feet and ankles, change in your bowel or bladder habits, or skin ulcers?

In a patient with a known history of diabetes, the likelihood of her foot drop representing neuropathy is high. It is important to ask about other neurologic symptoms however, since cerebrovascular accident is in the differential diagnosis of a focal neurologic deficit such as this. Polydipsia, polyphagia, and polyuria might indicate that her blood sugar has been elevated. There are many possible causes of rash especially in the diabetic patient including bacterial and fungal infections, dermopathy, and eruptive xanthomatosis. Further questions about symptoms of diabetic end-organ effects including ischemic heart disease with congestive heart failure, gastrointestinal motility disorders, genitourinary motility, and infectious complications, and skin ulcers are vital to the patient's overall care.

QUESTION #2

SUGGESTED SOLUTIONS	RATIONALE

- Why did you go to the doctor at the time you were diagnosed with diabetes?
- What was your blood sugar at that time?
- Why did you not follow-up with the care recommended at that time?
- Do you have a family history of diabetes?
- Have you gained any weight recently?
- What kind of diet to you have?
- Do you exercise regularly?

Finding more about how advanced the patient's diabetes might have been at the time of the previous diagnosis might give insight into the progression of the disease since that time. The patient's commitment to her own care is vital to adequate management of this complex disease. Identifying risk factors and recent changes in weight, diet, and exercise habits may provide insights into important management modalities.

QUESTION #3

SUGGESTED SOLUTIONS	RATIONALE

- Do you have any history of heart disease, lung disease, kidney disease, or vascular disease?
- Do you have any eye problems?
- Have you ever been in the hospital or had surgery?
- Do you smoke or do you use alcohol?
- Are you on any medication?
- Do you have any allergies?

A fairly detailed history of the patient's overall health history can provide further information about possible diabetic end-organ effects, and any other potential problems that this patient might encounter during her therapy.

QUESTION #4

SUGGESTED SOLUTIONS	RATIONALE
• Obesity • Elevated blood pressure • Skin with scaling rash in skin fold areas • Fundi with early vascular changes • Rest of exam negative for evidence of cardiac, pulmonary, gastrointestinal, or vascular disease except for mild decrease in pedal pulses. • Neurological exam normal except for right foot drop and mild bilateral pedal sensory deficits, including light touch, vibration, and proprioception.	*Her elevated blood pressure during this exam is pertinent given her history of probable previous diagnosis of hypertension. In the absence of previous medical records, this part of the exam will need to be repeated on at least two other occasions to confirm the diagnosis (see Chapter 1). The vascular changes in her eyes may be hypertensive or diabetic in nature and will need prompt opthamologic evaluation. Her exam is otherwise normal except for an isolated motor weakness in her right foot and a stocking-like bilateral sensory deficit both characteristic of diabetic neuropathy.*

QUESTION #5

SUGGESTED SOLUTIONS	RATIONALE
• Serum chemistries including BUN and Cr, calcium, and magnesium • Hemoglobin A1C • Lipid profile (preferably when she returns to fasting) • Urinalysis and start 24-hour urine for protein • Stain and wet prep of smear from rash • ECG • Electromyography of both lower extremities	*This patient has not followed through on a previous effort to evaluate her diabetes. It makes sense to go ahead and get her laboratory work started even though she is not fasting at this time. The diagnosis of diabetes can be confirmed on random glucose testing if her values exceed certain levels, and she can be asked to return for a fasting blood glucose and lipid profile. She needs evaluation for her hypertension as well, including calcium and magnesium and electrocardiogram. Urinalysis will help with assessing for diabetic and/or hypertensive renal dysfunction, and a 24-hour quantitative urine analysis for protein can document microalbuminuria that is below the level detectable by dipstick. A stain and wet prep of a smear from the rash will help to determine if this is bacterial or fungal in origin. Finally, electromyography of the lower extremities can confirm a peripheral neuropathy, especially in a patient with unilateral neurologic findings.*

QUESTION #6

SUGGESTED SOLUTIONS	RATIONALE
• Repeat BP if still hypertensive; ECG suggests significant hypertension for a long time with evidence of left ventricular hypertrophy. • Random glucose, fasting glucose, and HGB A1C all exceed the criteria for diagnosis of diabetes. • Urinalysis negative for protein, but 24-hour urine confirms microalbuminuria at a level that indicates risk for nephropathy and cardiovascular mortality. • Lipid profile consistent with diabetic dyslipidemia and significant cardiovascular risk. • Wet prep indicated candidal skin infection. • EMG consistent with peripheral neuropathy.	*The patient has clear evidence of long-standing hypertension and will need medication if lifestyle intervention is unsuccessful. She far exceeds the criteria for diagnosis of diabetes and may require aggressive management. Her lipid profile, in addition to her hypertension and diabetes, puts her at very high risk for atherosclerotic cardiovascular and cerebrovascular disease. She also has microalbuminuria, which puts her at risk for increased cardiovascular mortality and end stage renal disease. The EMG confirms peripheral neuropathy without evidence of upper motor neuron deficit.*

QUESTION #7

SUGGESTED SOLUTIONS

- Schedule the patient for a comprehensive diabetic education program to begin as soon as possible.
- Begin caloric restriction with diabetic diet and reduce salt, fat, and alcohol intake.
- Advise smoking cessation.
- Begin supervised exercise program with careful monitoring for evidence of cardiac ischemia.
- Either continue lifestyle management for 3 months and reassess, or begin either sulfonylurea or metformin and begin home serum glucose monitoring as well as arrange for frequent office follow-up visits.
- Goal for glycemic control should be obtained within 6 months or add an additional hypoglycemic agent from another class of drugs.
- Ophthamologic referral for optimal management of retinopathy.
- Make neurologic referral for advice on the optimal management of her foot drop.
- Recheck BP and consider pharmacologic management if lifestyle modification ineffective.
- Administer antifungal for candidal rash.
- Monitor skin, cardiovascular, cerebrovascular, renal, and neurological exams regularly.

RATIONALE

The management of this patient is complex. Of primary importance to the success of any intervention is the patient's full understanding of the severity of her illness and her clear commitment to helping in its management. Obvious interventions include diet modification, supervised exercise, and smoking cessation. What is less clear is whether to institute these lifestyle modifications alone and recheck her blood pressure and blood sugars after 3 months, or to begin oral hypoglycemics immediately. The standard of care for many patients would be to try the lifestyle changes first, but some authors would argue that in a person who has increased blood sugars to the level of this patient and with significant end-organ effects, more aggressive treatment including oral hypoglycemics should be instituted immediately. If the decision is to begin oral hypoglycemics, there are four possible choices: sulfonylureas (glipizide, glimepiride), biguanides (metformin), α-glucosidase inhibitor (acarbose), or thiaxolidinedione (troglitazone). In the moderately obese patient, sulfonylureas are often effective and are inexpensive. There is, however, a significant risk of hypoglycemia with these agents, and metformin can be safer and quite effective in the obese patient. Should single agent therapy be inadequate, the addition of another oral agent from another class is recommended. If this is still ineffective, she may need to add night-time insulin injections. Although most of the diabetic care in the United States can be ably supplied by primary care providers, consideration should be given to neurologic referral to optimize her neuropathy care, and certainly ophthamologic referral to diagnose, treat, and monitor her retinopathy. Her blood pressure will almost certainly also need pharmacologic treatment unless lifestyle modification is hugely successful, she should almost certainly be treated with an angiotensin converting enzyme inhibitor which is protective against end-stage renal disease. She needs careful follow-up in the office, and most authors would suggest that she begin home glucose monitoring.

CHAPTER 12

QUESTION #1

SUGGESTED SOLUTIONS

- When did you first notice the shortness of breath and fatigue?
- Have you had any chest pain, cough, orthopnia, edema, wheezing, or respiratory infections?
- How long have you had your gastrointestinal symptoms?
- Have you had any vomiting, regurgitation, vomiting blood, diarrhea, blood per rectum, or black tarry stools?
- Is there anything that makes your symptoms worse or better?
- How much alcohol do you drink and for how long?

RATIONALE

With this limited history, the differential diagnosis is extremely long, and initial questions should begin to extract more detail about the named symptoms. Cardiac and pulmonary disease are likely causes of dyspnea and fatigue so that questions about symptoms of ischemic heart disease, congestive heart failure, airways disease, or infections are logical. With his history of alcohol abuse, gastrointestinal (GI) symptoms like his are commonly associated with gastroesophageal reflux, peptic ulcer disease, or pancreatitis, so that questions looking for evidence of these problems are also reasonable.

QUESTION #2

SUGGESTED SOLUTIONS

- Have you ever been diagnosed with heart, lung, or gastrointestinal disease?
- Have you ever had any surgery?
- Do you smoke?
- Are you on any medications?
- Do you have any allergies?

RATIONALE

A more thorough past medical history of previously diagnosed illnesses is essential. Given his history of significant alcohol intake, combined with symptoms suggestive of upper GI blood loss, he may carry a diagnosis of peptic ulcer disease and may have had upper GI surgery in the past.

QUESTION #3

SUGGESTED SOLUTIONS

- Pale appearing with pale sclera
- No evidence of upper respiratory infection
- No adenopathy
- Lungs clear
- Cardiac exam normal except for a systolic murmur
- Abdomen with epigastric tenderness but nonacute exam
- No hepatic enlargement, no ascites, no spider angiomata
- Stool heme positive
- No edema
- No neurologic abnormalities

RATIONALE

Pale sclera and skin with a flow-like systolic murmur are common findings in significant anemia. This patient with a documented history of peptic ulcer disease has exam findings consistent with ulcer persistence or recurrence after incomplete past therapy, now with evidence of upper GI blood loss. There is no evidence of alcoholic liver disease by exam. He has no evidence of pulmonary, cardiac, neoplastic, or infectious disease on his exam.

QUESTION #4

SUGGESTED SOLUTIONS

- Peptic ulcer disease with evidence of chronic hemorrhage
- Anemia
- Pancreatitis
- Esophageal erosions
- Esophageal varices

RATIONALE

As outlined above, the patient's past medical history, his current complaints, and his physical exam are most consistent with peptic ulcer disease with upper GI bleeding and anemia. Given the gradual increase in his dyspnea and with no history of acute hematemesis or hematochezia, it is likely that his GI blood loss has been slow. Pancreatitis or esophageal disease have not been ruled out but are less likely.

QUESTION #5

SUGGESTED SOLUTIONS

- CBC with differential, RBC indices, and RBC distribution width (RDW)
- Reticulocyte count
- Peripheral blood smear
- PT and PTT
- Liver function tests
- Electrolytes and amylase
- Upper gastrointestinal endoscopy

RATIONALE

With his history of blood loss, assessing his hematocrit is essential, but further evaluation of his blood count, reticulocyte count, peripheral blood smear, coagulation indices, and liver function tests are indicated due to his history of heavy alcohol abuse.

QUESTION #6

SUGGESTED SOLUTIONS

- His WBC and platelets are normal, indicating an isolated RBC defect and not marrow aplasia or neoplastic marrow replacement.
- Anemia is confirmed; indices are fairly normal, but RDW is increased, indicating a possible mixed anemia.
- Reticulocyte count is low, indicating inadequate erythropoiesis, especially given the history of blood loss.
- Smear confirms a mixed microcytic/hypochromic anemia consistent with iron deficiency anemia, and a macrocytic/normochromic anemia consistent with megaloblastic anemia, and/or direct toxicity from alcohol.
- Confirmatory tests should include serum iron studies, bone marrow biopsy, and serum folate and B_{12} studies.

RATIONALE

The automated RBC indices give an <u>average</u> of the cell sizes and color; the RDW is the clue to the presence of both microcytes and macrocytes. This is confirmed on the smear. The normal WBC and platelet counts and appearance make primary marrow disease much less likely. With a history of chronic blood loss and microcytic hypochromic RBC, iron deficiency anemia is likely. Alcoholics are also at risk for malnutrition and folate and B_{12} deficiency, which lead to megaloblastic changes in the bone marrow and a macrocytic normochromic anemia. Alcohol directly decreases serum folate levels, and can also exert a direct toxic effect on marrow also manifested by a macrocytic anemia. The documented continued blood loss but inability of the marrow to respond with an increase in reticulocytes indicates a significant defect in erythropoiesis. Serum studies to evaluate iron, folate, and B_{12} levels should be complimented by a bone marrow biopsy to ascertain whether the macrocytosis is megaloblastic in origin.

QUESTION #7

SUGGESTED SOLUTIONS

- Iron deficiency anemia
- Folate deficiency with megaloblastic anemia
- Duodenal ulcer with chronic blood loss; *Helocobactor pylori (H. Pylori)* positive

RATIONALE

The laboratory findings confirm iron deficiency and folate deficiency with combined marrow disorders of decreased iron stores and megaloblastic changes contributing to inadequate erythropoiesis. His peptic ulcer disease is active with continued risk of hemorrhage requiring adequate therapy and close follow-up.

QUESTION #8

SUGGESTED SOLUTIONS

- Treatment of the duodenal ulcer with omeprazole, tetracycline, and clarithromycin (see Chapter 15).
- Avoid transfusion unless the patient developed increased GI blood loss and symptoms of severe anemia, such as chest pain, neurologic symptoms, or symptoms of congestive heart failure.
- Oral iron replacement (ferrous sulfate 325 mg 3 times a day between meals).
- Patient education about side effects of iron replacement.
- Oral folate supplementation 1 mg per day
- Referral to an appropriate professional to manage discontinuation of alcohol.
- Careful follow-up of duodenal ulcer, stool guaiacs, HCT, and reticulocyte counts.

RATIONALE

As described in Chapter 15, H. pylori *duodenal ulcer requires triple drug therapy for adequate healing and to reduce recurrence. As long as his bleeding is controlled and he does not develop further symptoms of his anemia, transfusion should be avoided. Oral iron replacement is associated with significant GI side effects including nausea, abdominal cramping, epigastric distress, and diarrhea in up to 20% of patients, until this patient's ulcer improves he may require a reduction to 1 to 2 doses of iron per day. Folate supplementation is not associated with side effects but will likely be ineffective unless his alcohol consumption is eliminated. Significant improvements in his hematocrit should be expected in 4 to 8 weeks. Careful follow-up of his peptic and hematologic conditions is vital.*

CHAPTER 13

QUESTION #1

SUGGESTED SOLUTIONS

- Previous medical and surgical history
- Current home medications
- Allergies
- Course during surgery
- Current status

RATIONALE

This information is vital to the full assessment of this patient's likelihood for postoperative complications and for planning the most effective postoperative care.

QUESTION #2

SUGGESTED SOLUTIONS

- Volume status (vital signs, central venous pressure, urine output, physical exam)
- Laboratory values: hemoglobin, HCT, PLTs, PT, and PTT
- Chest x-ray

RATIONALE

It is important to assess for potential hypovolemia due to postanesthesia status and moderate blood loss. Lab values should be obtained rapidly to assess for anemia as well as to obtain basic coagulation values. The chest x-ray will assess for endotracheal tube placement, chest tube placement, and postsurgical lung expansion.

QUESTION #3

SUGGESTED SOLUTIONS

- Significant anemia
- Mild thrombocytopenia
- No detectable coagulopathy
- No evidence of postoperative respiratory complication

RATIONALE

His hemoglobin and hematocrit are decreased. His PT/PTT are both normal. His platelets are mildly decreased. His electrolytes are typical of a patient who is postop from a major procedure during which he received considerable IV fluids. The patient does not appear hypovolemic and there is no evidence of other major respiratory postoperative complications. Thus, these values represent a significant anemia and loss of oxygen-carrying capacity related to blood loss during and after surgery, as well as some degree of hemodilution from crystalloid fluid infusion during the operation.

QUESTION #4

SUGGESTED SOLUTIONS

- Excessive postoperative bleeding

RATIONALE

The most common cause of bleeding in the immediate postoperative period is a surgical cause. Surgical bleeding can generally be managed medically without further surgical intervention. Occasionally, reoperation may be necessary to control and correct the bleeding problem.

QUESTION #5

SUGGESTED SOLUTIONS

- Transfusing packed red blood cells
- Transfusing fresh frozen plasma and platelets
- Normalize his body temperature
- Replace calcium
- Increase the PEEP (positive end-expiratory pressure) to 7.5 mmHg

RATIONALE

Maintenance of adequate oxygen carrying capacity is vital to the postoperative patient. Optimizing coagulation studies with plasma and platelets will promote effective clotting and control of bleeding. Hypothermia can impede proper clotting mechanisms. Mr. H. was only mildly hypothermic at 35.8 ° C rectally. Normalizing his body temperature may help control and improve his body's abilities to properly clot off the bleeding problem. Calcium ion is an important factor in the intrinsic clotting cascade. Fluid shifts during anesthesia and surgery can lead to aberrations in electrolyte values. Normalizing the ionized calcium can help improve the body's ability to properly form blood clots. In addition, citrate present in banked blood binds with calcium ion after transfusion, and can lead to calcium ion depletion, hence impeding the body's ability to properly maintain hemostasis. Increased intrathoracic pressure with PEEP can assist in tamponading a thoracic bleeding source.

QUESTION #6

SUGGESTED SOLUTIONS

- Mr. H. is having severe and potentially life-threatening bleeding complication after his surgery.
- In addition to a possible surgical bleeding problem, he is demonstrating a developing coagulopathy.

RATIONALE

After receiving packed red blood cells, Mr. H.'s hemoglobin and hematocrit remained essentially unchanged. More concerning, however, is the drop in his platelet value after the platelet transfusion, as well as his increasingly abnormal clotting times (PT, PTT).

QUESTION #7

SUGGESTED SOLUTIONS

- Fibrinogen level
- Fibrin degradation (split) products
- D-dimer

RATIONALE

A fibrinogen level will assess Mr. H.'s supply of fibrinogen that is necessary to make fibrin clot. In a postsurgical patient, this value may be mildly decreased. A significant decrease would represent abnormal clotting activity. Measuring fibrin degradation (split) products will assess the degree to which Mr. H.'s body is making and concurrently breaking up fibrin clots. If Mr. H. is experiencing accelerated clotting activity, followed by the normal fibrin degradation process, this value will be markedly elevated. D-dimer is a specific antigen which is a byproduct of fibrin clot lysis, and will be markedly elevated in accelerated coagulation/degradation.

QUESTION #8

SUGGESTED SOLUTIONS

- Disseminated intravascular coagulation (DIC)

RATIONALE

Mr. H.'s lab results indicate that he has developed a coagulopathy in which he is using clotting factors and platelets at an accelerated rate, leading to depletion of clotting factors and fibrinogen, increased clot lysis, and production of fibrin degradation by-products, and subsequent continued bleeding. The presence of increased fibrin degradation products further exacerbates the bleeding problem by providing an anticoagulation effect.

QUESTION #9

SUGGESTED SOLUTIONS

- Possible transfusion reaction
- Tissue injury from the surgery

RATIONALE

Although the exact cause of DIC is not known, there are many events/risk factors that can precipitate this problem. The common theme in the development of DIC includes acute shock/anoxia as seen in conditions such as burn injuries, septicemia, transfusion reactions, obstetric emergencies, and tissue injuries. Causes of coagulopathy in this case most likely include a possible transfusion reaction as well as tissue injury from the surgery.

QUESTION #10

SUGGESTED SOLUTIONS

- Repeat rectal temperature
- Blood smear
- Urine for hemoglobin
- BUN and Cr

RATIONALE

The possibility of a transfusion reaction must be explored that requires evaluation for evidence of fever, hemolysis, hemoglobinuria, and changes in renal function. He should also remain well hydrated with intravenous fluids in the event of a transfusion reaction.

QUESTION #11

SUGGESTED SOLUTIONS

- Withhold the transfusion of blood products
- Consider heparin administration

RATIONALE

Continued replacement of clotting factors and platelets may only exacerbate the accelerated coagulation problem and are, therefore, not recommended. Transfusion of packed red blood cells may also exacerbate the accelerated coagulation problem due to (1) presence of citrate in stored blood, and (2) the possibility of transfusion reaction as the etiology for Mr. H.'s coagulation problem. Blocking the accelerated coagulation process with heparin is controversial.

CHAPTER 14

QUESTION #1

SUGGESTED SOLUTIONS

- Initial UTI
- Recurrent UTI
- Persistent UTI
- Hemorrhagic UTI
- Pyelonephritis (febrile UTI)

RATIONALE

This woman has the classic symptoms of a UTI, including suprapubic discomfort, urinary frequency, urgency to urinate, and dysuria. Since she does not have a fever, pyelonephritis (febrile UTI) is not likely. However, we cannot exclude other causes of her symptoms, including interstitial cystitis or pelvic pain until we know more about the patient's urine.

QUESTION #2

SUGGESTED SOLUTIONS

- Have you ever had a urinary tract infection before?
- Have you ever been diagnosed with any congenital or acquired conditions affecting the urinary system?
- Are your urinary symptoms related to intercourse?

RATIONALE

Additional questions include any history of previous urinary tract infections and congenital or acquired conditions affecting the urinary system. Because the patient is a young adult and a community-dwelling woman, she should be questioned about any relationship between UTI occurrence and intercourse.

QUESTION #3

SUGGESTED SOLUTIONS

- UTI limited to the lower urinary tract

RATIONALE

All of the historical evidence strongly suggests a UTI limited to the lower urinary tract. This event is similar to previous episodes and it is not associated with a fever or any atypical symptoms suggesting a complicated UTI.

QUESTION #4

SUGGESTED SOLUTIONS

- Dipstick urinalysis
- Microscopic urinalysis
- Urine culture

RATIONALE

A dipstick urinalysis and microscopic examination should be performed on ALL individuals with a history suspicious of UTI. A urine culture is justified in this patient because of recurrence of her infections.

QUESTION #5

SUGGESTED SOLUTIONS

- None

RATIONALE

*An imaging study would be justified if this patient had a first time **febrile** urinary tract infection or persistent urinary infection despite appropriate culture and sensitivity driven antibiotic therapy. If her culture reveals a Proteus, Klebsiella, or other urea-splitting organism, an imaging study of the upper urinary tract should be performed to rule out urinary calculi. Unless you are comfortable with selecting and obtaining upper urinary tract imaging studies, the referral to a urologist is appropriate. The referral should include a history of previously documented UTI as well as culture and sensitivity reports.*

QUESTION #6

SUGGESTED SOLUTIONS

- Nitrofurantoin or trimethoprim-sulfamethoxazole BID
- Vaginal antifungal agent

RATIONALE

An antibiotic is selected based on the sensitivity report, knowledge of the patient's drug allergies, and clinical judgment. For this woman, Macrobid has the advantages of a "BID" dosage schedule and minimal risk of vaginitis. TMX-SMZ offers the advantage of a "BID" dosage and inexpensive cost. Since the risk of secondary vaginitis is greater, treatment should be supplemented with an antifungal vaginal agent in the susceptible patient. Ciprofloxacin or another fluoroquinolone is not recommended for this noncomplicated UTI.

QUESTION #7

SUGGESTED SOLUTIONS

- Consider self-start therapy
- Patient education about voiding after intercourse, proper hydration, and avoiding constipation

RATIONALE

Because this patient has relatively infrequent episodes, self-start therapy may or may not be justified. She should be taught to urinate immediately following intercourse, and she should be counseled about the importance of adequate hydration and avoiding constipation.

CHAPTER 15

QUESTION #1

SUGGESTED SOLUTIONS

- Duodenal ulcer
- Gastric ulcer
- Gastroesophageal reflux
- Pancreatitis
- Cholelythiasis
- Cholecystitis
- Appendicitis
- Diverticulitis
- Intestinal ischemia
- Infectious cholitis
- Ischemic heart disease

RATIONALE

Dyspeptic symptoms are nonspecific and can be an indication of many abdominal inflammatory or infectious processes. Given the limited history so far, any of the listed possibilities must be considered, although PUD is the most common cause of the described symptoms. Occasionally, the pain of ischemic heart disease can be confused with that of upper gastrointestinal (UGI) disease and should be considered.

QUESTION #2

SUGGESTED SOLUTIONS

- Is it a pressure or a burning pain?
- What makes it worse or makes it better?
- Does the pain radiate to your back or have you had any other symptoms such as vomiting blood or blood in your stools, fever, weight loss, or loss of appetite?
- Do you have any pain after eating fatty foods?
- Any change in your bowel movements?
- Have you had any trouble with your liver, such as jaundice, increasing abdominal girth, or easy bruising?
- Any pain or shortness of breath with exercise?

RATIONALE

Symptoms commonly associated with PUD include burning epigastric pain relieved with food but recurring 2 to 3 hours after meals, nausea, and belching. "Alarm" symptoms include radiation to the back, GI bleeding, fever, weight loss, and anorexia. Fatty food intolerance might indicate biliary disease, and change in stool might indicate colonic disease. Symptoms of jaundice, ascites, and coagulopathy would indicate hepatic disease. Shortness of breath and pain with exercise might indicate ischemic heart disease.

QUESTION #3

SUGGESTED SOLUTIONS

- Have you been taking any aspirin or ibuprofen?
- Do you drink alcohol?
- Do you smoke?
- Have you had any recent unusual stress?
- Do you have any history of abdominal or heart disease?
- Are you on any medications?
- Do you have any allergies?

RATIONALE

PUD remains at the top of the list, and NSAID use is one of the most common causes. Alcohol is a risk factor for PUD and liver disease. Smoking and stress are risk factors for PUD. A history of previous abdominal or cardiac disease can help sort out the likelihood for the other possibilities. Current medications and allergy history are, of course, important in all patients.

QUESTION #4

SUGGESTED SOLUTIONS

- Afebrile, no evidence of severe systemic illness
- Mildly hypertensive
- No evidence of retinopathy
- No evidence of cardiopulmonary disease
- No ileus, no hepatosplenomegaly
- Epigastric tenderness without evidence of peritonitis
- No hemorrhoids; stool heme positive

RATIONALE

The patient is in no distress and vital signs reveal no evidence of systemic illness such as sepsis or organ failure. There is no evidence of hypertensive end-organ involvement. Abdominal exam remains nonspecific (epigastric tenderness is consistent with many of the entities in the differential diagnosis) but does not indicate peritonitis or severe abdominal involvement. Lack of hemorrhoids is reassuring but does not rule out increased portal pressures. Heme positive stool indicates an upper or lower GI source of bleeding.

QUESTION #5

SUGGESTED SOLUTIONS

- Chemistries including calcium and renal function
- CBC with differential
- Liver function tests with bilirubin
- Bilirubin
- Amylase
- ECG
- Abdominal x-ray
- Endoscopy

RATIONALE

Electrolyte abnormalities are common with significant GI disorders, particularly pancreatitis and bowel ischemia. A CBC would evaluate for signs of infection (e.g., appendicitis) and anemia. Liver function tests would be helpful in evaluating for hepatic dysfunction and biliary disease. Amylase is useful for diagnosing pancreatitis or bowel infarction. The ECG is to assess for myocardial ischemia. An abdominal film is unlikely to give more information at this time, but should be done if the patient develops increasing pain or an ileus.

QUESTION #6

SUGGESTED SOLUTIONS

- Endoscopy with biopsy and culture

RATIONALE

A choice must be made between an empiric therapeutic trial for presumed PUD, noninvasive H. pylori *testing, or endoscopy with definitive identification of any ulcers with the possibility of biopsy. This patient's heme positive stool is a definite "alarm" that requires aggressive evaluation. In addition, this patient's age makes it more likely that he will have side effects from prescribed medications and makes it more important to rule out gastric cancer. Although the NSAID use may be exacerbating what is a primary* H. pylori-*related problem, empiric therapy for* H. pylori *is not indicated without definitive diagnosis. Endoscopy would allow for cultures as well as histology.*

QUESTION #7

<table>
<tr><td>

SUGGESTED SOLUTIONS

- Discontinue NSAID
- Discontinue smoking and alcohol
- Avoid foods that exacerbate dyspeptic symptoms
- 4 to 6 weeks of therapy with an H2 receptor antagonist or PPI
- Educate the patient about symptoms that might indicate complications from his ulcer.
- Follow with maintenance therapy of H2 blocker at half-therapeutic dose at bedtime for up to 2 to 5 years.

</td><td>

RATIONALE

In this patient who is taking NSAIDs for a relatively insignificant indication, stopping the medication is vital. If he should ever require NSAIDs in the future, he should be placed on simultaneous misoprostol. Discontinuation of smoking and alcohol will promote healing and reduce the risk of recurrence. The choice between H2 blockers and PPIs is somewhat arbitrary; H2 blockers are readily available without a prescription but achieve healing somewhat slower than the expensive PPIs. Maintenance therapy is important, especially if he does not quit smoking, as recurrence rates may approach 100%.

</td></tr>
</table>

CHAPTER 16

QUESTION #1

SUGGESTED SOLUTIONS

- Where is the abdominal pain?
- Have you noticed any yellowing of your skin or eyeballs?
- Have you had any easy bruising?
- Have you had any increasing abdominal girth?
- Have you had any swelling of your feet?
- Has there been any change in your stools or any bleeding from the rectum?
- Have you had any rashes or aching, swollen, hot joints?
- Have you had any dyspnea, decrease in urination, or skin lesions?

RATIONALE

In inquiring further into this man's symptoms, evidence of fulminant hepatic failure must be sought. This would include questions about the manifestations of jaundice, coagulopathy, ascites, or edema. Clay colored stools would be an indication of jaundice, and blood in the stool might indicate variceal or hemorrhoidal bleeding consistent with portal hypertension. HBV and HCV can be associated with extrahepatic disease in both the acute and chronic phases of infection. HBV can be associated with a serum sickness-like syndrome of rashes and arthralgias. HCV is associated with autoimmune diseases such as pulmonary fibrosis, membranous glomerulonephritis, and skin changes.

QUESTION #2

SUGGESTED SOLUTIONS

- How long have you used IV drugs?
- Are you gay or do you have multiple heterosexual partners?
- Have you recently immigrated from another country or been in contact with an immigrant or someone else with known hepatitis?
- Have you had recent unprotected sex?
- Do you drink alcohol?
- Have you had any illness or hospitalizations in the past?
- Are you on any medications?
- Do you have any allergies?

RATIONALE

This patient has an obvious risk factor for hepatitis and for HIV, but other questions about risk factors need to be asked. Alcohol is a cofactor for liver damage in infectious hepatitis, and can itself be the cause of noninfectious hepatitis. A past medical history might indicate previous hepatic disease as well as the possibility of nosocomial exposures to pathogens such as HBV, HCV, HIV, and CMV. Some medications are associated with liver toxicity including isoniazid, rifampin, and acetaminophen.

QUESTION #3

SUGGESTED SOLUTIONS

- Mildly febrile
- No jaundice, rashes, or ecchymoses
- No thrush or other mouth lesions; no adenopathy
- No evidence of cardiopulmonary disease
- No ascites
- Liver slightly enlarged and tender
- Spleen not palpable
- No hemorrhoids or blood on rectal exam
- No joint involvement
- No confusion or neurologic symptoms

RATIONALE

Patient has evidence of acute hepatic involvement with hepatomegaly, right upper quadrant tenderness, and fever, but he does not show evidence of other significant systemic disease. Jaundice and rashes can occur with acute as well as chronic HAV, HBV, or HCV but are the exception rather than the norm with HBV and HCV. There is no evidence of hepatic failure (ascites, coagulopathy, hemorrhoids, GI bleeding, confusion) nor of the extrahepatic manifestations of HBV, HCV, HIV, or EBV (no thrush, no pharyngitis, no adenopathy, no lung or joint involvement, no splenomegaly).

QUESTION #4

SUGGESTED SOLUTIONS

- Hepatitis A
- Hepatitis B
- Hepatitis C
- Other viral hepatitis (EBV, CMV, HSV, coxsackievirus)
- Alcoholic hepatitis
- Toxic effect on liver
- Acute HIV infection or chronic with hepatic parasite
- Alcoholic cirrhosis
- Cholelithiasis/cholecystitis
- Biliary cirrhosis
- Sclerosing cholangitis
- Hemochromatosis

RATIONALE

Although the symptoms are nonspecific, the liver enlargement is suggestive of an acute hepatitis from either infectious, alcoholic, or toxic etiology. Alcohol ingestion is rarely associated with an acute hepatitis picture but it does occur. Toxic effects from acetaminophen are still possible since many patients do not consider this a medication. This patient is at risk for HIV and could have an opportunistic infection, or he is at risk for having HBV or HCV simultaneously with HIV since many of the risk factors are shared. Alcoholic cirrhosis is on the list and may underlie a bout of more acute alcoholic hepatitis. Cholelithiasis or cholecystitis usually present with more episodic and severe right upper quadrant pain but are still possible. Biliary cirrhosis and sclerosing cholangitis must be considered but generally present with more jaundice. Hemochromatosis may present with symptoms of chronic hepatic involvement and must be ruled out by labs.

QUESTION #5

SUGGESTED SOLUTIONS

- CBC with differential
- Chemistries
- Liver function tests
- Total bilirubin
- PT/PTT
- Serum ferritin
- Acetominophen level
- Hepatitis screen
- HIV PCR and anti-HIV ELISA

RATIONALE

Obtain CBC with differential to look for evidence of significant bacterial infection, chemistries to evaluate renal function and albumin. Liver function tests look for liver inflammation and hepatocyte injury. Bilirubin evaluates for biliary obstruction. PT/PTT evaluates liver function. Serum ferritin is used to rule out hemochromatosis. Acetaminophen level is used to look for the most common hepatotoxin. Hepatitis screen looks for acute or chronic HAV or HBV infection. HCV RNA PCR to look for acute HCV infection. HIV RNA PCR looks for acute HIV infection, anti-HIV ELISA looks for past HIV infection.

QUESTION #6

SUGGESTED SOLUTIONS

- WBC may indicate viral infection.
- Normal chemistries with albumin and normal coagulation studies do not indicate significant hepatic or renal dysfunction.
- Elevated LFTs with the ALT>AST is consistent with nonalcoholic hepatitis.
- No evidence of hemochromatosis.
- Lack of significant increase in bilirubin or alkaline phosphatase argues against acute biliary disease or cholangitis.
- Hepatitis screen is consistent with acute HBV.
- No current evidence of HAV, HCV, or HIV.

RATIONALE

Rationale for these is included with the suggested solutions at the left.

QUESTION #7

SUGGESTED SOLUTIONS

- The patient should be advised to notify all contacts of the need for testing and to receive immunoprophylaxis if indicated.
- Notify the health department.
- The patient should be advised on how to limit exposure of others in the future.
- He should be referred to a drug rehabilitation counselor for management of his IV drug addiction.
- It should be explained to the patient that no antiviral medication is needed at this time, but that he will need to be followed closely to make sure he does not develop liver problems or chronic infection.
- The patient should be advised to discontinue alcohol, to get plenty of rest, and to eat healthy meals.
- He should avoid Tylenol.

RATIONALE

The patient has probably exposed several people through either sexual, household, or contaminated needle contact. These people need to be identified and evaluated for immunoprophylaxis. Notification of the health department is required and can help in locating contacts. The patient should be educated about avoiding contact of others with body fluids or contaminated needles. He should be referred to a counselor about his IV drug addiction to reduce the likelihood that he will continue to expose others to HBV and to limit his risk of contracting other viruses such as HIV or HBC. At this time, he has no evidence of significant hepatic necrosis, and antivirals are not indicated for acute infection, so management is primarily supportive. He needs to be followed closely to see if he develops significant hepatic failure (coagulopathy, ascites, jaundice, encephalopathy, hypoalbuminemia, etc.). Repeat hepatitis serology will need to be completed after 6 months to see if he has become immune, or if he has developed the carrier state.

QUESTION #8

SUGGESTED SOLUTIONS

- Liver function tests
- PT/PTT
- Chemistries including albumin
- Hepatitis serology
- HIV serology

RATIONALE

Since the patient received no follow-up after his acute infection, it is important to assess his liver function, evidence for ongoing hepatic necrosis, evidence for carrier state or HBV immunity, and HIV serology as he is at significant risk for coinfection given his risk factors.

QUESTION #9

SUGGESTED SOLUTIONS

- No evidence of acute hepatic necrosis or dysfunction
- No evidence of HIV infection
- HBsAg indicates carrier state
- HBV DNA at low levels

RATIONALE

Patient is a carrier with little evidence of active hepatitis. He must be advised of his probable lifelong infectivity and the need for continued care in preventing exposure of others. There is no indication for interferon at this time since his liver function is normal and HBV DNA is low, but he should be followed regularly.

CHAPTER 17

QUESTION #1

SUGGESTED SOLUTIONS

- Alcoholic cirrhosis
- Portal hypertension with varices
- Spontaneous bacterial peritonitis
- Hepatitis (viral or toxic)
- Nonalcoholic steatohepatitis
- Hemochromatosis
- Primary biliary cirrhosis
- Peptic ulcer disease

RATIONALE

Although we have little data to accurately diagnose Mr. Z's problem, the combination of large tender abdomen, melena, and encephalopathy strongly suggests cirrhosis of the liver and its major sequelae. However, we do not have a complete history and must consider other potential etiologies such as infection and cancer, in addition to acute neurological events.

QUESTION #2

SUGGESTED SOLUTIONS

- Does Mr. Z have a history of liver or gallbladder problems?
- Has he ever had hepatitis?
- How much alcohol does Mr. Z consume? For how many years? When did he last drink?
- What OTC and/or prescription drugs does Mr. Z take? Recent use of same?
- Does Mr. Z smoke?
- Has Mr. Z had fever, nausea, vomiting, diarrhea, yellow skin, excessive bruising?
- Has Mr. Z ever experienced black stools and/or any bloody vomiting episodes in the past?
- Does Mr. Z have any cardiac problems?
- Any recent infections, illnesses, falls?

RATIONALE

Since M. Z is confused, questions are directed to his wife. Questions are used to explore related symptoms, duration, and severity of symptoms, and to further evaluate etiology.

QUESTION #3

SUGGESTED SOLUTIONS

- No history of other related etiologies (infection, hepatitis, toxins, cardiac or gallbladder disease).
- Consumption of large amounts of ethanol daily for years.
- Recent bleeding history coincides with encephalopathy.

RATIONALE

The history strongly points to alcoholic liver disease and related sequelae: gastrointestinal bleeding, ascites, and encephalopathy. Although you still need to differentiate between alcoholic hepatitis, alcoholic cirrhosis, and biliary cirrhosis, at this point, a biliary etiology is unlikely. Primary biliary cirrhosis has a >90% female preponderance and commonly presents first with pruritus. Bleeding and ascites are uncommon. Secondary biliary cirrhosis is usually associated with history of biliary obstruction for >1 year. Alcoholic cirrhosis is commonly associated with variceal bleeding from gastric or esophageal sources.

QUESTION #4

SUGGESTED SOLUTIONS

Pertinent positives:
- Confused
- Spider angiomas, jaundice, palmer erythema
- Gynecomastia
- Large tender abdomen with fluid wave and shifting dullness
- Passing maroon stools, vomiting blood
- Splenomegaly
- Nystagmus
- Asterixis
- Hyperreflexia

Significant negatives:
- Afebrile, not orthostatic
- Absence of bruises, masses, or deformities on head
- Cranial nerves intact (exception cranial nerve VI)
- No adenopathy
- No gallops, rubs, murmurs

RATIONALE

The pertinent positives found on examination include confusion in conjunction with findings associated with liver disease such as ascites, spider angiomas, gynecomastia, splenomegaly, asterixis, and hyperreflexia. The absence of obvious head injury is an important significant negative, and further suggests encephalopathy as the etiology of confusion as does the intact cranial nerve exam (except for CN VI, nystagmus is common in alcoholic encephalopathy). It is important that the cardiac exam demonstrates no signs of fluid overload or failure so that a cardiac source of hepatic failure may be ruled out. Active bleeding is occurring, yet cardiovascular status is only moderately compromised at this time. However, if bleeding continues at this rate, cardiovascular collapse will ensue. Hypersplenism is often present with portal hypertension and esophageal varices.

QUESTION #5

SUGGESTED SOLUTIONS

- Pulse oximetry
- IVs (two 16 gauge), NS at 100/hr (increase with hypotension)
- ECG
- Chest x-ray
- Labs: ABG, CBC with differential, HCT, electrolytes (full panel), PT/PTT, cholesterol, liver enzymes, ammonia level, type and cross 4 units packed red blood cells (PRBC), blood cultures
- Admit

RATIONALE

Mr. Z is actively bleeding. His stools have changed from black to maroon. Transfusion with PRBC and fresh frozen plasma is indicated immediately. It is likely that Mr. Z will require an ICU admission versus admission to a floor. Although endoscopy will be necessary, it will be accomplished once in the ICU. Stabilization of bleeding and restoration of blood volume takes precedence over all other therapy and diagnostic tests.

QUESTION #6

SUGGESTED SOLUTIONS

- Elevated PT
- HCT = 27
- PaO_2 = 62 mmHg
- Give fresh frozen plasma (FFP) and PRBCs
- O_2—2L NP
- Replace electrolytes

RATIONALE

Mr. Z will have to be stabilized prior to endoscopy. Two to 3 units of fresh frozen plasma (FFP) in needed to correct coagulopathies (1 unit of FFP will increase clotting factors by 2% to 3%). Three units of PRBCs should be given (each unit will increase HCT by 3%). O_2 is indicated, especially since Mr. Z has mental status changes. Aim for SaO_2 >90%. A mild respiratory alkalosis is common. Common electrolyte abnormalities in patients with ascites include low serum sodium and potassium. Hypomagnesemia and hypophosphatemia are also common. They should be replaced.

QUESTION #7

SUGGESTED SOLUTIONS

- Ratio of AST:ALT is approximately 3

RATIONALE

The AST:ALT ratio suggests alcoholic hepatitis and/or alcoholic cirrhosis (in alcoholic cirrhosis not complicated by alcoholic hepatitis, the AST is normal to moderately elevated). In viral hepatitis ALT is equal to/or exceeds AST, and in biliary cirrhosis AST is elevated, but moderately so.

QUESTION #8

SUGGESTED SOLUTIONS

- To decrease portal pressure and control bleeding

RATIONALE

Octreotide (somatostatin) and/or vasopressin both decrease portal pressure and can be given to decrease bleeding from varices. However, octreotide is associated with fewer negative side effects than is vasopressin.

QUESTION #9

SUGGESTED SOLUTIONS

Pharmacologic:
- Vitamin K
- Folate thiamine, pyridoxine
- Lactulose

Laboratory:
- Follow hemoglobin and hematocrit, PT/PTT
- Ammonia

Ascites management:
- Diagnostic paracentesis
- Diuresis

RATIONALE

Mr. Z's labs demonstrate acute hepatocellular injury (increased AST/ALT, increased bilirubin) and synthetic dysfunction (decreased albumin, increased PT/PTT, decreased cholesterol). Vitamin K is given to correct PT. A poor response to Vitamin K demonstrates poor synthetic dysfunction. Mr. Z is an alcoholic, therefore thiamine is given to prevent Wernickes syndrome. Folate and pyridoxine are also given since vitamin deficiencies are common. Lactulose is given orally (preferably by nasogastric tube) or rectally to produce osmotic diarrhea (get rid of toxins). Ammonia levels may or may not correlate with improvement in neurologic status.

Mr. Z's admission symptoms included abdominal pain. Spontaneous bacterial peritonitis (SBP) must be ruled out. Of hospitalized cirrhotic patients, 25% have SBP. SBP tends to occur in patients with preexisting ascites, abdominal pain, distension, and encephalopathy. Common organisms are Escherichia coli, pneumococcus, and streptococcus. Acute ascites management generally includes gentle diuresis and consideration for therapeutic paracentesis if pulmonary status is affected. If done, paracentesis must be done extremely cautiously. The most common cause of in hospital hepato-renal failure is over zealous diuresis and vigorous paracentesis, which may exacerbate a preexisting, prerenal state (intravascularly dry).

QUESTION #10

SUGGESTED SOLUTIONS

- Continue to closely monitor mental status, hemoglobin and hematocrit, electrolytes, PT and PTT
- Continue lactulose
- Ascites management: spironolactone, sodium restriction
- Repeat EGD with sclerotherapy (if rebleeds)
- Delirium tremens (DT) prophylaxis
- Consult addiction services

RATIONALE

Mr. Z is still at risk for a rebleed and should be monitored closely. Delirium tremens prophylaxis is indicated; however, given Mr. Z's encephalopathy, this must be cautiously done recognizing that benzodiazepines (the drugs of choice) are metabolized in the liver. Spironolactone acts on the distal tubule and causes natriuresis with sparing of potassium. If the patients fails to respond, furosemide may be gently added. Unless ascites are "tense" and cause breathing problems, paracentesis is not indicated.

QUESTION #11

SUGGESTED SOLUTIONS

- Stop drinking—strongly suggest attendance at Alcoholic Anonymous (AA) or other agency
- Follow-up with gastrointestinal service in 1 week
- Return immediately if symptoms/signs recur
- Continue lactulose (to attain one soft stool daily) until seen by gastrointestinal service
- Continue spironolactone; taper benzodiazepine

RATIONALE

Continued alcohol abuse reduces 5 year survival to 40%. Survival is 60% or greater however, in those who abstain. It is important that Mr. Z get help with his addiction. Referral to AA (or other agency that works with addictions is indicated). Lactulose may not be required long term but should be continued until seen again in clinic. Mr. Z's encephalopathy was likely a product of acute on chronic hepatic failure and gastrointestinal bleed (with increased ammonia). Benzodiazepine withdrawal is dangerous; a taper is recommended.

CHAPTER 18

SUGGESTED SOLUTIONS	RATIONALE

QUESTION #1

- Migraine headache
- Tension headache
- Cluster headache
- Meningitis
- Sinus congestion
- Tumor
- Injury
- Subarachnoid hemorrhage (SAH)
- Cerebrovascular accident (CVA)
- Temporal asterixis

Generalized dull headaches are generally not severe in nature; however, without a full, detailed history, we cannot rule out the life-threatening causes of headache such as meningitis, SAH, tumor, or intracranial bleeding.

QUESTION #2

- Where is the headache located?
- Has the headache interfered with your daily activities?
- Does the pain wake you up at night?
- Have you experienced nausea or vomiting?
- Have you experienced fever or chills?
- Have you noticed numbness or tingling in your arms or legs?
- Have you noticed any changes in your vision?
- Is there related symptomatology such as neck or shoulder pain or neck stiffness?
- Have you had any photosensitivity or decreased level of consciousness?
- Have you had any nasal congestion or postnasal drainage?

Additional questions must focus on the severity and exact location of the pain as well as the associated symptomatology in order that the differential list be narrowed. Headache location (global, unilateral, or localized) may suggest a likely cause. Nausea and vomiting, paraesthesias, and changes in vision are common with migraine, but can occur with structural or infectious central nervous system (CNS) disorders as well. Neck stiffness, photophobia, and fever might indicate infectious causes or possibly subarachnoid hemorrhage. Nasal symptoms are common with sinusitis.

QUESTION #3

- Have you had any injury to your head?
- Is there a lot of stress in your life right now?
- How much alcohol do you drink daily?
- Do you have a family history of headaches?
- When was your last menstrual period?
- Are you presently taking OCPs or estrogen?

Additional information including past medical history and lifestyle questions as well as a menstrual and hormonal history can help further elucidate the likely cause of headaches. A history of trauma might indicate posttraumatic headache. Stress and alcohol are associated with tension-type headache. Family history is most common with migraine but can occur with tension-type. Changes in headache frequency or severity is common with changes in hormonal status.

QUESTION #4

- Patient is alert, in no distress
- Afebrile
- BP slightly elevated
- No facial tenderness
- Tympanic membranes clear
- PERRL, no photosensitivity
- Fundi without papilledema or hemorrhages
- No cranial nerve palsies
- Good visual acuity
- No nasal or postnasal drainage
- Neck supple
- No adenopathy
- Neurologic exam without evidence of focal neurologic disease
- No meningismus

The patient demonstrates no decreased level of consciousness, no evidence of increased intracranial pressure, and no focal neurologic findings. This is reassuring that this patient likely does not have a focal structural CNS lesion. In addition, the lack of fever, meningismus, or cranial nerve palsies make meningitis or subarachnoid hemorrhage less likely. There is no evidence of sinusitis. This level of BP elevation is consistent with her immediate stress and is unlikely to be the source of her headache.

QUESTION #5

- None

In the absence of any focal neurologic signs or evidence of infection, no further diagnostic studies such as CT, MRI, lumbar puncture, spinal x-rays, or blood studies would be indicated at this time.

QUESTION #6

- Episodic tension-type headache

Tension headaches are bilateral, often described as a tight band around the head. They are frequently associated with increases in stress, fatigue, and depression. Episodic tension headaches generally increase in severity as the day goes on and the stresses mount. There are no focal neurologic signs associated with a tension headache, nor any signs of infectious process.

QUESTION #7

- Pharmacotherapy: aspirin or acetaminophen in combination with caffeine; nonsteroidal antiinflammatory drugs
- Physical therapy: increasing aerobic exercise; massage, hot/cold packs; stretching exercises
- Psychological therapy: stress management; relaxation therapy

Treatment plans for the episodic tension headache must focus first on pain reduction, and second on the prevention of a reoccurrence of future headaches.

QUESTION #8

- Maintaining a headache log or diary including:
    - Psychological and physical triggers (food, drink, events, emotions, menses)
    - Frequency of headaches
    - Severity of headaches
    - Amount of medication needed to relieve the headache
    - Success of other therapies

Monitoring future headaches can be a valuable tool in assessing the aggravating and relieving factors associated with the headache. Armed with this information, a clinician will be more effective in prescribing preventive therapies. Additionally, a diary can alert you to changing patterns of which the patient may not be aware. Overuse of medication can also be monitored with an accurate log.

CHAPTER 19

QUESTION #1

SUGGESTED SOLUTIONS

- Ischemic stroke
- Intracerebral hemorrhage
- Brain neoplasm
- Intracerebral abscess
- Subdural hematoma
- Epidural hematoma
- Neuropsychiatric disorder
- Hypoglycemia

RATIONALE

We know that the patient is elderly and had the sudden onset of symptoms referable to dysfunction of the left cerebral hemisphere. His symptoms have lasted greater than 20 minutes. We still have no past medical history, so we cannot rule out other underlying brain disorders or an infectious process.

QUESTION #2

SUGGESTED SOLUTIONS

- Have you ever experienced symptoms of weakness and numbness before?
- Do you have high blood pressure?
- Do you have diabetes mellitus?
- Do you have high cholesterol?
- Do you remember hitting your head recently?
- Have you had a recent respiratory, sinus, or inner ear infection?
- Have you had headache or morning vomiting?
- Do you have any heart problems?
- Do you have a family history of stroke and/or heart disease?
- Do you smoke?

RATIONALE

Additional questions should include a history of underlying brain diseases, infectious symptoms, family history, or history of comorbidity that are considered risk factors.

QUESTION #3

SUGGESTED SOLUTIONS

- Ischemic stroke with a history of transient symptoms (transient ischemic attacks)
- History of risk factors such as uncontrolled hypertension, hyperlipidemia
- Family history of cerebral infarction
- No history of head trauma, infectious process, or headache

RATIONALE

The historical evidence suggests stroke due to the sudden onset of symptoms and the previous transient events. The symptoms do not clearly point to an ischemic vs hemorrhagic origin, and more information will need to be obtained.

QUESTION #4

SUGGESTED SOLUTIONS

- These studies should be ordered STAT:
  - 12-lead ECG
  - Serum glucose
  - PT, PTT, CBC, platelets
  - Head CT scan without contrast

RATIONALE

*A rapid assessment of his neurological symptoms to determine improvement or worsening and an evaluation of other conditions that cause hemiparesis and dysarthria will direct the course of therapy for acute stroke. The Acute Stroke Intervention Team should be notified to determine acute stroke therapy if the patient's symptom onset was less than 3 hours prior to evaluation. A further evaluation of the cardiac arrhythmia would rule out acute myocardial infarction (AMI) and provide some insight into the possible etiology of the stroke. Hypoglycemia has been known to cause stroke symptoms. Prolonged bleeding times might indicate clotting abnormality and possible hemorrhagic causes. It is important to remember that these tests are performed to screen patients for thrombolytic therapy which must be delivered within 3 hours of symptom onset. There must be an absence of hemorrhage on head CT scan, as well as no history of recent surgery, trauma, rectal bleeding, bleeding ulcers, or anticoagulation to minimize the risk of hemorrhage. In addition, definite time of onset must be established to deliver thrombolytic therapy safely. **Further evaluation would potentially delay treatment.***

QUESTION #5

SUGGESTED SOLUTIONS

- A beta-blocker IV over 1 to 2 minutes to gradually lower the BP to <180/110 must be administered before thrombolytic therapy may be given. The dose may be repeated or doubled every 10 to 30 minutes up to 150 mg total.
- If a beta-blocker is contraindicated (e.g., congestive heart failure) or is ineffective, use an ACE inhibitor. Repeat in 10 minutes if there is no response.
- 2 L O_2 per nasal prongs
- Aspirin 325 mg PO

RATIONALE

Controlled lowering of the blood pressure is important to prevent hemorrhage and increased intracranial pressure while avoiding hypoperfusion. Beginning with small doses of a beta-blocker followed by repetitive dosing allows for careful management of the BP. Maximizing PaO_2 is important in maximizing O_2 delivery to ischemic tissue. Recent published results have shown that aspirin when given in the acute period improves overall outcome at 3 months when compared to no aspirin.

QUESTION #6

SUGGESTED SOLUTIONS

- Worsening of cerebral ischemia
- Increased weakness—patient is deteriorating
- Cerebral infarction is not present on CT for up to 24 hours after the event. This is not a hemorrhage or expanding mass lesion.
- No. His cerebral ischemia threshold may be higher than normal due to his chronic hypertension.

RATIONALE

It is clear from his examination and increasing right hemiparesis that the patient's ischemic penumbra (area of marginal perfusion) is succumbing to the prolonged ischemia and extending the infarction. The lowering of his blood pressure too drastically may exceed his high perfusion threshold, and normalizing his pressure would contribute to his infarction. BP should be managed conservatively during the acute period to maintain perfusion above the ischemic threshold. BP should be lowered by 10% increments with continued assessment for signs of ischemia.

QUESTION #7

SUGGESTED SOLUTIONS

- Time lapsed since onset the of symptoms is 90 minutes.
- rt-PA (activase), 0.9 mg/kg to a maximum dose of 90 mg
- Give 10% bolus over 21 minute, and infuse the remainder over the next hour. Assess for worsening or improvement of neurologic symptoms.
- Monitor vital signs Q 15 minutes for 2 hours; Q 30 minutes for 2 hours; and Q 1 hour for the next 24 hours.
- Monitor for symptoms of hemorrhagic conversion (projectile vomiting, sudden neurologic deterioration), sudden hypotension or systemic hemorrhage.
- If clinical deterioration occurs, notify the attending physician immediately and order a STAT head CT to rule out hemorrhage.

RATIONALE

*When Activase is introduced into the systemic circulation, it binds to fibrin in a thrombus and converts the entrapped plasminogen to plasmin. This initiates local fibrinolysis with limited systemic proteolysis. Activase is clot specific and dissolves emboli in the cerebral arteries to restore circulation and promote recovery of the ischemic penumbra. Thrombolytic therapy for ischemic cerebral infarction results in complete recovery 30% of the time when given within 3 hours of onset of symptoms. Activase may cause nuisance bleeding such as gingival bleeding or oozing at venipuncture sites, or more importantly, may cause hemorrhagic conversion of the ischemic infarction or bleeding into other sites. Hemorrhagic complications may occur in 6 % of treated cases and may result in death, however, morbidity and mortality rates are similar to that of all other treatments available for ischemic stroke. **The 3-hour treatment window and dosage must be strictly adhered to minimize the risk of hemorrhagic complications.** If the patient does not meet the time or other treatment criteria, all other interventions continue to apply.*

QUESTION #8

SUGGESTED SOLUTIONS

- Monitor closely through the night for recurrence of symptoms of ischemia or hemorrhage.
- Treat hypertension if BP ≥185/110; do not overtreat
- Repeat head CT 24 hours after treatment.
- Consider diagnostics for stroke etiology and appropriate therapy (echocardiogram, carotid doppler).
- Withhold anticoagulation therapy for 24 hours after activase treatment and after review of the follow-up CT scan.
- Identify and treat comorbid conditions (hypertension, atrial fibrillation, hyperlipidemia, smoking cessation).
- Initial assessments and interventions of clinical pathway

RATIONALE

Despite the obvious improvement in his exam, this was clearly a life-threatening event and he should be observed closely for 24 hours. Continued hypertension is associated with an increased incidence of hemorrhagic conversion. The second CT scan rules out silent intracranial hemorrhage that may be aggravated by anticoagulation. The cause of the stroke should be determined and appropriate treatment should be initiated to prevent a second event. The patient's risk factors should be evaluated and treated for secondary prevention. The multidisciplinary team (neurologist, neuro-nurse, rehabilitation nurse, physical therapist, speech therapist, social worker) should initiate the critical stroke pathway to expedite recovery.

QUESTION #9

SUGGESTED SOLUTIONS

- Aspirin 325 mg PO daily
- Digoxin 0.125 mg PO Q A.M.
- Cholesterol-lowering agent as adjunct to low-cholesterol diet
- Antihypertensive mediation (observe for interaction with digoxin)
- Stop smoking
- Recognize symptoms of stroke and transient ischemic attack (TIA), weakness/numbness on one side of the body, blurred vision, and difficulty with speech.
- See primary care provider for continued follow-up and control/treat risk conditions.

RATIONALE

Although this patient should be seen by his primary care provider soon after discharge, it is important for him to understand his risk factors and to continue his medications to reduce his risk for a second event (5% chance of second stroke within 1 year). His long-term care should include continued assessment of his carotid and cardiac status, and monitoring of his hypertension and hyperlipidemia. Treatment of hypertension alone could reduce annual stroke incidence by 50%.

QUESTION #10

SUGGESTED SOLUTIONS

- He should avoid salt and fat in his diet.
- He should exercise 30 to 40 minutes daily (walking).
- He should stop smoking and take his prescribed medications to lower his risk of second stroke.
- He should know the symptoms of stroke and seek emergency treatment if he experiences a second event.

RATIONALE

Salt contributes to fluid retention and can aggravate essential hypertension. High circulating lipid levels contribute to atherosclerosis and thickening of the arterial intimal layer. This ultimately leads to end-organ damage (heart disease, kidney disease, and cerebrovascular disease). Regular follow-up visits with his primary care provider allows close monitoring of his blood pressure, serum lipid levels, and progression of vascular disease, improves compliance with his treatment regimen, and reinforces important lifestyle changes. Treatment of these conditions can result in significant improvement in overall health and quality of life.

CHAPTER 20

QUESTION #1

SUGGESTED SOLUTIONS

- Delirium
- Depression
- Cognitive impairment related to a general medical condition: metabolic abnormality, endocrine disorder, cardiovascular disease, neurological disorder, infection, hematological cause, hypersensitivity
- Neurological injury
- Cognitive impairment related to medication
- Dementia: Alzheimer disease, Parkinson disease, Huntington disease, pseudodementia

RATIONALE

We know that the patient is elderly and was not feeling "well." Her symptoms suggest cognitive/perceptual dysfunction of unknown duration and onset. We still have no past medical history so we cannot rule out an underlying medical, neurological, or psychological disorder known to contribute to delirium, dementia or depression. Many physiological and psychosocial changes occur across the lifespan that can potentially affect memory and cognition; however intellectual and cognitive decline is not a normal part of aging.

QUESTION #2

SUGGESTED SOLUTIONS

- Has this type of confusion ever happened before?
- Does the patient have underlying medical diseases or psychological illness?
- Does the patient have a history of stroke, myocardial infarction, or trauma?
- Does the patient have any current or recent infectious symptoms?
- What medications is the patient taking?
- Does the patient have a family history of psychological illness or dementia?
- Does the patient have increased difficulty with any of the activities listed below:
    - Learning and retaining new information such as trouble with recent memory of events or conversations?
    - Handling complex tasks, such as cooking a meal or balancing a checkbook?
    - Reasoning ability, such as knowing what to do when a pot boils over on the stove?
    - Spatial ability and orientation, such as finding her way around familiar places?
    - Language, such as finding words to express ideas and following conversations?
    - Behavior, such as appearing more passive and less responsible, or more irritable or suspicious?

RATIONALE

Delirium is a cognitive disorder characterized by acute onset of impairment of cognition, perception, and behavior. The course usually fluctuates throughout the day and night, the duration is brief, and death may ensue if the underlying pathological processes are not resolved. Depression is of gradual onset. Although depression is the most common psychiatric illness in older persons, it is often underdiagnosed. When taking the history, look for symptoms such as changes in sleep patterns or appetite, weight loss, fatigue, withdrawal, behavioral slowing, sad affect, and/or complaints of diminished ability to think or concentrate. Dementia is a gradual, continuous, or fluctuating decline from previous levels of functioning and impairment in multiple cognitive domains. Determine whether a patient's symptoms are indicative of delirium, depression, or dementia. During the focused history, look for evidence of an acute confusional state or delirium and for dysphoric mood suggesting depression. These conditions can be mistaken for, or coexist with, dementia. Delirium and depression need to be addressed promptly and explicitly. If symptoms suggesting dementia remain after the patient has been treated for delirium or depression, continue the assessment for dementia. There are many causes of delirium, with the most common being intoxication from certain medications, metabolic abnormalities, endocrine disorders, cardiovascular diseases, organic neurological disease or trauma, neurological or systemic infection, anemia, allergy, or physical trauma.

QUESTION #3

SUGGESTED SOLUTIONS

- History of gradual functional and cognitive decline.
- Positive family history for Alzheimer disease.
- No history to suggest other metabolic, infectious, or medical/neurological disease process.

RATIONALE

The historical evidence suggests a progressive dementia. However, as discussed in this chapter, the conditions of delirium, depression, and dementia overlap in their presentation and pathophysiology. The DSM IV diagnostic criteria classify delirium and dementia as cognitive disorders with physiological etiology while depression is classified under mood disorders with or without physiological etiology.

QUESTION #4

SUGGESTED SOLUTIONS

- Head CT scan without contrast
- Chemistry, hematology, and metabolic laboratory tests
- Mini-Mental State Examination (MMSE)
- Geriatric Depression Scale (GDS)

RATIONALE

The head CT scan will determine any organic cause of the cognitive dysfunction. Multiple infarctions, chronic hematoma, hydrocephalus, tumor, and infection are all possible causes of changes in cognition. Serum chemistry, hematology, and metabolic screens can detect liver, kidney, and endocrine gland disorders that can contribute to delirium and dementia. Delirium is a medical emergency requiring immediate further evaluation and treatment for full recovery. It is not appropriate to administer cognitive testing in a person who displays sudden onset of cognitive impairment, disorientation, a decline in the level of consciousness, and hallucinations as this person is likely to have delirium rather than uncomplicated dementia. No single mental status test is clearly superior for determining the degree of impairment, and may in fact be insensitive to mild impairment. MMSE is the most widely and easily used brief mental status test. The finding of impairments in memory and at least one other cognitive domain is consistent with dementia. The GDS was developed specifically for older adults and should include information from both a patient self-report and a caregiver.

QUESTION #5

SUGGESTED SOLUTIONS

- Place patient in a quiet environment with good lighting; allow a family member to stay with her.
- Be patient and supportive when listening, and provide information about what is happening.
- Consult neurologist for thorough neurological evaluation.
- Consult neuropsychiatry schedule for formal neuropsychological testing.

RATIONALE

Once delirium is ruled out, further evaluation of the etiology of dementia can proceed at a less emergent pace. The neurologic and neuropsychiatric evaluation can rule out the presence of other illnesses that can result in dementia, and establish a baseline. Testing may be done to specifically identify cognitive deficits that may not be apparent. These tests may take several hours and provide more in-depth information than the mental status exams. Information gained from these tests will also direct more long-term intervention.

QUESTION #6

SUGGESTED SOLUTIONS

- Alzheimer dementia does not produce abnormalities on CT scan.

RATIONALE

Neurofibrillary tangles and neuritic plaques are isodense and are not detected by the CT scan.

QUESTION #7

SUGGESTED SOLUTIONS

- Condition is probably not delirium, as patient is stable with no altered level of consciousness.
- Findings are highly suggestive of Alzheimer dementia, at the forgetfulness stage.

RATIONALE

A family history, particularly in women, is highly predictive of Alzheimer dementia. No other definitive causes have been found. On close examination, many more symptoms may be discovered. The forgetfulness stage is characterized by short-term memory loss, compensation with memory aides, lists, and routines. The patient expresses awareness of problems and is concerned about abilities. The patient may become depressed, which confounds and aggravates the symptoms. The illness may not be diagnosable at this stage. Within the confusion stage, the patient is more dependent as memory decline progresses and interferes with all abilities. Day care and in-home assistance are commonly needed.

QUESTION #8

SUGGESTED SOLUTIONS

- Newly approved therapy for Alzheimer dementia is available upon definitive diagnosis by neuropsychiatry and neurology.
- Discuss with the family and the patient special services for special needs and the disease trajectory.
- Plans for regular and continued follow-up for health maintenance and functional assessment can be initiated in collaboration with the primary care provider.

RATIONALE

Although several pharmacologic agents have been approved for the management of Alzheimer disease, each of these drugs has significant potential for side effects, and the clear diagnosis of Alzheimer dementia is required. It is impossible to be certain of the speed of disease progression in any individual patient, but it is important to make the family aware of the likely needs the patient will have, and the services available to help address those needs. Regular follow-up supports the patient and the family.

QUESTION #9

SUGGESTED SOLUTIONS

- Begin treatment with tacrine initially 10 mg four times daily, then increase by 40 mg/day in intervals of at least 6 weeks in four equally divided doses. Monitor liver enzymes every other week for 16 weeks, then monthly for 2 months, then every 3 months, and at least 6 weeks following increased dosage.
- Make an appointment with the primary care provider.
- Contact the daughter or neighbor regularly.
- Continue to take antihypertensive and aspirin.

RATIONALE

If there are no contraindications, the new therapies for arrest of Alzheimer disease should be initiated. A routine to assist the patient in remembering to take her medications is important to establish, and a regular contact can assess safety issues and provide social support. This patient should be seen soon after discharge by her primary care provider. It is important to continue her antihypertensive and antiplatelet therapy and to recognize the potential adverse effects of Alzheimer medications. Adverse reactions to tacrine are increased serum transaminases, jaundice, seizures, gastrointestinal (GI) disturbance, myalgias, anorexia, ataxia, rhinitis, and rash. It also potentiates theophylline and increases the risk of GI bleeding with concomitant nonsteroidal antiinflammatory drugs.

QUESTION #10

SUGGESTED SOLUTIONS

- The patient and her daughter should assess the home environment.
- Health care providers should help the patient to adapt by identifying potential risk and taking appropriate precautions, rather than teaching and reteaching.
- The patient's activities may need to be simplified. Break activities into simple steps and take plenty of time to complete them.
- Support the patient's needs; allow and encourage independence, social interaction, and meaningful activity.
- Be realistic about what can be done. Obvious safety issues can be prevented, but all problems cannot be prevented.

RATIONALE

When an individual with Alzheimer disease is at home, safety and accessibility can be important concerns. The person may experience changes in judgment, orientation, behavior, physical ability, and sensory interpretation. With some creativity, flexibility and problem-solving, the home can be adapted to support these changes.

CHAPTER 21

QUESTION #1

SUGGESTED SOLUTIONS

- Epileptic seizure
- Subarachnoid hemorrhage
- Arteriovenous malformation
- Pseudoseizure
- Brain tumor
- Metabolic disorder
- Drug toxicity
- Vasovagal faint
- Cardiac syncope
- Transient ischemic attack
- Hyperventilation and anxiety

RATIONALE

We know that the patient is young and developed symptoms during physical exertion. His unusual irritability preceding the event suggests he was not feeling normal. We still have no past medical history and we cannot rule out an underlying organic disorder that precipitated the event.

QUESTION #2

SUGGESTED SOLUTIONS

- Do you remember what happened?
- Have you ever had a seizure before?
- Have you taken any drugs of alcohol?
- Have you had any recent upper respiratory or other infections recently?
- Do you have a history of birth injury or head injury of any kind?
- Do you ever have headaches or vomiting without nausea?
- Are you under any stress at school or at home?
- Does anyone in your family have epilepsy or a seizure disorder?

RATIONALE

History should include information to help determine what type of seizure has occurred. It is important to question witnesses; explore precipitating factors, description of onset, duration, characteristics, and setting to determine if loss of consciousness, presence of aura, antegrade amnesia, and postictal period occurred. Additional questions should include a history of underlying brain injury and chemical or organic processes that would present with seizure. Because epilepsy is a syndrome associated with several conditions and disease, it is important that an aggressive search be made for the underlying cause of seizure activity. A cause and effect relationship is not always apparent, and there may be an extensive interlude before seizures occur. In most of the possible predisposing conditions, signs and symptoms are present that suggest an organic process. With the many causes of seizure activity, diagnosis can become a very complex problem. The differential diagnosis listed above are but a few of the common conditions associated with seizure activity.

QUESTION #3

SUGGESTED SOLUTIONS

- Friend describes tonic/clonic motor activity with loss of consciousness; no evidence of aura, incontinence, antegrade amnesia, and postical period of about 5 minutes.
- Normal pregnancy, birth, and delivery
- A previous history of head trauma with a loss of consciousness is often associated with late onset epilepsy.
- Familial history of predisposition
- Now with increased stress in school and adolescence
- No symptom history to suggest other etiologies

RATIONALE

Most epileptic seizures arise from a few abnormally hyperactive and hypersensitive neurons that form an epileptogenic focus. These cells are abnormal physically, physiological, and chemically and are hyperactive even when quiet. Injury to an area of the brain caused by concussion, chemical irritation, infection, abnormal vascular supply, abnormal cell growth, anoxia, high fever, or even stress can stimulate the abnormal cluster of cells to fire erratically and recruit surrounding neurons as well. Given the right circumstances (physical or chemical stressors), anyone can be subject to seizures, however, some individuals have a genetic predisposition in which the seizure threshold of the brain is lower than normal. In these people, stimuli that are benign for most other people will precipitate seizures, and there appears to be a genetic tendency toward cerebral dysrhythmias. This boy's seizure may be a combination of mild head injury and stress during adolescence.

QUESTION #4

SUGGESTED SOLUTIONS

- Complete blood count.
- Urinalysis
- Blood chemistries, fasting glucose, calcium, blood urea nitrogen, and electrolytes
- Liver enzyme studies
- Consider lead level if ingestion is possible
- Urine and serum drug screen if history is questionable
- computerized tomography (CT) head scan or magnetic resonance image (MRI)
- EEG

RATIONALE

The studies are performed to help identify systemic or central nervous system disease that is triggering the seizure activity and that is amenable to treatment. For many patients, an extensive search for underlying etiology will not yield results. A rapid assessment of serum hematology and chemistries may rule out metabolic or toxic causes. The CT scan or MRI will rule out intracranial lesions such as tumor, blood, or infection. The EEG identifies patterns of electrical activity that can be correlated with particular types of seizures and aid in localizing an epileptogenic focus. In many causes, the EEG may be normal.

QUESTION #5

SUGGESTED SOLUTIONS	RATIONALE

SUGGESTED SOLUTIONS

- Be prepared for subsequent seizure activity and supportive therapy.
  - Maintain clear airway by turning patient on side with head down.
  - Do not pry tight jaws open to place an object between the teeth.
  - Protect patient from injuries.
  - Administer oxygen if cyanotic.
- Consult physician for all first-time seizures.
- Patients at increased risk include those with previous neurologic insults, positive family history, abnormal findings on neurologic exam, abnormal CT scan or MRI, or abnormal EEG.
- Is there a provoking factor that can be corrected?
- Estimate the risk of recurrence with first time seizure. Do the benefits of antiepileptic drug therapy outweigh the risks?
- In an unprovoked first seizure, no antiepileptic treatment is given.

RATIONALE

As with any patient, protection from injury with adequate ventilation and oxygenation is of immediate concern. Antiepileptic drug therapy is not without risk, therefore it is important to use caution when considering treatment after a first seizure.

QUESTION #6

SUGGESTED SOLUTIONS

- Phenobarbital 30 mg IM now (CIV—physician's order required)
- The phenobarbital 30 mg PO BID
- Oxygen per nasal cannula if the patient was cyanotic
- Monitor respirations
- Allow the patient to sleep on his side
- Reorient the patient when he awakens

RATIONALE

The rule is to begin with one drug and use it until therapeutic blood levels are reached and seizure control is obtained. Phenobarbital is effective in tonic/clonic seizures and has a limited side-effect profile, the IM phenobarbital will provide rapid establishment of blood levels that would prevent yet another seizure. Phenobarbital depresses respirations and causes drowsiness warranting close evaluating during initial treatment. If maximal therapeutic drug levels do not achieve control, or signs of toxicity occur, a second drug should be added to achieve therapeutic levels without discontinuing the first drug. Never abruptly withdraw any drug, always gradually taper, as this may stimulate seizure activity.

QUESTION #7

SUGGESTED SOLUTIONS

- Admit to the hospital
- Monitor closely through the night
- Continue phenobarbital

RATIONALE

Although seizures appear to be temporarily arrested, he should be osbserved in the hospital until therapeutic phenobarbital levels are reached (approximately 24 hours). A comprehensive teaching plan should be initiated to help the patient adjust to the condition.

QUESTION #8

SUGGESTED SOLUTIONS

- Warn family of drowsiness.
- Refer to specialist for titration of dosage and additive therapy if seizures continue.
- Teach family about the fundamentals of emergency management of seizures.
- Review precipitating factors such as stimulants, alcohol, caffeine, inadequate sleep, inadequate nutrition, or fever.
- Review state laws concerning driving an automobile.
- Teach patient and family about the actions and side effects of phenobarbital.
- Instruct to see a specialist as soon as possible for monitoring of blood levels every 2 to 4 weeks initially, CBC and LFTS annually.
- Patients at high risk should be treated for 2 years. If during that time they are seizure-free, they should be reevaluated for continued therapy.

RATIONALE

A teaching plan is based on a systematic assessment of patient needs. Social, psychological, vocational, and physical needs should be considered, particularly in the areas of self-concept and lifestyle adaptation in the adolescent years. A drug-teaching plan should be provided with discussion of side-effects and drug interactions that may occur. If the patient has good control of seizures, minimum restrictions are needed such as swimming with a buddy or wearing a helmet in some sports. Emotional problems occur in the family related to chronic sorrow, stress, social stigma, and unpredictability of seizure activity and need to be discussed. The diagnosis of seizure disorder carries social stigma and social limitations (such as restriction from driving) that require improved public education and awareness of the true nature of epilepsy to dispel the misconceptions and fears associated with this health problem.

CHAPTER 22

QUESTION #1

SUGGESTED SOLUTIONS	RATIONALE

SUGGESTED SOLUTIONS

- Have you had any neck pain or stiffness?
- Are you sleepy or having any trouble thinking?
- Does light hurt your eyes or has there been any change in your vision?
- Have you had any chills, rashes, nausea, or other associated symptoms?
- Has anyone around you been ill recently?
- Have you traveled recently?
- Have you had any chest pain or shortness of breath?

RATIONALE

This patient developed headache, productive cough, and fever after near-recovery from what sounds like a viral prodrome. This raises two primary possible concerns, meningitis and pneumonia. Meningitis is commonly characterized by stiff neck, decreased consciousness, and photophobia with blurred or double vision (due to cranial nerve palsy). A common type of meningitis in this age group is meningococcal meningitis which is frequently associated with a petechial rash, is quite contagious, and is associated with localized epidemics, especially in colleges and army barracks. Travel to foreign countries might indicate the possibility of a viral hemorrhagic fever such as Dengue Fever. Pneumonia is commonly characterized by shortness of breath or pleuritic chest pain, and chills might indicate bacteremia from a pulmonary source of infection that might lead to hematogenous spread of infection to the meninges.

QUESTION #2

SUGGESTED SOLUTIONS	RATIONALE

SUGGESTED SOLUTIONS

- Have you ever been ill or hospitalized before?
- Specifically, have you ever had meningitis or neurologic injury or condition in the past?
- Have you ever had pneumonia or other severe infections?
- Have you ever had a disease that attacked your immune system?
- Have you ever been tested for HIV?
- Are you on any medications?
- Do you have any allergies?
- Do you smoke?
- What immunizations have you had?

RATIONALE

Neurologic injury and disease may indicate increased risk for meningitis. A previous history of pneumonia or other infections, especially if there is also a history of immunocompromise such as HIV, would also indicate an increased likelihood that her current complaints are due to infectious causes. A medication history might reveal immunocompromising drugs or other medical conditions not mentioned by the patient. A smoking history would indicate increased risk for pneumonia. Finally, her immunization history is important in determining her vulnerability to certain infections such as Hemophilus influenza.

QUESTION #3

SUGGESTED SOLUTIONS	RATIONALE

SUGGESTED SOLUTIONS

- Well-built and well-nourished
- Fever, tachypnea, cough, and tachycardia without hypotension
- No rashes or cyanosis
- No papilledema
- Meningismus
- Right lower lobe consolidation on pulmonary exam
- No murmurs
- Extremities without lesions or rashes
- Neurological exam with lethargy without focal findings

RATIONALE

The patient's general well appearance is consistent with her negative past medical history; there is no obvious suggestion of underlying disease. Fever, tachypnea, and tachycardia are all consistent with an infection, and her cough suggests a possible pulmonary source. There is no evidence of shock. The absence of rashes is of particular importance as meningococcal meningitis is associated with a petechial rash. A stiff neck occurs in 85% of patients with meningitis. The positive Kernig (with the patient supine, flex the hip with the knee bent, then extend the knee—look for pain in the hamstrings and resistance to knee extension) and the Brudzinski (with the patient supine, flex the neck—look for hip flexion) confirm meningeal irritation. The absence of papilledema reduces the likelihood of increased intracranial pressure. The pulmonary exam is consistent with pneumonia; this can be a source for bacteremia and hematogenous spread of infection to the meninges. There are no murmurs or extremity findings to suggest cardiac disease. Lethargy is common in acute illness but is especially common in meningitis. Her lack of focal neurologic findings makes a space-occupying cranial lesion (such as an abscess) less likely.

QUESTION #4

SUGGESTED SOLUTIONS	RATIONALE

SUGGESTED SOLUTIONS

- Viral meningitis
- Bacterial meningitis
- Pneumonia
- Influenza
- Subarachnoid hemorrhage?
- Endocarditis?
- Rocky Mountain spotted tick fever?
- Vasculitis, hemolytic-uremic syndrome, thrombotic thrombocytopenia purpura

RATIONALE

The history and physical examination are suggestive of both meningitis and pneumonia. The meningitis could be viral or bacterial. Occasionally, a severe influenza will cause myalgias severe enough to mimic meningismus. Subarachnoid hemorrhage must be considered in a patient with severe headache and meningismus but the gradual onset of this headache, the viral prodrome symptoms, and the lack of physical exam evidence of increased intracranial pressure make this diagnosis unlikely. Bacterial endocarditis with associated bacteremia can result from pneumonia and cause widespread systemic symptoms, but is unlikely in this patient due to her lack of murmurs, rashes, or splinter hemorrhages on examination. Rocky Mountain spotted tick fever can give symptoms very similar to the ones this patient is experiencing, but the time of year (winter) and the lack of rashes makes this less likely. Noninfectious causes of meningeal symptoms include vasculitis (often idiopathic inflammatory involvement of vessels most commonly in brain, lungs, and kidneys), hemolytic-uremic syndrome (usually follows diarrheal illness caused by Shigella or E. coli), and thrombotic thrombocytopenic purpura (idiopathic hematologic syndrome that presents with fever, renal and neurologic findings, anemia, and thrombocytopenia) that are possible, but usually demonstrate physical findings consistent with more widespread tissue involvement.

QUESTION #5

SUGGESTED SOLUTIONS

- Place IV catheter and draw CBC and serum chemistries
- Draw blood cultures
- Begin empiric antibiotic treatment
- Sputum gram stain and culture lumbar puncture
- Chest x-ray
- Consider oxygen via nasal cannulae

RATIONALE

In a patient with suspected meningitis, beginning antibiotics as soon as possible is crucial to optimizing outcome and decreasing complications. An IV should be placed immediately with blood taken for serum chemistries and CBC, and blood cultures should be taken from two sterile sites. Empiric antibiotic therapy should be begun as soon as possible without waiting for further diagnostic studies to be completed. It is desirable to obtain blood cultures prior to beginning antibiotics as these are less likely to identify bacteremia if the patient has already received IV antibiotics. In contrast, CSF and sputum cultures are likely to be positive for a short time even after antibiotics have been administered, and these studies should not be allowed to delay appropriate treatment. Evaluation should then proceed with sputum and cerebrospinal fluid stains and culture. A CT scan prior to lumbar puncture is not indicated in a patient without evidence of increased intracranial pressure or focal neurologic findings. A chest x-ray can be performed after instituting antibiotics to confirm a localized infiltrate consistent with an infectious pneumonia. Arterial blood gases are not indicated in this otherwise healthy patient in little respiratory distress, although administration of oxygen may provide some comfort. Other studies not yet routinely performed but that could be considered in future patients include cerebrospinal fluid C-reactive protein, TNFα, IL-6, and polymerase chain reaction studies.

QUESTION #6

SUGGESTED SOLUTIONS

- No evidence of electrolyte disturbance.
- Serum leukocytosis consistent with bacterial infection.
- Sputum consistent with bacterial infection, most likely *streptococcus pneumoniae.*
- Chest x-ray confirms lobar pneumonia.
- Lumbar puncture/cerebrospinal fluid analysis consistent with bacterial meningitis; gram stain suggests *streptococcus pneumoniae.*
- No evidence of blood or fungi in the cerebrospinal fluid.

RATIONALE

Meningitis can result in electrolyte disturbances, most commonly due to the syndrome of inappropriate antidiuretic hormone (SIADH). The leukocytosis with predominance of polymorphonucleocytes is consistent with bacterial infection; this is confirmed by the sputum stain revealing pneumococcus. Pneumonia is confirmed on chest x-ray; there is no evidence of pulmonary vasculitis. On lumbar puncture, increased opening pressure with elevated protein and lactate, decreased glucose, and PMNs in the CSF are consistent with bacterial meningitis. Gram stain is consistent with pneumococcus most likely from hematogenous seeding of the meninges due to the pulmonary infection. There is no evidence of subarachnoid hemorrhage. Cultures of sputum and CSF are pending to confirm the bacterial identification and to determine antibiotic sensitivities.

QUESTION #7

SUGGESTED SOLUTIONS

- Ceftriaxone or meropenem plus vancomycin

RATIONALE

Approximately 35% of patients with pneumococcal meningitis will have organisms resistant to penicillin, and 15% will be resistant to cefotaxime. Until the cultures with antibiotic sensitivities are completed, empiric therapy for meningitis requires ceftriaxone plus vancomycin to provide adequate coverage for possible resistant organisms. Meropenem has just been approved for use with vancomycin for empiric therapy as well. If this patient's cultures confirm that her pneumococcal infection is penicillin sensitive, she can be switched to this less toxic antibiotic at that time.

QUESTION #8

SUGGESTED SOLUTIONS

- Increased intracranial pressure (ICP)
- Hydrocephalus
- Seizures
- Septic shock
- Disseminated intravascular coagulation
- Syndrome of inappropriate antidiuretic hormone (SIADH)

RATIONALE

Inflammation of the meninges can involve the underlying brain tissue leading to cerebral edema. This, plus the accumulation of CSF that can result from ineffective CSF reabsorption by inflamed arachnoid villi, can result in increased intracranial pressure. The onset of decreased consciousness, change in vision, and nausea with vomiting would suggest this possibility and would require rapid CT evaluation. Seizures are common in meningitis and should be controlled quickly to avoid further increases in ICP. Septic shock is a real possibility in this patient with two sites of infection; careful monitoring of blood pressure and tissue perfusion is essential. Disseminated intravascular coagulation (bleeding, thrombocytopenia, abnormal coagulation times, and increased fibrinogen degradation products) can also be seen in meningitis. SIADH resulting in hyponatremia can result in seizures. Children with meningitis are at risk for hearing loss, mental retardation, and paresis. The mortality of meningitis remains high especially in the very young and the very old. Despite all of these potential complications, with rapid and appropriate treatment, this patient should do well and be eventually discharged without complications.

CHAPTER 23

QUESTION #1

SUGGESTED SOLUTIONS

- Acute vertebral fracture
- Musculoskeletal strain
- Osteoporotic compression fracture
- Endocrine-related osteopenia (e.g., hyperthyroid, Cushings disease, hyperparathyroid)
- Intervertebral disc herniation
- Neoplasm
- Rheumatoid arthritis
- Osteomyelitis
- Metabolic bone disease

RATIONALE

The differential diagnosis of back pain in broad, and includes traumatic, neoplastic, rheumatic, and infectious causes of musculoskeletal disease. Other possibilities include osteopenia due to osteoporosis, endocrine, or metabolic causes. The presence of a vertebral fracture can be difficult to differentiate from muscle strain by history alone.

QUESTION #2

SUGGESTED SOLUTIONS

- Have you had any back injury?
- Have you lost any height or weight?
- Have you had any unusual bleeding?
- Any fever or chills?
- Any heat or cold intolerance?
- Any change in your hair, skin, or nails?

RATIONALE

A history or trauma would, of course, reduce the likelihood that this represents a neoplastic or infectious cause for her back discomfort. It would not rule out osteopenia due to osteoporosis, endocrine, or metabolic causes, and other questions should be asked to look for evidence for these etiologies. Loss of height is consistent with osteopenic fracture and/or osteoporosis of the spine.

QUESTION #3

SUGGESTED SOLUTIONS

- Are you taking any medications at this time? If so, what kind?
- Have you ever taken a medicine in the past for a long time?
- How long have you been postmenopausal and are you on hormone replacement therapy?
- Have you ever had thyroid or other endocrine diseases?
- Have you ever had kidney disease?
- Have you ever been diagnosed with breast cancer?

RATIONALE

The past medical history can help establish the likelihood of endocrine or metabolic causes of her osteopenia. Of great interest is her medication history, especially those taken for a prolonged period (e.g., hydrochlorothiazide, steroids, or thyroid replacement). Menopausal osteoporosis is common in women, and the risk is greater if the patient has not been on hormone replacement therapy. A history of thyroid disease, renal dysfunction, or breast cancer would point to other possible specific causes of osteopenia and possible vertebral fracture.

QUESTION #4

SUGGESTED SOLUTIONS	RATIONALE

- What kind of diet do you have?
- Do you get much exercise?
- Do you go outdoors regularly?
- Do you smoke or drink alcohol?
- How much caffeine do you generally drink in a day?
- Do you take calcium or vitamin D supplements?

Menopausal osteoporosis remains one of the most likely causes of this woman's symptoms given her lack of trauma or medical history. Many of the risk factors for osteoporosis can be determined by a detailed past and present history.

QUESTION #5

SUGGESTED SOLUTIONS	RATIONALE

- Patient is white and of small stature
- Cervical lordosis without tenderness or decreased range of motion
- No thyromegaly or masses
- Lungs with normal excursion
- Motor and sensory neurologic exam without deficits
- No evidence of meningitis
- Tenderness over L1 and L2
- Decreased flexion and extension without pain on lateral bending
- No dowager hump
- No joint involvement

Menopausal osteoporosis is more common in thin Caucasian women due to decreased trabecular bone and decreased endogenous estrogen production. There is no evidence of cervical spine involvement. There is no evidence of thyroid disease. There is no limitation on lung expansion due to kyphosis or pain. There is no evidence of spinal cord or radicular injury or dysfunction. Tenderness and range of motion findings consistent with anterior/posterior injury to the L1 or L2 vertebrae. No evidence of severe kyphosis or arthritis.

QUESTION #6

SUGGESTED SOLUTIONS	RATIONALE

- Plain x-ray of the lumbosacral spine

In a patient with tenderness and decreased range of motion, vertebral fracture is possible. Osteoporotic fractures are most common in trabecular bone where bone turnover is rapid. The plain film is relatively insensitive for finding osteopenia; approximately 30% of the bone must be lost before osteopenia become evident.

QUESTION #7

SUGGESTED SOLUTIONS	RATIONALE

- Chemistries including BUN and Cr, calcium, and phosphate
- CBC
- Thyroid functions
- Rheumatoid factor (RF)
- Alkaline phosphatase (serum and 24-hour urine)
- Erythrocyte sedimentation rate (ESR)
- Serum protein electrophoresis
- Dual energy x-ray densitometry or quantitative CT.

Although menopausal osteoporosis is the most likely cause for this patient's osteopenia and compression fracture, other metabolic, hormonal, rheumatic, and neoplastic causes have not been ruled out. The chemistries evaluate for evidence of endocrine or metabolic disease. The CBC, alkaline phosphatase, and serum protein electrophoresis evaluate for neoplasms. The RF and ESR evaluate for rheumatic disease. Finally, the densitometry or CT will quantitate the amount of osteopenia.

QUESTION #8

SUGGESTED SOLUTIONS

- Compression fracture of L2
- Menopausal osteoporosis

RATIONALE

Menopausal osteoporosis is often not diagnosed until a patient presents with signs of a fracture. Our patient's history gives a strong indication that she is at high risk. She is menopausal, and never took protective estrogens because of her family history of breast cancer. She is inactive and a cigarette smoker. She has never replaced calcium in her diet and has eaten a high-protein diet all of her life. She has taken a diuretic for her hypertension for 15 years. Her laboratory studies also make other causes of osteopenia unlikely.

QUESTION #9

SUGGESTED SOLUTIONS

- Compression fracture management:
  - Pain medications
  - Rest back to avoid bending and lifting
  - Fit with back brace
  - Physical therapy referral for strengthening exercises
- Prevent further bone loss:
  - Nutrition: balanced diet with moderation of protein and fat, increase calcium sources and decrease phosphorous intake
  - Calcium supplementation of 1500 mg/day, and vitamin D 50,000 units twice a month
  - Encourage weight-bearing exercise and strength training
  - Biphosphonates and calcitonin
  - Change anithypertensive medication to a nondiuretic
  - Smoking cessation

RATIONALE

Initial management must concentrate on the pain of the compression fracture. After stabilization of that fracture, the goal must be focused on preventing future fractures and disability. Prevention techniques which maximize bone density, minimize future bone loss, and help prevent future falls must be the foundation of your treatment plan.

QUESTION #10

SUGGESTED SOLUTIONS

- Yearly monitoring for height loss
- Watch for constipation and respiratory difficulties associated with postural changes
- Monitor for gastrointestinal intolerance to calcium
- Avoid the future use of osteopenic medications
- Consider the future use of estrogen analogues

RATIONALE

Continued monitoring of this patient's osteoporosis, looking for the response and side effects of management, is key to success. Continued preventative measures are also important. Estrogen analogues that provide all of the benefits of estrogen for bone and the cardiovascular system, but are not associated with increased breast cancer risk, are being evaluated for future use.

Chapter 24

QUESTION #1

SUGGESTED SOLUTIONS

- Has the pain in your knees gotten worse gradually or more suddenly?
- Are there other joints that are affected?
- Do your joints ever get swollen, hot, or red?
- Do you have any joint deformity?
- Have you ever had any knee trauma?
- Are there things other than the weather that make your symptoms better or worse?
- Has you back pain gotten worse?
- Is it associated with any weakness, numbness, or shooting pains in the legs?
- Does your hip still hurt?
- Do you take any medications for your joint and back pain?

RATIONALE

Further information about the nature of the patient's joint complaints is vital to differentiating between the numerous potential causes of musculoskeletal disease. Widespread noninflammatory joint disease that has had a gradual increase in severity is characteristic of the most common cause of rheumatologic disease, OA. A history of joint trauma may indicate secondary OA. OA tends to get symptomatic when the weather changes. OA is characterized by joint stiffness after inactivity with restoration of full movement in less than 30 minutes of mobilizing the joint. Her back pain may be caused by OA, but could also be the result of intervertebral disc disease, trauma, or osteoporosis with possible compression fracture. Evidence of radicular involvement with leg numbness or weakness may indicate significant vertebral disc disease, and the knee pain could be referred from L4-L5. Response to medications is important to quantifying the severity of symptoms and planning care.

QUESTION #2

SUGGESTED SOLUTIONS

- Have you ever been diagnosed with arthritis?
- Have you ever been told you have osteoporosis?
- Have you ever had any lung, heart, or kidney disease?
- Have you ever had an ulcer or blood in your stool?
- Have you ever been hospitalized?
- Have you ever had surgery?
- Have you ever taken hormone replacement therapy?
- Are you taking any medications?

RATIONALE

Further questions about the patient's overall medical and surgical history can provide further insights into the current complaint as well as predict possible responses to care. A history of heart, lung, or kidney disease could potentially suggest a systemic collagen vascular disease such as systemic lupus erythematosus. A gastrointestinal history is important in an elderly patient taking NSAIDs as the risk for ulceration and bleeding is high in this age group. A history of oophorectomy or hormone replacement would help to identify the risk of OA.

QUESTION #3

SUGGESTED SOLUTIONS

- Are you physically active now?
- What is your diet like? Do you get enough calcium?
- Do you smoke or drink alcohol?
- Do you live alone?
- Does your house have stairs?

RATIONALE

Documenting the patient's level of activity can be useful to assessing limitations as well as designing interventions. Questions about diet, smoking, and alcohol may provide insight into risks for osteoporosis as well as her general health. Ascertaining her living situation is useful in understanding her limitations and in considering treatment options.

QUESTION #4

SUGGESTED SOLUTIONS

- Primary osteoarthritis
- Secondary osteoarthritis
- Osteoporosis with possible vertebral compression
- Other collagen vascular disease such as systemic lupus erythematosus or anklyosing spondylitis
- Gout

RATIONALE

Although this patient gives a fairly classic history for primary OA, it is possible that her knee pain is primarily a result of previous trauma and could therefore be called secondary OA. She may also have osteoporosis given her age and her poor diet. Rheumatoid arthritis and the other collagen vascular diseases are in the differential, but they are much less common and are usually associated with a more inflammatory joint picture as well as evidence of other systemic organ effects. Gout is usually monoarticular and it is associated with severe pain and inflammation and thus is unlikely.

QUESTION #5

SUGGESTED SOLUTIONS

- She has mild systolic hypertension.
- With exception of the musculoskeletal exam, her exam is entirely normal.
- Her musculoskeletal exam results:
  - Noninflammatory joint deformity in the form of bony protuberances at the DIP (Heberdens nodes) and PIP (Bouchards nodes).
  - Decreased range of motion in all of the affected joints.
  - Most of these findings are symmetrical, except at the knee where the right knee is more affected than the left, and at the right hip that was previously fractured.

RATIONALE

Aside from her mild systolic hypertension (which would need to be evaluated as well), the patient has no evidence of systemic disease to indicate an underlying inflammatory collagen vascular disease such as systemic lupus erythematosus. Her musculoskeletal exam is entirely consistent with OA. The lack of joint deformity such as ulnar deviation of the metacarpal phalangeal (MCP) joints, wrist and elbow involvement, and no evidence of inflammation makes rheumatoid arthritis less likely. Her more severe symptoms and exam findings in the right knee may indicate some secondary OA related to her past sports injury or trauma during her hip fracture. The residual decrease in range of motion at the hip may be the result of her previous fracture or may indicate secondary OA from the trauma of the fracture.

QUESTION #6

SUGGESTED SOLUTIONS

- Chemistries including BUN, Cr, calcium, and phosphate
- CBC
- Liver function tests
- Thyroid function tests
- X-ray of knee and lumbosacral spine

RATIONALE

The patient's history and exam are classic for OA and a case could be made for pursuing no further evaluation. Because this patient has risk factors for osteoporosis and a history of hip fracture, it is reasonable to evaluate serum chemistries and thyroid function tests, as well as both the knee and lumbosacral spine x-rays to rule out pathologic fracture. A CBC is prudent given the patient's history of long-term nonsteroidal antiinflammatory drugs and upper GI symptoms to rule out chronic blood loss and anemia. Liver function testing is indicated prior to consideration of acetaminophen therapy if this patient has OA as is suspected.

QUESTION #7

SUGGESTED SOLUTIONS

- Osteoarthritis

RATIONALE

The blood studies show no evidence of systemic disease or metabolic causes of osteoporosis. The plain x-ray is a very insensitive measure of bone density, but it is useful in ruling out compression fracture as a cause of her pain.

QUESTION #8

SUGGESTED SOLUTIONS

- She should have diet counseling with a goal of gradual weight loss, maximizing calcium intake, and reducing phosphate intake.
- She should be enrolled in a supervised exercise and physical therapy program to support range of motion, muscle strength, and joint stability.
- She should discontinue nonsteroidal antiinflammatory drugs and substitute them with acetaminophen up to a dose of 4000 mg/day with follow-up monitoring of symptoms and liver function.
- Discuss the potential benefits of chondroprotective drugs such as combinations of chondroitin sulfate and glucosamine sulfate.
- Future consideration would be for orthopedic surgery if the knee pain should be progressive and resistant to conservative therapy.
- Consider bone density measurement and possible initiation of hormone replacement therapy or estrogen analogue.

RATIONALE

Management of OA includes a combination of physical therapy and exercise with analgesic medication. This patient is already engaged in regular physical activity and has no history of cardiovascular disease. so it is reasonable to enroll her in a supervised exercise and physical therapy program. Weight loss is indicated especially with her knee involvement. Maximizing her calcium and minimizing phosphate will reduce her risk of osteoporosis. Her lack of previous response to NSAIDs and potential GI side effects makes discontinuation of these drugs prudent. Acetaminophen has been found to be equally effective as NSAIDs in many patients and is safer as long as liver function is normal. The chondroprotective drugs have been shown to be helpful in many patients and have a low risk of significant side effects. If her knee pain progresses despite conservative therapy, consideration for one of the many possible orthopedic procedures may be necessary. Finally, further evaluation and possible management of osteoporosis is important especially with her history of hip fracture.

CHAPTER 25

QUESTION #1

SUGGESTED SOLUTIONS	RATIONALE

- Have your symptoms developed gradually or more suddenly?
- How often do you get hot flashes?
- Do they wake you up at night?
- Are your vaginal symptoms associated with any abdominal pain or dysuria?
- Have you had any vaginal infections in the past?

Although this patient's history is classic for menopausal estrogen deficiency, questions about the onset and severity of symptoms can give clues to more acute problems and how bothered the patient is by her symptoms. Consideration must be given to the other causes of her vaginal symptoms, especially the possibility of infectious causes.

QUESTION #2

SUGGESTED SOLUTIONS	RATIONALE

- Do you have any other health problems?
- Have you ever had migraines, gallbladder disease, blood clots, or liver disease?
- Have you ever had breast cancer?
- Has anyone in your family had breast cancer?
- Have you ever had trouble with your cholesterol or heart disease?
- Have you ever considered hormone replacement therapy?

A careful past medical history can help to determine other likely causes of her symptoms, as well as identify indications and contraindications to hormone replacement therapy.

QUESTION #3

SUGGESTED SOLUTIONS	RATIONALE

- What is your diet like?
- Do you exercise regularly?
- Do you smoke?
- Do you drink alcohol?

A lifestyle history can help identify risks for osteoporosis and atherosclerotic disease thus providing more information as to indications for hormone replacement.

QUESTION #4

SUGGESTED SOLUTIONS	RATIONALE

- Skin is dry and thick
- No evidence of cardiac, pulmonary, or hepatic disease
- No evidence of deep venous thrombosis
- Pelvic with perivaginal and vaginal dryness and atrophy
- Breast exam without masses, nipple discharge, or axillary adenopathy

The patient's exam with vaginal atrophy and with skin dryness is consistent with postmenopausal estrogen deficiency. Mild kyphosis may be the result of vertebral osteoporosis. The rest of her exam is completely normal with no evidence of systemic disease or contraindications to hormone replacement. Her breast and axillary exam is normal.

QUESTION #5

SUGGESTED SOLUTIONS

- FSH
- Chemistries including calcium and phosphate
- CBC
- Liver function tests
- Lipid profile
- Thyroid-stimulating hormone (TSH)
- Mammogram
- Dual energy x-ray densitometry

RATIONALE

Although her history leaves little doubt as to the cause of her symptoms, a serum FSH will confirm a normal postmenopausal state. With her risks for osteoporosis, a chemistry profile including calcium is indicated before considering hormone replacement. Her fatigue may be due to estrogen deficiency, but a hematologic profile and TSH are reasonable. Liver function testing and mammography will help determine if she has any contraindications to hormone replacement. Her lipid profile and bone mineral density testing will help pinpoint indications for hormone replacement in addition to her symptoms.

QUESTION #6

SUGGESTED SOLUTIONS

- Discuss the pros and cons of HRT.
- If patient decides to try hormone replacement, treat with 0.625 mg/day as conjugated estrogen orally or via a transdermal patch.
- Begin medroxyprogesterone acetate 2.5 mg/day orally.
- Instruct in the necessity of immediate notification of vaginal bleeding, but discuss with patient the likelihood of occasional spotting for the first few months of therapy.
- Instruct in the necessity of continued yearly pelvic and breast exams and mammograms.
- Instruct in proper diet for increasing calcium intake and lowering LDL cholesterol. Suggest a recheck of the lipid profile in 6 months.
- Encourage exercise for relief of postmenopausal symptoms, an increase in bone density, and an increase in HDL.

RATIONALE

The patient has several indications for hormone replacement including hot flashes, vaginal atrophy, dyslipidemia, and decreased bone mineral density. She has no contraindications for estrogen treatment including no evidence of deep venous thrombosis, migraines, breast cancer, endometrial cancer, or ovarian masses. Although a newer estrogen analog has been approved for the treatment of osteoporosis, this new class of drugs tends to increase hot flashes and their effect on lowering cardiovascular risk remains unproven. In this patient with no contraindications to estrogen, it remains the best choice for hormone replacement therapy. In a patient with an intact uterus, daily progesterone must be added to avoid the risk of endometrial cancer.

NOTES

NOTES

NOTES

NOTES

NOTES

NOTES

NOTES

NOTES

NOTES

NOTES